Health Metrics and the Spread of Infectious Diseases

Health Metrics and the Spread of Infectious Diseases: Machine Learning Applications and Spatial Modelling Analysis with R is an introductory guide to health metrics and infectious diseases. It demonstrates how to calculate these metrics to compare the health status of different countries and explores the world of infectious diseases. It tests various machine learning tools for analyzing trends and relationships among key variables, aiming to prevent unexpected outcomes. Through detailed explanations and practical examples, readers will gain a comprehensive understanding of Disability Adjusted Life Years (DALYs) and their components.

Key Features:

- Structured into four main sections—foundational health metrics, machine learning applications, data visualization, and real-world case studies
- Integrates real-world case studies with data visualization and machine learning techniques, including spatial modelling with the R programming language
- Covers specific infectious diseases such as COVID-19 and malaria, providing insights into their spread and control
- Includes detailed explanations, practical exercises, and clear illustrations to enhance understanding and application
- Adopts a practical approach, making advanced concepts accessible to a wide audience

The book is primarily aimed at researchers, data scientists, and public health professionals who seek to leverage data to improve health outcomes. By blending theoretical knowledge with practical applications, the book equips readers with the tools to make informed decisions and produce meaningful data analyses in public health.

Health Metrics and the Spread of Infectious Diseases

Machine Learning Applications and Spatial Modelling Analysis with R

Federica Gazzelloni

CRC Press
Taylor & Francis Group
Boca Raton London New York

CRC Press is an imprint of the
Taylor & Francis Group, an **informa** business
A CHAPMAN & HALL BOOK

First edition published 2025
by CRC Press
2385 NW Executive Center Drive, Suite 320, Boca Raton FL 33431

and by CRC Press
4 Park Square, Milton Park, Abingdon, Oxon, OX14 4RN

CRC Press is an imprint of Taylor & Francis Group, LLC

ISBN: 978-1-032-62578-2 (hbk)
ISBN: 978-1-032-62592-8 (pbk)
ISBN: 978-1-032-62593-5 (ebk)

DOI: 10.1201/9781032625935

Typeset in Latin Modern font
by KnowledgeWorks Global Ltd.

Publisher's note: This book has been prepared from camera-ready copy provided by the authors.

In loving memory of my dear brother,
whose dedication and simplicity will forever live on in our hearts.

Contents

Preface

This book will teach you about health metrics such as Disability Adjusted Life Years (DALYs), Years of Life Lost (YLLs), Years Lived with Disabilities (YLDs), and others. It explains how to calculate these metrics and discusses their components in detail. You will explore the machine learning framework and learn how to apply the influence of infectious disease dynamics on trends in these metrics. The book equips you with all the necessary tools for data collection, analysis, visualisation, and modelling.

Think of it as a toolbox for assessing the health of a country and comparing it with others. You will also learn how to select the best tools for predicting health trends using statistics, visualising data, and working with maps in the R programming language.

Consider this book as your guide to understanding the health status of a population at both global and country levels, leveraging expertise in managing various statistical tools.

Audience and Utility of the Book

This book serves as both a manual and a textbook for introductory courses in health metrics data analysis. Additionally, it provides valuable source code for practitioners and data scientists. The book offers a comprehensive set of tools for analysing various models through tailored case studies. It focuses on health data, providing an overview of the burden of diseases to facilitate comparisons between populations' health status. By combining theoretical insights with practical applications, the book aims to equip readers with the necessary skills to conduct health data analyses and make informed decisions.

Prerequisites

Before delving into the book, it is beneficial for readers to have a basic understanding of health concepts and terminologies. Familiarity with fundamental statistical concepts can aid in comprehending the metrics discussed. Additionally, a grasp of basic epidemiological principles and awareness of global health challenges will enhance the reader's engagement. However, it is important to note that if this knowledge is not already in place, a dedicated section in the book provides the necessary background.

A basic knowledge of the R programming language is required for those interested in the technical aspects of health data analysis, which cover a large part of this book. An open mindset and curiosity about the evolving field of health metrics are key prerequisites, as the book covers a spectrum from historical perspectives to modern machine learning applications.

Overall, a multidisciplinary approach, combining aspects of health sciences, statistics, and technology, will enrich the reader's experience.

Acknowledgements

A big thank you to all my friends and colleagues for their support throughout this journey. Your encouragement and belief in my work have been invaluable.

This book is the result of nearly four years of dedicated work, research, and continuous learning in the field of data science and public health. My journey began as a consequence of the COVID-19 outbreak. Witnessing the global impact of this pandemic inspired me to investigate the spread of infectious diseases and contribute to the understanding and management of public health crises.

I would also like to acknowledge the invaluable assistance of ChatGPT, an AI language model developed by OpenAI, which provided essential inputs, helped refine complex ideas, and offered suggestions that greatly enhanced the content of this book. The ability to leverage such advanced technology has significantly contributed to the clarity and depth of the material presented.

Finally, I would like to express my profound gratitude to the researchers, data scientists, and public health experts whose work and insights have been referenced and built upon throughout this book. Your pioneering efforts and dedication to improving public health have laid the foundation for the analyses and models discussed herein. Your contributions have been a source of inspiration and guidance.

How to Cite This Book

To cite this book in publications, please use:

> Federica Gazzelloni (2024). *Health Metrics and the Spread of Infectious Diseases: Machine Learning Applications and Spatial Modelling Analysis with R.* CRC Press, Boca Raton, FL, USA. ISBN: .

About the Author

The author of this book is *Federica Gazzelloni*[1], Actuary and Statistician by education and training. She is also a collaborator[2] at the *Institute for Health Metrics and Evaluation (IHME)*, which inspired this work to serve as a manual providing formulas and code for working with health metrics. Federica began focusing on modelling health data, particularly infectious diseases, following the COVID-19 outbreak, when this deadly disease was rapidly spreading worldwide. Before that, she briefly worked in corporate and academic environments, serving as a research practitioner actuary and teaching mathematics to high school students

[1] To learn more about the author's ongoing projects, please visit here: https://www.federicagazzelloni.com

[2] If you'd like to know more about who are GBD Collaborators, have a look here: https://www.healthdata.org/research-analysis/gbd/collaborator-network

and computer science to university students. She is actively involved with the open source tech community, collaborating with organisations such as Actex Learning, the Carpentries, Bioconductor, and the R Consortium. More about her ongoing projects here: https://federicagazzelloni.com/

Data Sources

All data used in this book are from the **Institute for Health Metrics and Evaluation (IHME). GBD Results**. Seattle, WA: IHME, University of Washington, 2020 (https://vizhub.healthdata.org/gbd-results/ - accessed January 2023), the **World Health Organization (WHO), Global Health Observatory data repository** (https://apps.who.int/gho/data/), and the **European Centre for Disease Prevention and Control (ECDC)** (https://opendata.ecdc.europa.eu/covid19/).

In particular, for reproducibility all data used throughout the book is collected in the `{hmsidwR}` R package, years span from 2000 to 2021, and both the GBD 2019 and 2021 is used. Careful consideration is to be done when data is extracted before the next GBD study data is released, as then all data is updated to consider the estimates of the latest GBD study. In some parts of the book the data is extracted from the IHME API, the GHO, and Athena WHO API – the code is provided in the book.

Author

Federica Gazzelloni is an Actuary and Statistician with a focus on health metrics, machine learning, and data visualization. Her collaboration with the Institute for Health Metrics and Evaluation (IHME) inspired her to create this book as a practical guide for analyzing health metrics data, bridging complex methodologies with real-world applications.

Prior to her work in public health, she gained experience in both corporate and academic settings, where she served as a research-oriented actuary, taught mathematics to high school students, and instructed university students in computer science. This varied background enables her to bridge complex statistical concepts with real-world applications, making data-driven insights accessible to broader audiences.

A dedicated advocate for open-source technology and inclusivity, Federica is an active contributor to organizations such as the Data Science Learning Community (DSLC), Actex Learning, The Carpentries, Bioconductor, and the R Consortium. As the lead organizer of R-Ladies Rome, she fosters a supportive space for underrepresented groups in technology to develop skills in data science and visualization. Her passion for turning complex data into clear, actionable visual narratives is reflected throughout her work.

For updates on her latest projects and initiatives, visit federicagazzelloni.com.

1

Introduction

1.1 The Concept of Health

The concept of being "well" has evolved over the years and is not solely confined to physical health. Traditionally, health metrics focused on factors like life expectancy, mortality rates, and the prevalence of diseases. However, the understanding of well-being has expanded to include broader dimensions, incorporating mental health, social factors, and overall life satisfaction.

In recent years, there has been an increased emphasis on holistic well-being, recognizing that health is not merely the absence of disease but a state of complete physical, mental, and social well-being. This perspective aligns with the 1946 *World Health Organization*'s constitution principles[1] of health which states: **"a state of complete physical, mental, and social well-being and not merely the absence of disease or infirmity."**

1.1.1 The Culture

The cultural context significantly influences the values, norms, and expectations within a society, and these, in turn, contribute to people's understanding of what constitutes a good life. Education, media, legal systems, and community practices all play pivotal roles in shaping individuals' perceptions of well-being. Cultural norms and values often define what is considered acceptable or taboo, influencing individuals' behaviours and aspirations. Understanding these cultural nuances is crucial when developing health metrics and policies that aim to capture and improve well-being. It emphasises the need for a holistic approach that considers not only physical health but also the social, cultural, and psychological dimensions of individuals and communities.

Achieving a global mean or standard for well-being involves considering, not just the diversity of cultures but also acknowledging the common elements that contribute to human happiness and health. Behavioural education, more specifically the process of teaching individuals how to modify their behaviours in order to improve their overall well-being, plays a pivotal role in this process. Promoting positive behaviours that are conducive to both individual and societal well-being can be a universal goal. Understanding what constitutes "good behavior" in the context of health and happiness is, indeed, central to standardising well-being metrics.

[1] "Constitution of the World Health Organization," n.d., https://www.who.int/about/accountability/governance/constitution.

DOI: 10.1201/9781032625935-1

Moreover, this aligns with the idea that *health is closely tied to happiness.* Cultivating positive behaviours, such as maintaining a healthy lifestyle, fostering social connections, and contributing to one's community, can significantly impact both health and happiness. These behaviours can be universal, yet their interpretation and emphasis might vary based on cultural contexts.

1.1.2 A Global Perspective

In essence, achieving global standardisation in well-being requires a multi-faceted approach that includes education, social support systems, and a collective effort to reshape cultural narratives. It's a complex task, but incremental changes in education and social structures can contribute to a more harmonised vision of well-being across diverse cultures.

The aim of this book is to provide extensive information about the way this well-being can be statically measured. Public health metrics, such as **Years of Life Lost (YLL)** and **Years lived with Disability (YLD)**, are examples of the key metrics discussed and used throughout this book. They are expressed in *number of years of life lost* or *years lived with disabilities*, and their sum represents a crucial value named **Disability Adjusted Life Years (DALYs)**. DALYs are generally used for ranking the health status of a population. The book covers the history of the development of the health metrics and aims at stimulating reasoning to suggest alternatives by providing a comprehensive manual to make reference to if you get lost among the plethora of information. The hope is to provide insights for health researchers and policymakers.

To be more specific, the book compares the metrics used to summarise the health status of a population across different locations. It tests prediction levels using key models. The initial tools are `{tidymodels}` and `{INLA}` for modelling, but other machine learning packages like `{mlr3}` and `{caret}` are also tested as alternative tools.

In practice, the data will include information about humanity such as age, sex, life expectancy, mortality, and risk levels. The interesting part is related to the identification of insights from past outbreaks to predict and manage future ones. This is done through a process called *model transfer*. Imagine each outbreak as a story with unique but similar events, like the spread patterns and impacts of diseases. By studying these *stories*, models can be built to capture key factors influencing outbreaks, such as transmission rates, environmental triggers, and population behaviours.[2]

A focus on the impact of recent infectious disease outbreaks, such as SARS-Covid19, on the state of health of the population, will be provided along with the most affected locations to compare results of both *deterministic* and *stochastic* (Bayesian) models. Risk factor analysis is another important aspect covered in this book. It aims at identifying connections that could lead to an increase in the number of DALYs for specific populations. Additionally, it looks at providing suggestions for public health policy and practice.[3]

[2]Kirstin Roster, Colm Connaughton, and Francisco A. Rodrigues, "Forecasting New Diseases in Low-Data Settings Using Transfer Learning," *Chaos, Solitons, and Fractals* 161 (August 2022): 112306, doi:10.1016/j.chaos.2022.112306.

[3]Theo Vos et al., "Global Burden of 369 Diseases and Injuries in 204 Countries and Territories, 1990–2019: A Systematic Analysis for the Global Burden of Disease Study 2019," *The Lancet* 396, no. 10258 (October 2020): 1204–22, doi:10.1016/s0140-6736(20)30925-9.

1.2 The Structure of the Book

The book is structured with an alternation of text and chunks of code, primarily in the R programming language; hints for translations in Python are provided in Appendix C. The book encourages readers to actively engage with real-world case studies, transforming theoretical concepts into practical skills. This hands-on approach enables readers to become practitioners, applying the methods learned directly to relevant scenarios.

The material supports full exploratory data analysis and model visualisation, offering code for generating compelling spatial visualisations using packages such as `{ggplot2}`, `{leaflet}`, `{sf}`, and `{terra}`, among others, which allow for extensive user customization. The inclusion of these tools is intended to unlock the full potential of the R language, broadening the reader's understanding of both spatial and health metrics.

To ensure reproducibility, the book-project employs the `{renv}` package, which provides a snapshot of the specific versions of all packages used during the writing of the book Appendix B. This enables readers to restore all R package libraries to the exact versions they were in at the time of writing, ensuring that all code examples work as intended regardless of future package updates. This detail is crucial for readers who wish to recreate the analysis or adapt it to their own datasets.

This book is designed for practitioners at early stages of their careers and graduate students in STEM fields, yet it remains a valuable resource for experts who seek to have all the tools in one place for quick reference. The overarching goal of this book is to contribute to the scientific development of health metrics and evaluation, providing a comprehensive resource that supports both learning and application in this important field.[4]

1.2.1 Navigating the Chapters and Key Concepts

First Section: Metrics and Evaluation

The **Metrics and Evaluation** section introduces the foundational concepts of health metrics. Chapter 2 (**Introduction to Health Metrics**), provides an overview of the definitions, historical context, and development of health metrics over time. Chapter 3 (**Methods and Calculations**) is a first level calculation of the metrics, including Disability-Adjusted Life Years (DALYs) and their components: Years of Life Lost (YLLs) and Years Lived with Disability (YLDs), along with Healthy Life Expectancy (HALE), which represents an advanced development in assessing population health. Chapter 4 (**Metrics Components**) examines essential building blocks for maintaining consistency in population health calculations, covering life tables, life expectancy, mortality rates, incidence, prevalence, and disability weights. This chapter is complemented by Appendix A, where detailed calculations are further explained. Chapter 5 (**Causes and Risks**) evaluates the factors influencing these metrics and identifies major threats that increase YLLs and YLDs, stimulating exploration of preventive strategies and policy development.

Second Section: Machine Learning

The **Machine Learning** section offers a deeper dive into evaluating health metrics using modelling techniques and provides an overview of R packages. Chapter 6 (**Introduction to

[4]Christopher JL Murray and Julio Frenk, "Health Metrics and Evaluation: Strengthening the Science," *The Lancet* 371, no. 9619 (April 5, 2008): 1191–99, doi:10.1016/S0140-6736(08)60526-7.

Machine Learning) guides readers on how to utilise machine learning models in health metrics analysis. Chapter 7 (**Techniques for Machine Learning Applications**) covers various types of models appropriate for health data. Chapter 8 (**Essential R Packages for Machine Learning**) lists useful R packages for modelling, paired with case study applications to illustrate practical use. Chapter 9 (**Predictive modelling and Beyond**) focuses on applying predictive models to forecast health outcomes and trends.

Third Section: Data Visualisation

The **Data Visualisation** section equips readers with the knowledge to create and customise plots and maps in R. Chapter 10 (**Introduction to Data Visualisation**) discusses the history and application of data visualisation techniques in R. Chapter 11 (**Interpreting Model Results Through Visualisation**) provides detailed methods for tailoring visual representations to enhance data interpretation. Chapter 12 (**Spatial Data Modelling and visualisation**) instructs on how to create informative maps, while Chapter 13 (**Advanced Data Visualisation Techniques**) presents practical examples to reinforce learning.

Fourth Section: Infectious Diseases

The **Infectious Diseases** section starts with Chapter 14 (**Introduction to Infectious Diseases**) setting the stage for detailed case studies. Chapter 15 (**COVID-19 Outbreaks**) and Chapter 16 (**The Case of Malaria**) provide in-depth analysis of COVID-19 and malaria, illustrating how these diseases impact population health metrics. The section concludes with Chapter 17 **(Summary: The State of Health)**, comparing countries and regions to evaluate health status.

Conclusion

The tools and methods introduced in this book serve as a foundation for a deeper understanding of health metrics and evaluation. The book aims to empower readers to apply these concepts to real-world scenarios, fostering a culture of data-driven decision-making in health policy and practice. By combining theoretical knowledge with practical skills, readers can develop a comprehensive understanding of health metrics and their applications, contributing to the advancement of public health research and policy.

Part I

Health Metrics

2

Introduction to Health Metrics

> **"The concept of health also has highly subjective connotations, precisely because it is conditioned by the personal view of happiness." René Dubos[1]**

Health metrics are key variables to understanding the state of health of a population. In this first section of the book we'll explore the history of these metrics, how to calculate them, and how to account for their variation due to causes and risks. We will examine the components of these metrics and the challenges in providing standardised values for global comparison. Additionally, in the following sections, we will learn how to build a model, evaluate the effect of infectious disease spread on health metrics, and how it impacts the overall health status of a population.

2.1 The History of Health Metrics

The history of health metrics is a fascinating journey that spans centuries, evolving from rudimentary observations to sophisticated statistical methods, as illustrated by Figure 2.1.

One of the earliest forms of health metrics can be traced back to the work of *John Graunt*, an Englishman, in the 17th century.[2] In 1662, Graunt published a landmark work titled "Natural and Political Observations Made upon the Bills of Mortality." Graunt, defined as the **father of human demography**, was largely self-educated, and his interest in mortality data was driven by the Bills of Mortality, which were weekly and annual records of deaths in London, and provided information on the number of births and deaths in the city. Graunt meticulously analysed this **mortality data** and produced **tables** that presented various patterns and trends. His work laid the foundation for modern demography and statistical analysis. Among his notable contributions were the concepts of **life expectancy** and **mortality rates**. One of Graunt's key observations was the consistent pattern of higher mortality among infants and young children. He noted the difference in life expectancy between males and females and provided insights into factors influencing mortality, such as epidemics and seasons.

Over time, advancements in mathematics, medicine, and statistics led to the development of more sophisticated health metrics. The 19th century saw the emergence of **life tables**, which provided a systematic way to analyse mortality and life expectancy.

[1] R Dubos, "The State of Health and the Quality of Life." *Western Journal of Medicine* 125, no. 1 (July 1976): 8–9, https://www.ncbi.nlm.nih.gov/pmc/articles/PMC1237171/.

[2] "John Graunt," January 24, 2024, https://en.wikipedia.org/w/index.php?title=John_Graunt&oldid=1198718407.

DOI: 10.1201/9781032625935-2

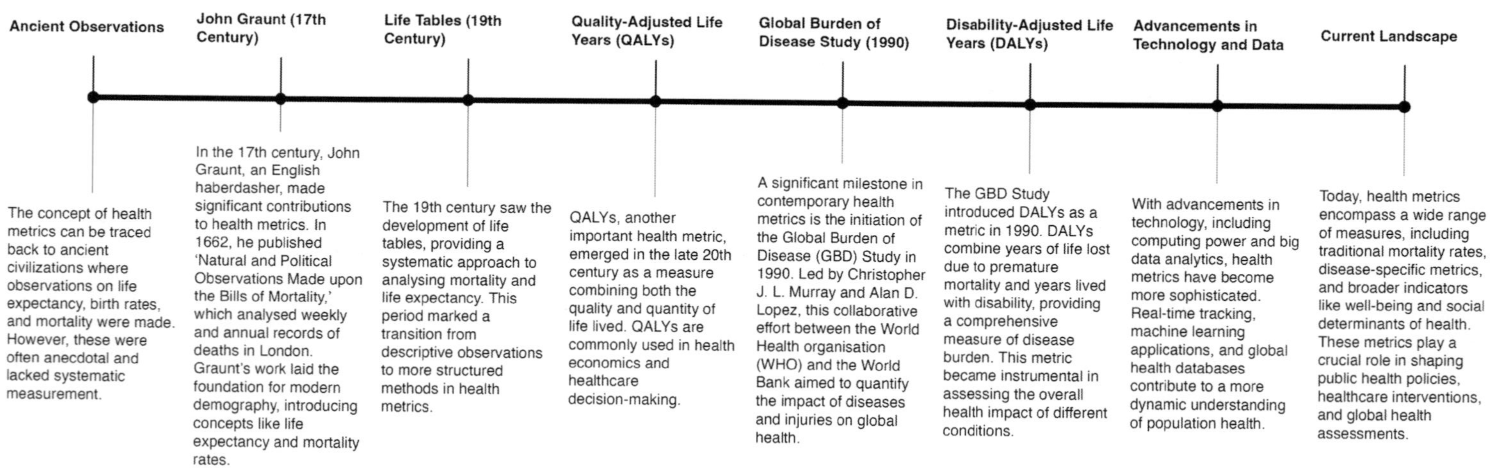

Figure 2.1 Health Metrics Development Timeline

More specifically, *Mary Dempsey* in 1940s wrote an article[3] for the National Tuberculosis Association about the concept of **Years of Life Lost (YLLs)**, assessing time-lost as a metric for health for the first time. She was then followed by other more advanced improvements spanning all throughout the rest of the century.

> **"The quality of life depends also on the state of "public health"-namely on factors that affect the biological welfare of the community as a whole."**[4]

The 20th century marked significant advancements in epidemiology, driving the expansion and refinement of health metrics. This period saw the widespread adoption of life tables and the modification of expected survival time to incorporate weighted metrics, such as disability-adjusted life years (DALYs). These developments enabled more comprehensive assessments of population health by accounting for both mortality and the quality of life, laying the foundation for modern health evaluation tools.

The term **Summary Measures of Population Health (SMPH)**[5] was established in the field, originating from the need to encapsulate both fatal and non-fatal health outcomes into a single, comprehensive measure, representing a significant evolution in health metrics. Used for various purposes, the SMPH compares the health of populations and includes the contributions of different diseases, injuries and risk factors to the total disease burden in a population. SMPH, also referred to as a composite indicator,[6] is divided into two broad families: health expectancies and health gaps.

Health expectancies are summary measures that combine information on mortality and morbidity to represent the average number of years that an individual can expect to live in good health. Such as **healthy life expectancy (HALE)** and the **quality adjusted life expectancy (QALE)** using health-related quality of life.

Health gaps, on the other hand, represent the difference between the current health status of a population and an ideal health situation, providing a measure of the potential for improvement in health outcomes. Divided into the **disability adjusted life years (DALYs)**[7] in the global burden of disease (GBD) study and the **quality adjusted life years (QALY)** used as the outcome index of the cost-utility analysis.

In the contemporary era, the integration of computing power and big data has further transformed health metrics. Today, we have complex models, machine learning algorithms, and global health databases that allow for real-time tracking of diseases and health outcomes.

John Graunt's work may have been modest in its origins, but it laid the groundwork for a scientific approach to understanding population health. From Graunt's early analysis of the *Bills of Mortality*[8] to the development of today's advanced health metrics, this journey reflects the ongoing effort to measure and understand the complexities of human health and disease.

---

[3] Mary Dempsey, "Decline in Tuberculosis," *American Review of Tuberculosis*, April 23, 2019, https://www.atsjournals.org/doi/epdf/10.1164/art.1947.56.2.157?role=tab.

[4] Dubos, "The State of Health and the Quality of Life." July 1976.

[5] Christopher J. L. Murray et al., eds., *Summary Measures of Population Health: Concepts, Ethics, Measurement and Applications* (World Health Organization, 2002).

[6] Adnan A. Hyder, Prasanthi Puvanachandra, and Richard H. Morrow, "Measuring the Health of Populations: Explaining Composite Indicators," *Journal of Public Health Research* 1, no. 3 (December 2012): 222–28, doi:10.4081/jphr.2012.e35.

[7] C. J. Murray, "Quantifying the Burden of Disease: The Technical Basis for Disability-Adjusted Life Years." *Bulletin of the World Health Organization* 72, no. 3 (1994): 429–45, https://www.ncbi.nlm.nih.gov/pmc/articles/PMC2486718/.

[8] "John Graunt," January 24, 2024, https://en.wikipedia.org/w/index.php?title=John_Graunt&oldid=1198718407.

2.1.1 Quality-Adjusted Life Years (QALYs)

The concept of **Quality-Adjusted Life Years (QALYs)** emerged in the late 1970s, originating from the idea of combining both the *quantity* and *quality* of life by *Joseph S. Pliskin*, then it became a widely used metric for evaluating the *cost-effectiveness* of healthcare interventions.[9] One *QALY* corresponds to one year in perfect health, it ranges from 1 (perfect health) to 0 (dead). However, this metric, used in various sectors such as health insurance, is somewhat criticised due to its lack of addressing disparities among individuals. It might result in discrimination against individuals with specific medical conditions or disabilities.

A controversial outcome emerged after 25 years of research and studies, raising concerns about the metric's validity and inclusiveness. Started in the early 1989s, to step in the 2010 with the *European Commission*[10] which started the largest-ever study specifically dedicated to testing the assumptions of the *QALY*,[11] ending in 2013 with the recommended "not using QALYs in healthcare decision making", arguing that patients with disabilities are valued less under a QALY-based system than individuals with no disabilities. This result has been further criticised and remains a topic of debate.

> **"Thus, medicine cannot by itself determine the quality of life. It can only help people to achieve the state of health that enables them to cultivate the art of life-but in their own way. This implies the ability to enjoy the fundamental satisfactions of the biological joie de vivre. It also implies the ability for each person to do what he wants to do and become what he wants to become, according to human values that transcend medical judgement" R.Dubos**[12]

Used in health policy to measure the value of medical interventions by balancing both the quantity and quality of life added, QALYs help decision-makers determine which treatments or programs offer the greatest health benefits relative to their costs. For example, a health policy might prioritise funding for treatments that deliver high QALYs per dollar spent, ensuring resources are allocated to maximise health outcomes across the population. This approach guides decisions in healthcare budgeting, insurance coverage, and prioritising interventions for chronic illnesses, preventive care, or new therapies.

2.1.2 Disability-Adjusted Life Years (DALYs)

In the 1990s, the World Bank financed a study at Harvard University to develop a sustainable index that considered not only the health status but also the identification of the level of disabilities concerned by disparities. This lead to a new way of comparing the overall health and life expectancy of different countries, released along with the Global Burden of Disease Study in 1990;[13] a project that involved *Christopher J. L. Murray*[14] and *Alan Lopez*,[15]

[9] "Quality-Adjusted Life Year," December 27, 2023, https://en.wikipedia.org/w/index.php?title=Quality-adjusted_life_year&oldid=1192021016.

[10] "Echoutcome," October 8, 2016, https://web.archive.org/web/20161008010513/http://echoutcome.eu/.

[11] David Holmes, "Report Triggers Quibbles over QALYs, a Staple of Health Metrics," *Nature Medicine* 19, no. 3 (March 1, 2013): 248–48, doi:10.1038/nm0313-248.

[12] R. Dubos, "The State of Health and the Quality of Life." *Western Journal of Medicine* 125, no. 1 (July 1976): 8–9, https://www.ncbi.nlm.nih.gov/pmc/articles/PMC1237171/.

[13] C. J. Murray, A. D. Lopez, and D. T. Jamison, "The Global Burden of Disease in 1990: Summary Results, Sensitivity Analysis and Future Directions." *Bulletin of the World Health Organization* 72, no. 3 (1994): 495–509, https://www.ncbi.nlm.nih.gov/pmc/articles/PMC2486716/.

[14] "Christopher J. L. Murray," January 1, 2024, https://en.wikipedia.org/w/index.php?title=Christopher_J._L._Murray&oldid=1192936044.

[15] "Alan Lopez," December 11, 2023, https://en.wikipedia.org/w/index.php?title=Alan_Lopez&oldid=1189335406.

in collaboration with the World Health organization (WHO). This effort resulted in the development of the Disability-Adjusted Life Years (DALYs),[16] a metric that combines **years of life lost due to premature death (YLLs)** and **years lived with disabilities (YLDs)**.

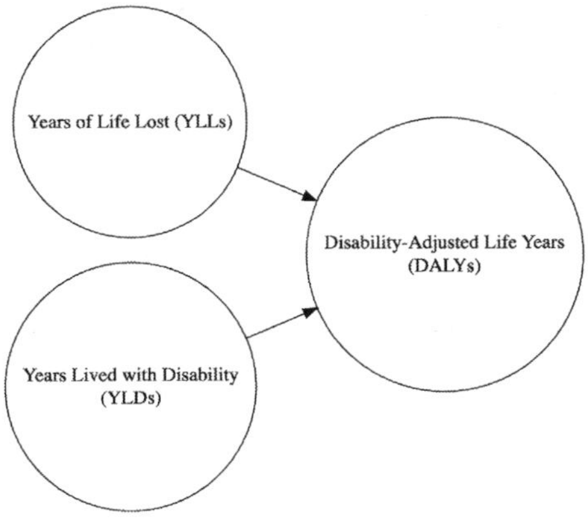

Figure 2.2 YLLs and YLDs components of DALYs

DALYs are connected with QALYs in that both metrics seek to quantify the impact of health on quality and length of life. However, while QALYs focus on the benefits with and without medical intervention, DALYs measure the overall burden of diseases.

The DALY metric is calculated by summing the **years of life lost (YLLs)** due to premature death and the **years lived with disabilities (YLDs)**. This metric provides a comprehensive measure of a population's health status by highlighting both mortality and disability. For example, consider a population with a life expectancy of 80 years. Individuals who die before reaching this age contribute to the YLLs, while those living with disabilities add to the YLDs. The sum of these values gives the total DALYs for the population, which can then be compared globally to assess health status and identify areas needing improvement in facilities, research, or investment.

2.1.3 Health-Adjusted Life Years (HALY)

Health Adjusted Life Years (HALY) is a metric that combines aspects of both DALYs and QALYs to provide a comprehensive measure of health outcomes in a population. HALYs quantify the burden of disease and the overall quality of life experienced by individuals, measuring the number of years of healthy life lived by a population while accounting for both mortality and morbidity. The information about the prevalence of diseases and disabilities, as well as the impact of these conditions on individuals' quality of life is incorporated in the calculation of HALYs.

HALYs adjust life expectancy levels based on the prevalence of health conditions and their associated disability weights. Disability weights reflect the severity of different health conditions and their impact on daily functioning. By applying these weights to the prevalence of each condition, researchers can estimate the overall burden of disease in terms of years of healthy life lost, similar to the calculation of DALYs. Unlike DALYs, which focus primarily on morbidity and mortality, HALYs incorporate measures of individuals' quality of life, allowing for a more comprehensive assessment of health outcomes.

[16] "Disability-Adjusted Life Year," December 8, 2023, https://en.wikipedia.org/w/index.php?title=Disability-adjusted_life_year&oldid=1188922629.

2.1.4 Health-Adjusted Life Expectancy (HALE)

Healthy Life Expectancy (HALE)[17][18] is a measure of overall health and well-being that accounts for both the quantity and quality of life. HALE combines years of life expectancy with the prevalence and severity of disability in a population, providing a more nuanced view of health outcomes than traditional measures of life expectancy.

HALE provides a more comprehensive view of health outcomes than other traditional measures of life expectancy, which only consider the quantity of life. The calculation of HALE typically involves estimating the number of years that an individual can expect to live in good health, taking into account the impact of diseases and injuries on quality of life. This information is then used to estimate the overall health status of a population. It is a useful tool for public health practitioners and policy makers, as it provides a more nuanced view of the health outcomes of a population. This information can help inform public health interventions and prioritise resources, as well as help track changes in health outcomes over time. Additionally, HALE can be used to compare the health outcomes of different populations and identify disparities in health outcomes, which can help inform targeted public health interventions.

Overall, the HALE metric provides a valuable perspective on the overall health and well-being of a population, combining information about both quantity and quality of life to provide a comprehensive view of health outcomes. It adjusts overall life expectancy by the amount of time lived in less than perfect health. This is calculated by subtracting from the life expectancy a figure which is the number of years lived with disability multiplied by a weighting to represent the effect of the disability[19].[20]

2.1.5 Healthy Life Years (HLY)

There is one more health metrics that is worth mentioning, the **Healthy Life Years (HLYs)** indicator, also known as **Disability-Free Life Expectancy (DFLE)** or **Sullivan's Index**.[21] It assesses the number of years an individual can expect to live in good health, free from significant health problems or disabilities. It is a measure of the *quality of life-adjusted life expectancy*, focusing on the years lived in full health rather than simply the total number of years lived. It specifically focuses on the number of years a person can expect to live without disability, providing valuable insights into overall health and well-being beyond just life expectancy. It takes into account both mortality and morbidity, providing a comprehensive picture of overall health and well-being.

HLYs differs from HALE in that it focuses on the number of additional years a person can expect to live in good health after reaching a certain age, typically 65. This makes HLYs especially relevant for assessing health in ageing populations and evaluating interventions that aim to improve the quality of life for older adults.

[17] **Variations in Terminology:** The terms "Health-Adjusted Life Expectancy" (HALE), "Healthy Life Expectancy" (HALE), and other variants are sometimes used interchangeably in this book.

[18] "Indicator Metadata Registry Details," n.d., https://www.who.int/data/gho/indicator-metadata-registry/imr-details/158.

[19] www.healthknowledge.org.uk

[20] "Healthy Life Expectancy (HALE)," n.d., https://www.who.int/data/gho/data/themes/topics/indicator-groups/indicator-group-details/GHO/healthy-life-expectancy-(hale).

[21] "Healthy Life Years," January 26, 2024, https://en.wikipedia.org/w/index.php?title=Healthy_Life_Years&oldid=1199224227.

Table 2.1 Health Metrics Overview

Metric	Purpose	Focus	Usage	Calculation
QALY (Quality-Adjusted Life Year)	Measures health benefits of interventions by combining quantity and quality of life gained	Health gains from interventions	Used in cost-effectiveness studies, healthcare resource allocation, and insurance	Calculated by adjusting life years gained for quality of life (e.g., 1 year at half quality = 0.5 QALY)
DALY (Disability-Adjusted Life Year)	Measures burden of disease by capturing premature death and disability impact	Health loss due to disease and disability	Used in public health to understand and compare disease burden globally	Calculated by summing years of life lost (YLL) and years lived with disability (YLD)
HALY (Health-Adjusted Life Year)	General measure combining health quantity and quality; similar to QALY but less common	Health gains or losses from interventions or disease impact	Used similarly to QALY, though less frequently in decision-making	Calculated by adjusting life years for health quality; similar to QALY
HALE (Healthy Life Expectancy)	Estimates life expectancy in 'healthy' years, adjusting for disability and illness	Overall healthy life expectancy at a population level	Primarily used in population health and public health reports for health expectancy	Calculated by adjusting total life expectancy based on age-specific disability prevalence
HLY (Health Life Years)	Measures the additional healthy years expected, often from a specific age like 65	Healthy life expectancy focused on ageing populations	Used in geriatric health assessments and interventions for ageing populations	Typically calculated by estimating additional years of good health beyond a baseline age
WAHE (Well-being Adjusted Health Expectancy)	Incorporates both physical and subjective well-being for life expectancy in 'full health'	Overall well-being and mental health as well as physical health	Applicable for holistic health assessments, incorporating quality of life and mental wellness	Calculated by weighting health states to reflect impact on well-being and quality of life

For example, an organisation focusing on elder care policy might use HLYs to measure program impact on older adults specifically, while a global health agency might prefer HALE for its applicability to general population health across all ages.

HLY is typically calculated by subtracting the number of years lived with disability from life expectancy at birth. The resulting figure represents the number of years an individual can expect to live in good health, free from significant health-related limitations. Unlike life expectancy, which focuses solely on the length of life, HLY incorporates measures of the quality of life by considering the impact of health conditions on individuals' ability to engage in daily activities and maintain independence.

2.1.6 Well-being-Adjusted Health Expectancy (WAHE)

Currently, **Well-being-Adjusted Health Expectancy (WAHE)** is still an emerging metric in health research that combines traditional health indicators with **well-being factors** to provide a more comprehensive assessment of population health. WAHE is calculated by estimating the number of life years equivalent to full health, taking into account both physical and psychological well-being.

WAHE aims to capture the overall health and well-being of individuals by incorporating measures of physical health, mental health, and social well-being. This metric goes beyond traditional health metrics like life expectancy and disability-adjusted life years to provide a more holistic view of health outcomes by considering factors like **happiness**, **life satisfaction**, and **social connectedness**.

Particularly relevant in the context of global health, WAHE provides a more holistic view of population health that can inform public health policies, healthcare interventions, and resource allocation decisions[22].[23].[24]

2.2 How the Metrics are Used in Global Health

These metrics are used alone or in combination with other health metrics in global health assessments conducted by organisations such as the **World Health Organisation (WHO)**, the **European Commission**, and the **Institute for Health Metrics and Evaluation (IHME)**. They provide a global perspective and insights into the health status of populations, helping to track progresses towards long-term health objectives over time. The metrics also inform public health policies, healthcare interventions, and resource allocation decisions, helping to prioritise health needs and target interventions effectively.

The investigation into finding updated metrics is a sustained commitment, aiming to develop new measures tailored to the evolving landscape of the health field. Recently, the new **Summary Measure of Population Health (SMPH)** proposed the **Well-being-Adjusted Health Expectancy (WAHE)** measure as an estimate of the number of life years equivalent to full health.[25] This approach reflects a growing recognition that health metrics should account for physical and clinical indicators and consider psychological and overall well-being.

2.3 Summary

Health metrics play a crucial role in understanding and improving population health. From John Graunt's early work in the 17th century to today's sophisticated metrics like DALYs,

[22] "Ipc2021," n.d., https://ipc2021.popconf.org/abstracts/210817.

[23] Magdalena Muszyńska-Spielauer and Marc Luy, "Well-Being Adjusted Health Expectancy: A New Summary Measure of Population Health," *European Journal of Population* 38, no. 5 (December 2022): 1009–31, doi:10.1007/s10680-022-09628-1.

[24] Well-Being Adjusted Health Expectancy - a New Summary Measure of Population Health | Population Europe," n.d., https://population-europe.eu/research/books-and-reports/well-being-adjusted-health-expectancy-new-summary-measure-population.

[25] Muszyńska-Spielauer and Luy, "Well-Being Adjusted Health Expectancy".

QALYs, HALYs, HALE, and HLY, these measures have evolved to provide a comprehensive view of health outcomes. They guide public health policies, healthcare interventions, and global health assessments, highlighting areas for improvement and helping to allocate resources effectively. As health metrics continue to evolve, incorporating both traditional and well-being indicators, they will remain essential tools in the quest to quantify and enhance the complexities of human health and disease.

What's next? In the next chapter we will investigate deeper into how DALYs break down health impacts into two powerful metrics—Years of Life Lost (YLLs) and Years Lived with Disability (YLDs). These calculations not only reveal the total toll of disease but drive critical decisions on where to focus resources and which interventions can most effectively boost population health.

3

Methods and Calculations

Learning Objectives

- Explore key health metrics and their significance in public health analysis
- Learn how to apply and interpret these metrics using real-world data
- Identify opportunities to improve health metrics and their use in decision-making

The objective of this chapter is to provide a first level calculation of the burden of diseases, focusing on disability and premature mortality, which are captured by DALYs and HALE. In Chapter 2, we defined the metrics to establish the theoretical framework for constructing them. In this chapter, we will proceed with a general calculation of YLLs and YLDs to obtain the DALYs. This step is essential for understanding the structure of the metric components, which will be further investigated in Chapter 4.

Used to measure the burden of disease and quantify the impact of diseases and injuries on individuals and populations, these metrics can help prioritise public health interventions and evaluate the effectiveness of public health programs.

3.1 YLLs Calculation

The **Years of Life Lost (YLLs)** is a metric that measures the number of years a person would have lived if they had not died prematurely due to a disease or injury. **YLLs are calculated by subtracting the age at death from the expected age at death in a population without the disease or injury**.

In the late 1940s (Chapter 2), **William Haenszel**[1] introduced the concept of **Standardized Rate for Mortality in units of Lost Years of Life**, marking an early attempt to quantify the impact of premature mortality. This approach emphasized the importance of considering the *age at death* and comparing it to the *expected life expectancy*, highlighting that early deaths have a greater impact than those occurring later in life. It was ascertained that accounting for the number of years lost for a group of people would help recognize the potential life lost for a certain cause. Since this first approach, some adjustments to the standard death rates were made, leading to a new calculation that considered standardised death rates applied to age-specific factors for specific causes of death.

[1] William Haenszel, "A Standardized Rate for Mortality Defined in Units of Lost Years of Life," *American Journal of Public Health and the Nations Health* 40, no. 1 (January 1950): 17–26, https://www.ncbi.nlm.nih.gov/pmc/articles/PMC1528498/.

DOI: 10.1201/9781032625935-3

Building on these ideas, **Mary Dempsey**[2] formalized the concept in 1947 to assess the burden of tuberculosis, coining the term **Years of Life Lost (YLLs)**. This metric was specifically designed to identify areas requiring improvement to reduce health loss and prevent premature death.[3] Her work established YLLs as a critical tool for understanding and addressing the disproportionate effects of early mortality on population health.

> The impact of premature losses on society extends beyond the grief of losing a loved one; it also includes the economic and social cost of losing productive members of the workforce. Such premature deaths lead to a significant burden on the community, affecting overall economic stability and societal well-being.

Standard Formula

$$YLL = N * le \tag{3.1}$$

In Equation 3.1, N is the number of premature deaths, and le is the standard life expectancy at the age of death. This calculation takes into account the number of deaths at each age and multiplies it by the standard life expectancy remaining at that age, using global life tables to determine life expectancy. More details about the components of YLLs are provided in the next chapter (Chapter 4), and a sample of the construction of a life table with relative estimations of the life expectancy can be found in Appendix A.

In general, the **Global Burden of Disease studies (GBD)** use standardised life tables, to consistently measure the impact of various diseases. This approach allows for reliable comparisons across different conditions and populations, providing a comprehensive assessment of disease burden on a global scale.[4] Additionally, country-specific life expectancies are valuable for investigating premature deaths resulting from health-related causes, such as fatal diseases. For instance, certain types of country-specific life expectancies are frequently recommended due to their ability to provide insight into longevity characteristics, which can inform policymakers and aid in prevention efforts, as exemplified by the Japanese life expectancy.[5] A G7 cross-country study demonstrated that Japan has the longest average life expectancy, primarily attributed to significantly low mortality rates from ischemic heart disease and cancer, which are the leading causes of death in most countries, as indicated by the GBD study.

3.1.1 Example: YLLs Due to Stroke

Stroke can be a consequence of several infectious diseases, such as COVID-19, Tuberculosis (TB), and Malaria. The impact of these diseases on the cardiovascular system can lead to stroke, as infections can cause inflammation, blood clot formation, or direct damage to blood vessels.

In the following example, we calculate the YLLs due to stroke in the year 2019 for the Global region. We use the data from the Global Burden of Disease (GBD) study, which

---

[2] Mary Dempsey, "Decline in Tuberculosis," *American Review of Tuberculosis*, April 23, 2019, https://www.atsjournals.org/doi/epdf/10.1164/art.1947.56.2.157?role=tab.

[3] Robert C. Reiner and Simon I. Hay, "The Overlapping Burden of the Three Leading Causes of Disability and Death in Sub-Saharan African Children," *Nature Communications* 13, no. 1 (December 6, 2022): 7457, doi:10.1038/s41467-022-34240-6.

[4] Brecht Devleesschauwer et al., "Valuing the Years of Life Lost Due to COVID-19: The Differences and Pitfalls," *International Journal of Public Health* 65, no. 6 (2020): 719–20, doi:10.1007/s00038-020-01430-2.

[5] Shoichiro Tsugane, "Why Has Japan Become the World's Most Long-Lived Country: Insights from a Food and Nutrition Perspective," *European Journal of Clinical Nutrition* 75, no. 6 (2021): 921–28, doi:10.1038/s41430-020-0677-5.

provides estimates of the **number of deaths due to stroke** in different regions. The data can be downloaded from the `{hmsidwR}` package, which contains the necessary datasets for this calculation. The `deaths2019` dataset comprises 2754 observations and 7 variables, containing the estimated number of deaths due to 9 causes, including stroke, across 6 regions: Global, France, Italy, Germany, the United Kingdom, and the United States. We also use the **Global Health Observatory Life Tables** to estimate the life expectancy at different ages, which is used to calculate the YLLs due to stroke.

```
install.packages("hmsidwR")
# install.packages("devtools")
devtools::install_github("Fgazzelloni/hmsidwR")
```

```
library(tidyverse)
library(hmsidwR)
```

```
unique(hmsidwR::deaths2019$cause)
#> [1] "Lower respiratory infections"
#> [2] "Stroke"
#> [3] "Chronic obstructive pulmonary disease"
#> [4] "Road injuries"
#> [5] "Diabetes and kidney diseases"
#> [6] "Colon and rectum cancer"
#> [7] "Tracheal, bronchus, and lung cancer"
#> [8] "Breast cancer"
#> [9] "Alzheimer's disease and other dementias"
```

Our specific task is to calculate the Years of Life Lost (YLLs) attributable to stroke in the year 2019 for the Global region. We filter the location to be "Global" and the cause to be "Stroke". The use of `str_detect()` is to match the cause of death containing a specific word, it is very useful when the cause of death is not exactly containing just one word.

```
deaths_stroke <- hmsidwR::deaths2019 %>%
  arrange(age)%>%
  filter(location == "Global",
         str_detect(cause, "Stroke")) %>%
  select(-location, -cause, -upper, -lower)

deaths_stroke %>% head()
#> # A tibble: 6 x 3
#>   sex    age      dx
#>   <chr>  <ord> <dbl>
#> 1 male   <1     3640.
#> 2 female <1     2404.
#> 3 both   <1     6044.
#> 4 male   01-04 2049.
#> 5 female 01-04 1505.
#> 6 both   01-04 3553.
```

Then, we visualise the number of deaths due to stroke by age group, with a `geom_boxplot()`. The boxplot shows the distribution of the number of deaths by age group, with the median, quartiles, and outliers. The plot is divided by age group and shows the variation in the number of deaths due to stroke between gender as it is stratified by gender, highlighting variations in stroke mortality between males and females. We can observe the difference in the number of deaths increases for older age groups.

```
deaths_stroke %>%
  filter(!sex == "both") %>%
  ggplot(aes(x = age,y = dx)) +
  geom_boxplot() +
  labs(title = "Male and Female Deaths due to Stroke",
       subtitle = "Year 2019",
       caption = "IHME GBD 2019 Data",
       x = "Age Group", y = "Deaths") +
  theme(axis.text.x = element_text(angle = 45, hjust = 1))
```

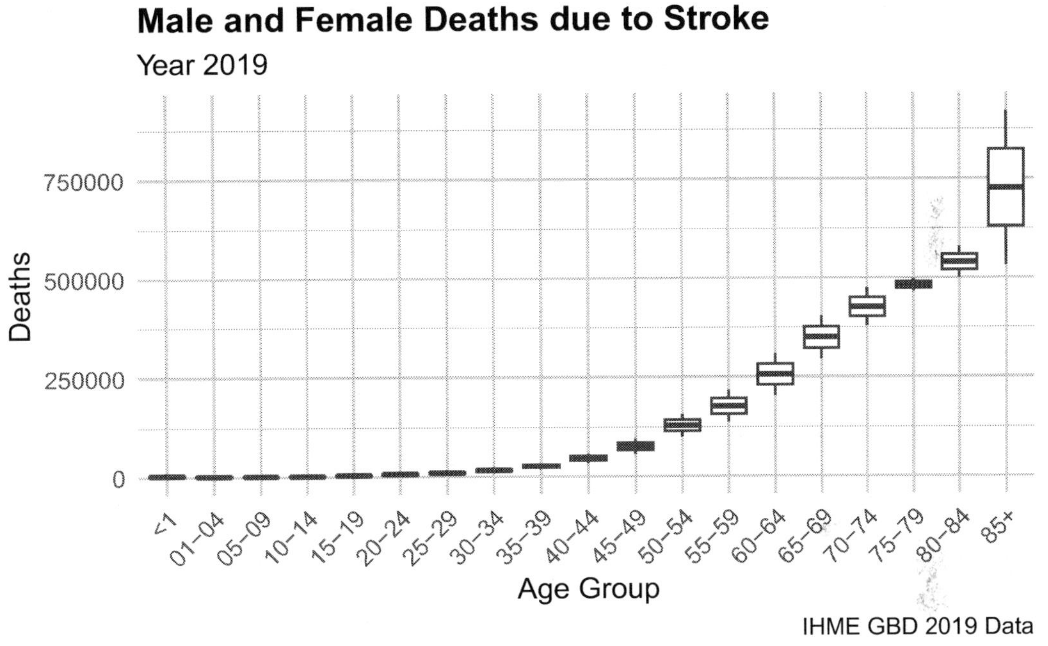

Figure 3.1 Boxplots showing male and female deaths variation due to Stroke by Age Group (2019)

Among the indicators available in the `hmsidwR::gho_lifetables` dataset, we specifically focus on the indicator denoted as e_x. The expectation of life at age x (e_x) refers to the *average number of additional years a person is expected to live*, given that they have already reached age x. This measure is commonly referred to as life expectancy at age x. This dataset is part of the Global Health Observatory (GHO) data repository, which is maintained by the World Health Organization (WHO). The dataset also contains life table indicators, such as the number of person-years lived above age x (l_x), the number of person-years lived between ages x and $x+n$ ($_nL_x$), the age-specific death rate between ages x and $x+n$ ($_nM_x$), the number of people dying between ages x and $x+n$ ($_nd_x$), and the probability of dying between ages x and $x+n$ ($_nq_x$).

Table 3.1 Life Table Indicators

Indicator	Description
Tx	person-years lived above age x
ex	expectation of life at age x
lx	number of people left alive at age x
nLx	person-years lived between ages x and x+n
nMx	age-specific death rate between ages x and x+n
ndx	number of people dying between ages x and x+n
nqx	probability of dying between ages x and x+n

We use the estimated value of the expected life for 5-year age groups, such as `<1, ... , 05-09, 10-14`, etc. for both females and males.

On the other hand, the standard life expectancy represents the *maximum number of years a person is expected to live from birth.* For example, according to estimates released in 2021 by the United Nations Population Division, the **Japanese life expectancy at birth** is approximately 84.6 years. This figure is significantly higher than the global average life expectancy of around 72.6 years.

To calculate the YLLs due to stroke, we need to use the life expectancy at different ages. We filter the `gho_lifetables` dataset to year 2019, which is the most updated year available for the life expectancy data, and select the indicator `ex` to get the life expectancy at different ages, renaming it as `le`.

```
ex2019 <- hmsidwR::gho_lifetables %>%
  filter( year == 2019, indicator == "ex") %>%
  select(-indicator, -year) %>%
  rename(le = value)

ex2019 %>% head()
#> # A tibble: 6 x 3
#>   age   sex      le
#>   <ord> <chr>  <dbl>
#> 1 <1    male    70.8
#> 2 <1    female  75.9
#> 3 <1    both    73.3
#> 4 01-04 male    72.0
#> 5 01-04 female  76.9
#> 6 01-04 both    74.4
```

Then we merge the `deaths_stroke` with the `ex2019` data to calculate the YLLs due to stroke in the Global region with the `full_join()` function, and group the data by age and sex before to create one more vector named `YLL`, which is the product of the number of deaths and the life expectancy at that age. These YLLs values are expressed in millions, and are not necessarily the real values, but estimated values. Their values are strongly dependent on the life expectancy and the number of deaths due to stroke, also other adjustments can be made to the life expectancy values to get more accurate results. In the past, the calculation of YLLs included the use of a discount rate, which is no longer used in the most recent calculations.

Table 3.2 YLLs due to Stroke in the Global region-5 years age groups

```
YLL_global_stroke %>% head()
#> # A tibble: 6 x 5
#>   sex    age      dx    le     YLL
#>   <chr>  <ord> <dbl> <dbl>   <dbl>
#> 1 male   <1    3640.  70.8 257916.
#> 2 female <1    2404.  75.9 182396.
#> 3 both   <1    6044.  73.3 443136.
#> 4 male   01-04 2049.  72.0 147563.
#> 5 female 01-04 1505.  76.9 115680.
#> 6 both   01-04 3553.  74.4 264428.
```

```
YLL_global_stroke <- deaths_stroke %>%
  full_join(ex2019) %>%
  group_by(age, sex) %>%
  mutate(YLL = dx * le) %>%
  ungroup()
```

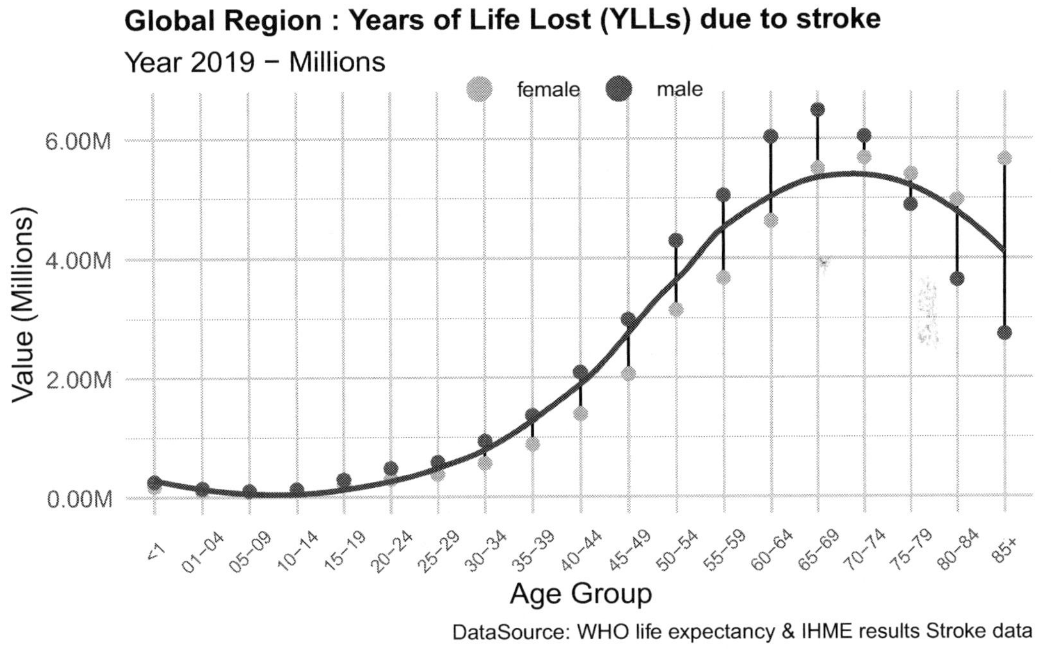

Figure 3.2 YLLs due to Stroke in the Global region

Based on these results, we can conclude that the components of YLLs due to stroke are essential measures of the impact of this condition on the quality of life of individuals in the Global region. The YLLs due to stroke are particularly high in older age groups, where the number of deaths is higher, and the life expectancy is lower. This indicates that stroke has a significant impact on the overall burden of disease in the Global region, particularly among older populations.

Table 3.3 All-Ages IHME Metrics for Stroke in the Global region for the year 2019

```
stroke_ihme %>%
  mutate(across(where(is.numeric), ~round(., 2))) %>%
  filter(year == 2019,
         age == "All ages") %>%
  select(metric, DALYs, YLDs, YLLs)
#> # A tibble: 3 x 4
#>   metric          DALYs        YLDs         YLLs
#>   <chr>           <dbl>       <dbl>        <dbl>
#> 1 Number  156261906.   14462764.   141799142.
#> 2 Percent          0.06        0.02         0.08
#> 3 Rate          2018.        187.        1831.
```

3.1.2 Exercise: All-Ages YLLs Estimation

Calculate the YLLs due to stroke in the Global region for **All-ages**, and compare the results with the IHME data for the year 2019.

The YLLs due to stroke in the Global region in 2019-IHME data can be downloaded from the healthdata.org, with 2019 data reflecting the updates of 2021 GDB releases.

The `stroke_ihme`[6] dataset contains the estimated values for the numbers, percent and rates of Deaths, DALYs, YLLs, and YLDs due to stroke in the Global region-All ages and Age-standardized, for years 2019 and 2021.

Filtering the data for the year 2019-All Ages, we can visualise only the values of all metrics due to stroke in the Global region, as shown below.

In the Global region, YLLs (Years of Life Lost) due to stroke for all age groups total 141.799 million years, accounting for 8% of the total disease burden. On average, approximately 1,830 years of life were lost prematurely due to stroke for every 100,000 people in the population.

To calculate the YLLs due to stroke in the Global region for **All-ages** use the Table 3.2 datasets, and compare the results with the IHME data for the year 2019. As estimated by the IHME for the year 2019, this calculation is based on the number of deaths caused by stroke and the corresponding life expectancy at different ages, which together determine the YLLs attributable to stroke.[7]

Note that the values are not necessarily the real values, but estimated values. Their values are strongly dependent on the life expectancy and the number of deaths due to stroke, also other adjustments can be made to the life expectancy values to get more accurate results. In the past, the calculation of YLLs included the use of a discount rate, which is no longer used in the most recent calculations.

[6] For reproducibility the `stroke_ihme` data is stored in the GitHub repository of the book (https://github.com/Fgazzelloni/hmsidR).

[7] Alize J. Ferrari et al., "Global Incidence, Prevalence, Years Lived with Disability (YLDs), Disability-Adjusted Life-Years (DALYs), and Healthy Life Expectancy (HALE) for 371 Diseases and Injuries in 204 Countries and Territories and 811 Subnational Locations, 1990–2021: A Systematic Analysis for the Global Burden of Disease Study 2021," *The Lancet* 403, no. 10440 (May 18, 2024): 2133–61, doi:10.1016/S0140-6736(24)00757-8.

3.2 YLDs Calculation

YLDs (Years Lived with Disability) measure the number of years a person lives with a disability due to a disease or injury. It is calculated by multiplying the **prevalence of a condition** by the **disability weight**, which reflects the **severity** of the disability.

The key factor of the disability weights (DW) is linked to the severity (mean of the range of health loss suffered to disease) of a non-fatal health condition due to disease or injury. DW ranges between 0 (equivalent to full health) and 1 (equivalent to death). The estimation of the disability weights is challenging and has been continuously changed by modifying and adapting methodologies in various studies.[8] The challenge is assigning disability weights to diseases with different levels of prevalence and severity, such as cases with high prevalence and low severity. People's experiences of the same condition can vary significantly, making it difficult to establish a Standardised weight that accurately reflects the global impact on quality of life. Furthermore, the results need to be reported to a year-based value.

Moreover, the calculation of YLDs has been updated over the years, shifting from an incidence to a prevalence-based approach. More in-depth analyses are in Chapter 4; for now, we will show how both types of calculations differ, but then we will focus on using the most updated approach based on values of prevalence estimated by the GBD2021, summarised in the `hmsidwR::incprev_stroke` dataset. This dataset specifically contains the estimated values for the incidence and prevalence of stroke in the Global region for the years 2019 and 2021.

3.2.0.1 Incidence-based Calculation

Standard Formula

$$YLD_i = I * DW * L \tag{3.2}$$

In Equation 3.2, I is the incidence of the condition, DW is the disability weight, and L is the average duration of the condition. The incidence takes into account the number of new cases of a disease or health condition that occur in a population over a specific period. The disability weight reflects the severity of the health condition, and the average duration of the condition is the average length of time a person lives with the condition.

3.2.0.2 Prevalence-based Calculation

Standard Formula

$$YLD_p = p * DW \tag{3.3}$$

In Equation 3.3, p is the prevalence, DW are the disability weights. While an incidence-based approach focuses on the number of new cases of a health condition, the prevalence-based approach considers the total number of cases in the population. The disability weight reflects the severity of the health condition and it is applied to the prevalence to calculate the YLDs, and the duration of the condition is not considered in the prevalence-based calculation.

[8] Xiaoxue Liu et al., "Disability Weight Measurement for the Severity of Different Diseases in Wuhan, China," *Population Health Metrics* 21 (May 2023): 5, doi:10.1186/s12963-023-00304-y.

3.2.1 Example: YLDs Due to Stroke

Since the release of GBD 2010, the WHO has decided to switch to a prevalence-based approach for the calculation of YLDs. The major impact of this shift is to distribute the weights of the YLDs more evenly across all age groups, rather than concentrating them at the age of incidence.

In the following example we use the `disability weights` and the `severity` levels extracted from a dataset in the GBD study. The `disweights` dataset is stored in the `{hmsidwR}` package and is made of 463 observations and 9 variables. It contains the estimated values for the disability weights, which are measured on a scale from 0 to 1, where 0 equals a state of full health and 1 equals death.

```
hmsidwR::disweights %>%
  filter(year == 2019) %>%
  group_by(cause1, severity) %>%
  reframe(dw = mean(dw)) %>%
  filter(cause1 == "Stroke")
#> # A tibble: 3 x 3
#>   cause1 severity     dw
#>   <chr>  <chr>     <dbl>
#> 1 Stroke mild      0.019
#> 2 Stroke moderate 0.193
#> 3 Stroke severe    0.57
```

The level of **severity** is assigned based on the **degree of disability** assessed by the National Institutes of Health Stroke Scale (NIHSS). The classification is used by healthcare providers to objectively quantify the impairment caused by a stroke. Here is assumed a sample population affected by a stroke, categorised as **mild**, **moderate**, or **severe** with assigned proportions.

Table 3.4 Level of disability by the National Institutes of Health NIH or more specifically by the **National Institutes of Health Stroke Scale (NIHSS)**.

Score	Stroke severity	Severity Level	Severity %
0-4	Minor stroke	Mild	50.3%
5–20	Moderate stroke	Moderate	25.3%
21-42	Severe stroke	Severe	24.4%

These levels are general for all ages; the values might vary for other specifications of the level of disability.[9]

```
dwsev2019 <- hmsidwR::disweights %>%
  select(cause1, severity, dw) %>%
  drop_na() %>%
  mutate(severity_n = case_when(
    severity == "mild" ~ 0.503,
    severity == "moderate" ~ 0.253,
    severity == "severe" ~ 0.244))
```

[9]Grant M. A. Wyper et al., "Prioritising the Development of Severity Distributions in Burden of Disease Studies for Countries in the European Region," *Archives of Public Health* 78, no. 1 (January 2020): 3, doi:10.1186/s13690-019-0385-6.

```
dwsev2019 %>% head()
#> # A tibble: 6 x 4
#>   cause1             severity    dw severity_n
#>   <chr>              <chr>    <dbl>      <dbl>
#> 1 Infectious disease mild     0.006      0.503
#> 2 Infectious disease moderate 0.051      0.253
#> 3 Infectious disease mild     0.006      0.503
#> 4 Infectious disease mild     0.006      0.503
#> 5 Infectious disease mild     0.006      0.503
#> 6 Infectious disease mild     0.006      0.503
```

The values for disability weights and severity are considered for all ages; in general, they differ by age, and for different types of stroke.

```
dw_stroke <- dwsev2019 %>%
  filter(cause1 == "Stroke") %>%
  group_by(severity, severity_n) %>%
  reframe(avg_dw = mean(dw))

dw_stroke
#> # A tibble: 3 x 3
#>   severity severity_n avg_dw
#>   <chr>         <dbl>  <dbl>
#> 1 mild          0.503  0.206
#> 2 moderate      0.253  0.293
#> 3 severe        0.244  0.632
```

Then, calculate the part of the population affected by a specific level of severity considering the prevalence (and/or the incidence) multiplied by the severity levels.

For instance, here we use the `incprev_stroke` and the `dw_stroke` datasets to calculate the YLDs due to stroke, and have a look at how incidence and prevalence differ from each other.

Health metrics values can be expressed as numbers, percentages or rates:

- If the prevalence of stroke is 1,541,506.96 for male with age between 34-39 and it is expressed in numbers, it means that there are approximately 1,541,507 individuals in the age group 35-39 who had a stroke.
- If the prevalence of stroke is 0.58 for male with age between 34-39 and it is expressed in percent value (%), it means 0.58% of the population within that age range had a stroke.
- If the prevalence of stroke is expressed as rate, it is the number of cases of stroke per 100,000 individuals in the population.

Percentages and numbers are related by the size of the population in that age group. To convert between these forms, you need to know the total population in the age group.

Let's consider the numbers of incidence and prevalence, and assign them as two separate vectors in a new dataset named `inc_prev_stroke_5y`. We use the `pivot_wider()` function to spread the data into a wider format, with the `measure` column as the key column and the `val` column as the value column.

```
inc_prev_stroke_5y <- hmsidwR::incprev_stroke %>%
  filter(year == 2019) %>%
  select(measure, sex, age, val) %>%
  pivot_wider(names_from = "measure", values_from = "val")
```

Let's check the values for the age group 35-39.

```
inc_prev_stroke_5y %>%
  arrange(sex) %>%
  filter(age == "35-39")
#> # A tibble: 3 x 4
#>   sex    age   Prevalence Incidence
#>   <chr>  <ord>      <dbl>     <dbl>
#> 1 both   35-39   3147689.   257815.
#> 2 female 35-39   1606182.   113831.
#> 3 male   35-39   1541507.   143984.
```

Then, multiply these values for the severity levels for stroke in the Global region. In this way we obtain three values, one for each severity level.

For calculating the prevalence-based YLDs, we use the `prevalence` values, the `severity` and the `average weights`, while for incidence-based YLDs, we also need to consider the `average duration` of the condition.

In particular, for stroke, the average duration of the condition can vary based on:

- duration for acute stroke: up to 28 days
- duration for chronic stroke: beyond 28 days, often modelled for long-term consequences, sometimes up to the lifetime of the patient depending on the model used.

In this example, we consider the average duration of the condition for 28 days. It does need to be converted to be year-based:

$$\hat{L}_{stroke} = \frac{28}{365} \tag{3.4}$$

These values strongly depend on the disability weights and the severity values assigned to the condition.

```
YLD_by_severity <- merge(inc_prev_stroke_5y, dw_stroke) %>%
  group_by(sex, age, avg_dw) %>%
  reframe(prev_sev = Prevalence*severity_n,
          inc_sev = Incidence*severity_n,
          yld_p = prev_sev* avg_dw,
          yld_i = inc_sev* avg_dw * 28/365)
```

Let's check the values for the age group 35-39.

```
YLD_by_severity %>%
  filter(age == "35-39")
#> # A tibble: 9 x 7
#>   sex    age   avg_dw prev_sev inc_sev    yld_p yld_i
#>   <chr>  <ord>  <dbl>    <dbl>   <dbl>    <dbl> <dbl>
#> 1 both   35-39  0.206 1583288.  129681.  326847. 2054.
#> 2 both   35-39  0.293  796365.   65227.  233379. 1466.
```

```
#> 3 both   35-39  0.632  768036.  62907. 485262. 3049.
#> 4 female 35-39  0.206  807910.  57257. 166781.  907.
#> 5 female 35-39  0.293  406364.  28799. 119087.  647.
#> 6 female 35-39  0.632  391908.  27775. 247616. 1346.
#> 7 male   35-39  0.206  775378.  72424. 160066. 1147.
#> 8 male   35-39  0.293  390001.  36428. 114292.  819.
#> 9 male   35-39  0.632  376128.  35132. 237646. 1703.
```

We can reverse the calculation to check the original values.

```
YLD_by_severity %>%
  filter(age == "35-39") %>%
  group_by(sex, age) %>%
  reframe(prev=sum(prev_sev),
          inc=sum(inc_sev))
#> # A tibble: 3 x 4
#>   sex    age       prev     inc
#>   <chr>  <ord>    <dbl>   <dbl>
#> 1 both   35-39 3147689. 257815.
#> 2 female 35-39 1606182. 113831.
#> 3 male   35-39 1541507. 143984.
```

And, finally calculate the total value for YLDs as:

$$\text{Total YLDs} = \text{YLD}_{\text{mild}} + \text{YLD}_{\text{moderate}} + \text{YLD}_{\text{severe}} \tag{3.5}$$

```
YLD_global_stroke <- YLD_by_severity %>%
  group_by(sex, age) %>%
  reframe(YLD_p = sum(yld_p),
          YLD_i = sum(yld_i))
```

For instance, for a male with age 34-39, the YLDs due to stroke calculated on the population of that age group who have the condition for three different severity levels, are shown below.

```
YLD_global_stroke %>%
  filter(sex == "male",
         age == "35-39")
#> # A tibble: 1 x 4
#>   sex   age     YLD_p YLD_i
#>   <chr> <ord>   <dbl> <dbl>
#> 1 male  35-39 512004. 3669.
```

This value is the sum of the severity levels of prevalence-based YLDs due to stroke; it strongly depends on the disability weights and the severity values assigned to the condition. Here we have considered estimated values, which do not necessarily correspond to the real values.

We note the difference in the YLDs if incidence or prevalence is used in the calculation. The magnitude of the YLDs is similar, but the values are distributed differently across the age groups.

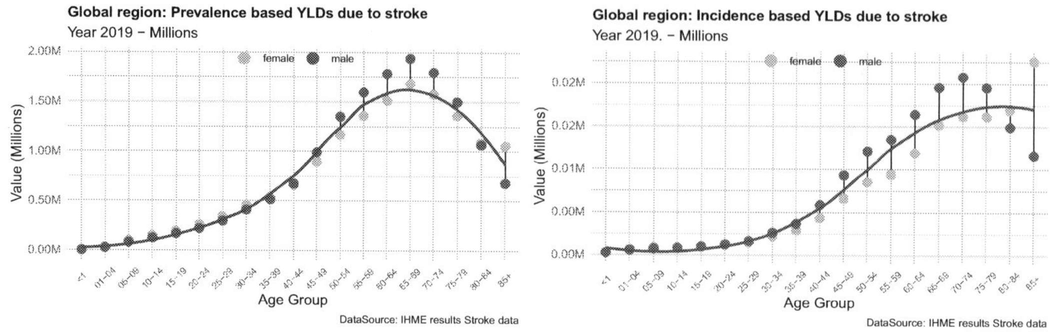

(a) YLDs calculated with prevalence **(b)** YLDs calculated with incidence

Figure 3.3 YLDs due to stroke in the Global region

In summary, the YLDs due to stroke are an important measure of the impact of this condition on the quality of life of individuals in the Global region. In this example we saw how the level of disability and the severity of the condition can affect the YLDs, and how the prevalence-based and incidence-based calculations can provide different results. The YLDs due to stroke are particularly high in older age groups, where the prevalence of the condition is higher, and the severity of the disability is more pronounced. This indicates that stroke has a significant impact on the overall burden of disease in the Global region, particularly among older populations.

3.2.2 Exercise: All-Ages YLDs Estimation

Calculate the YLDs due to stroke in the Global region for **All-ages**, and compare the results with the IHME data for the year 2019 as done for the YLLs. Use the IHME data provided in Section 3.1.2 Table 3.3 from the `stroke_ihme` dataset.

3.3 DALYs Calculation

As a measure of the overall disease burden, **Disability Adjusted Life Years (DALYs)** are used to quantify the sum of years of potential life lost due to premature death (YLLs) and years lived with disability (YLDs). The number of DALYs indicates the number of years of life lost due to premature deaths, disease, or injury. This metric takes into account both the **quantity** and **quality** of life.

DALYs are a generalisation of the well-known **Potential Years of Life Lost measure (PYLLs)**, which includes the loss of good health. We do not consider PYLLs in this book, but more information can be found in the references.[10]

Standard Formula

$$DALYs = YLLs + YLDs \tag{3.6}$$

One DALY is one lost year of healthy life. This measure is used to assess how diseases and injuries impact populations, providing a comprehensive picture of the overall burden of disease by combining YLLs and YLDs in different groups.

[10] "Global Health Estimates," n.d., https://www.who.int/data/global-health-estimates.

3.3.1 Example: DALYs Due to Stroke

The sum of YLLs and YLDs releases the overall value of DALYs due to stroke in the Global region.

```
DALY_global_stroke <- YLL_global_stroke %>%
  select(age, sex, YLL) %>%
  full_join(YLD_global_stroke %>%
              select(age, sex, YLD=YLD_p),
              by = c("age","sex")) %>%
  distinct() %>%
  mutate(DALY = YLL + YLD)

DALY_global_stroke %>%
  head()
#> # A tibble: 6 x 5
#>   age    sex        YLL   YLD    DALY
#>   <ord>  <chr>    <dbl> <dbl>   <dbl>
#> 1 <1     male   257916.  1475. 259391.
#> 2 <1     female 182396.  1696. 184092.
#> 3 <1     both   443136.  3170. 446307.
#> 4 01-04 male    147563. 25094. 172657.
#> 5 01-04 female  115680. 30047. 145728.
#> 6 01-04 both    264428. 55142. 319570.
```

Let's have a closer look at the 35-39 age groups.

```
DALY_global_stroke %>%
  filter(age == "35-39")
#> # A tibble: 3 x 5
#>   age   sex         YLL      YLD    DALY
#>   <ord> <chr>     <dbl>    <dbl>   <dbl>
#> 1 35-39 male   1363806.  512004. 1875809.
#> 2 35-39 female  879509.  533485. 1412994.
#> 3 35-39 both   2273474. 1045489. 3318963.
```

In summary, DALYs are a valuable metric for assessing the overall burden. The DALYs due to stroke provide a comprehensive measure of the impact of this condition on the quality of life of individuals, combining the years of life lost due to premature death and the years lived with disability.

DALYs can vary significantly between conditions, reflecting both the severity and impact of each disease on quality and length of life. For instance, stroke and diabetes, both prevalent globally, differ widely in their DALY contributions. Strokes tend to have high DALYs due to their immediate impact on mortality (Years of Life Lost or YLLs) and long-term disability (Years Lived with Disability or YLDs). On the other hand, diabetes, a chronic condition, has a lower YLLs but a higher YLDs, reflecting the long-term impact on quality of life.

3.3.2 Exercise: Total DALYs Estimation

Calculate the DALYs due to stroke in the Global region for **All-ages**, and compare the results with the IHME data for the year 2019 as done for the YLLs. Use the IHME data provided in Section 3.1.2 Table 3.3 from the `stroke_ihme` dataset.

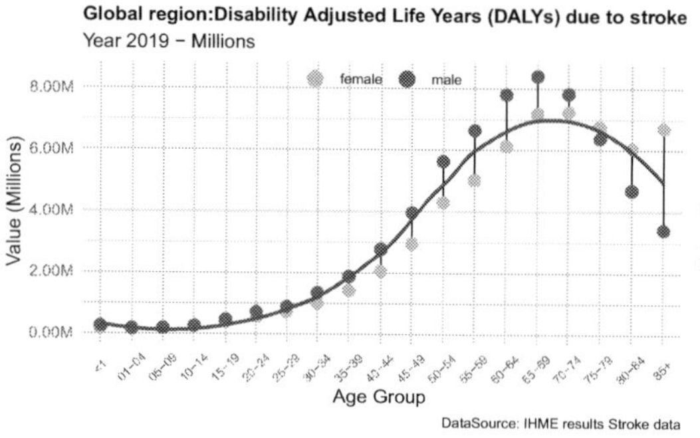

(a) DALYs due to stroke in the Global region for females and males.

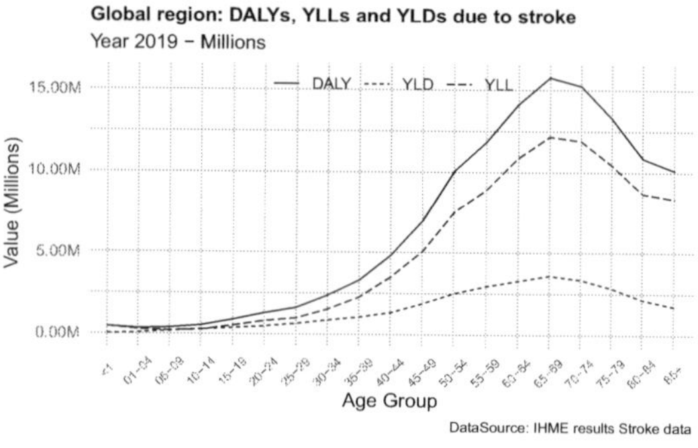

(b) DALYs, YLLs and YLDs due to stroke in the Global region

Figure 3.4 DALYs due to stroke in the Global region

3.4 How DALYs are Used

DALYs, YLLs, and YLDs can be used in several ways to help identify health priorities, evaluate the impact of diseases and injuries, and inform public health decision-making. Some common uses of these metrics include:

- **Prioritising public health interventions**: By calculating the overall burden of disease in a population, public health practitioners can prioritise which diseases and injuries to address first. This helps allocate resources and target interventions to the areas of greatest need.
- **Evaluating the impact of diseases and injuries**: These metrics can be used to measure the impact of diseases and injuries on individuals and populations and to track changes over time. This information can help inform public health decision-making and allocate resources more effectively.
- **Comparing the burden of disease across populations**: DALY, YLL, and YLD can be used to compare the burden of disease across populations and between different regions. This information can help identify disparities in health outcomes and inform targeted public health interventions.
- **Evaluating the effectiveness of public health programs**: These metrics can be used to evaluate the impact of public health programs and to assess the effectiveness of public health interventions. This information can help public health practitioners identify areas for improvement and make necessary changes to ensure that programs are achieving their goals.
- **Monitoring global health trends**: DALY, YLL, and YLD can also be used to monitor global health trends and track changes in the burden of disease over time. This information can be used to inform global health policies and allocate resources to address emerging health threats.

To mention the case of Rwanda, the GBD 2021 results released by the IHME showed that the country had made significant progress in reducing the burden of disease over the past decade.[11] By using DALYs, YLLs, and YLDs, public health leaders were able to

[11] Ferrari et al., "Global Incidence, Prevalence, Years Lived with Disability (YLDs), Disability-Adjusted Life-Years (DALYs), and Healthy Life Expectancy (HALE) for 371 Diseases and Injuries in 204 Countries

identify key areas for improvement and target resources to address the most pressing health challenges. For example, the government used the DALYs metrics to address the burden of non-communicable diseases (NCDs), public health leaders observed that conditions like cardiovascular disease and diabetes were contributing significantly to the country's overall disease burden, surpassing infectious diseases in certain demographics. This insight led to targeted policy shifts, including prioritising funding for NCD prevention and treatment programs, investing in training for healthcare providers on chronic disease management, and increasing public awareness of lifestyle risk factors like smoking and poor diet.

Overall, the health metrics of DALY, YLL, and YLD provide valuable information for public health practitioners, researchers, and policy makers to help prioritise and allocate resources, evaluate the impact of diseases and injuries, and inform public health decision-making.

3.4.1 General Application of DALYs

As an example here is shown how the DALY metric can be used for prevention. Suppose we have data on the number of cases of a particular disease, as well as the average number of years of life lost due to this disease. We can use this information to calculate the total number of DALYs lost due to this disease.

```
# Data frame with the number of cases and average years of life lost
df <- data.frame(
  YLL = c(5, 10, 15),
  YLD = c(1, 3, 4))

# Calculate the number of DALYs lost
df <- df %>% mutate(DALY = YLL + YLD)

# Sum the total number of DALYs lost
total_dalys <- sum(df$DALY)

total_dalys
#> [1] 38
```

In this example, the number of cases of the disease and the average years of life lost for each case are used to calculate the number of DALYs lost for each case. Finally, the total number of DALYs lost for the entire population.

This information can be used to inform public health interventions to prevent the spread of this disease and reduce the number of DALYs lost. For example, the information could be used to prioritise resources for disease control and prevention activities, such as health education campaigns, vaccination programs, and screening and treatment programs.

3.5 HALE Calculation

Healthy Life Expectancy (HALE) is a metric used to estimate the number of years a person can expect to live in good health, taking into account both mortality and morbidity factors. It is often used as a measure of overall population health and quality of life. It takes into account

and Territories and 811 Subnational Locations, 1990–2021".

the impact of both fatal and non-fatal health outcomes on overall life expectancy. HALE is typically calculated using data on mortality rates and health-related quality of life measures, such as disability-adjusted life years (DALYs) or quality-adjusted life years (QALYs). These measures allow for the estimation of the number of years lost due to premature death or disability.

It can be used to identify health disparities, assess the effectiveness of healthcare interventions, and inform public health policies. By measuring the number of years lived in good health, HALE offers a more nuanced understanding of population health rather than traditional life expectancy measures.

Standard Formula

$$HALE = \text{life expectancy} - YLD \tag{3.7}$$

HALE is obtained by subtracting the YLDs from the life expectancy of a population. However, if we consider more specifications such as comorbidities and other health factors that can occur in real life, the calculation can be adjusted by assuming different levels of prevalence based on disease sequelae with associated disability weights, and eventually accounting for comorbidity levels by using a Monte Carlo simulation approach.

We use age-specific mortality and YLDs per capita by location, age, sex, and year, and define the HALE as:

> the average number of years that a person at a given age can expect to live in good health, taking into account mortality and loss of functional health.

The process of calculating HALE for a specific population, considering factors such as sex, country, and year, involves computing the average health of individuals across different age groups within the population and integrating information on the prevalence of various health conditions and their associated disability weights. Comorbidity is addressed using a Monte Carlo simulation approach, assuming independence of comorbidities within each age group. Simulations are conducted to model exposure to different health conditions based on their estimated prevalence in each age group, resulting in a simulated population reflecting the prevalence of multi-morbidities.[12]

Positive health associated with each health condition is defined as one minus the disability weight $(1 - DW)$. The combined health for an individual in the simulated population is determined by multiplying these positive health values for all relevant health conditions present.

The **average health** values are then computed as one minus the Years Lived with Disability (YLD) $(1 - YLD)$ per person in the population, which are used to calculate health-adjusted person years. The **Sullivan method** is employed to incorporate these average health values into the life table. This involves adjusting the values in the nLx column of the life table by the corresponding average health values, recalculating the life table using these adjusted values, and then using an iterative process to estimate health-adjusted person-years for different age groups.

Finally, HALE is calculated by dividing the adjusted person-years for each age group by the proportion of a hypothetical birth cohort still alive at that age.

[12] Jeffrey D Stanaway et al., "Global, Regional, and National Comparative Risk Assessment of 84 Behavioural, Environmental and Occupational, and Metabolic Risks or Clusters of Risks for 195 Countries and Territories, 1990–2017: A Systematic Analysis for the Global Burden of Disease Study 2017," *The Lancet* 392, no. 10159 (November 2018): 1923–94, doi:10.1016/s0140-6736(18)32225-6.

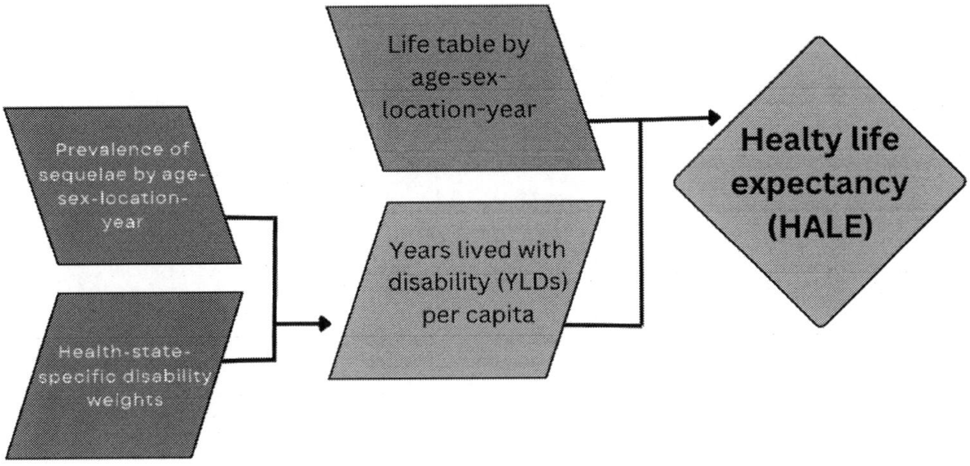

Figure 3.5 HALE - GLOBAL HEALTH METRICS VOLUME 392, ISSUE 10159, P1859-1922, NOVEMBER 10, 2018

3.5.0.1 Simulating Life Table Data

To understand the process of calculating HALE, we can simulate life table data. We'll define age intervals (e.g., every 5 years) and simulate survival probabilities for each age interval (between 0 and 1).

```
set.seed(040424)
age_intervals <- seq(0, 100, by = 5)
survival_probabilities <- runif(length(age_intervals),
                                min = 0.5, max = 1)
```

```
life_table <- data.frame(
  Age = age_intervals,
  Survival_Probability = survival_probabilities,
  nLx = 100000 - (age_intervals * survival_probabilities))

life_table %>% head()
#>   Age Survival_Probability       nLx
#> 1   0            0.5579497 100000.00
#> 2   5            0.9241893  99995.38
#> 3  10            0.8810716  99991.19
#> 4  15            0.9562922  99985.66
#> 5  20            0.6927314  99986.15
#> 6  25            0.5607459  99985.98
```

We then calculate adjusted T_x for each age group as the sum of health-adjusted person-years for all age intervals above the current age interval.

```
# Simulate prevalences
prevalences <- runif(length(age_intervals),
                     min = 0, max = 0.5)
```

```
# Simulate disability weights
disability_weights <- runif(length(age_intervals),
                            min = 0, max = 1)
# Calculate average health for each age group
average_health <- 1 - (prevalences * disability_weights)

# Adjust Tx for each age group
life_table$adjusted_px <- life_table$Survival_Probability * average_health

life_table %>% head()
#>   Age Survival_Probability       nLx adjusted_px
#> 1   0            0.5579497 100000.00   0.5345848
#> 2   5            0.9241893  99995.38   0.7786488
#> 3  10            0.8810716  99991.19   0.5781898
#> 4  15            0.9562922  99985.66   0.7392462
#> 5  20            0.6927314  99986.15   0.5813254
#> 6  25            0.5607459  99985.98   0.3603310
```

Let's make a function to calculate the **HALE**:

```
calculate_HALE <- function(age, px) {
  # Initialise a vector to store adjusted Tx for each age group
  adjusted_Tx <- numeric(length(age))
  # Iterate over each age interval to calculate adjusted Tx
  for (i in 1:length(age)) {
    # Calculate adjusted Tx for the current age group
    adjusted_Tx[i] <- sum(px[i:length(age)])
    }
  HALE <- numeric(length(age))
  # Calculate HALE for each age group
  for (i in 1:length(age)) {
    # Calculate HALE for the current age group
    HALE[i] <- adjusted_Tx[i] / px[i]
  }
  HALE
}
```

Now, we calculate HALE for the simulated life table data.

```
# Calculate HALE for the simulated life table data
HALE1 <- calculate_HALE(age_intervals, life_table$Survival_Probability)
HALE2 <- calculate_HALE(age_intervals, life_table$adjusted_px)
```

To visualise the HALE for both the standard and adjusted life table data we can plot the results with a line graph.

The difference between the two lines represents the impact of adjusting a life table for health conditions on the calculation of HALE. The adjusted life table data considers the prevalence of health conditions and their associated disability weights, providing a more accurate estimate of the number of years a person can expect to live in good health.

In general, HALE is a valuable metric for assessing the overall health of a population, by incorporating information on the prevalence of health conditions and their associated disability weights, HALE offers a more specific understanding of population health.

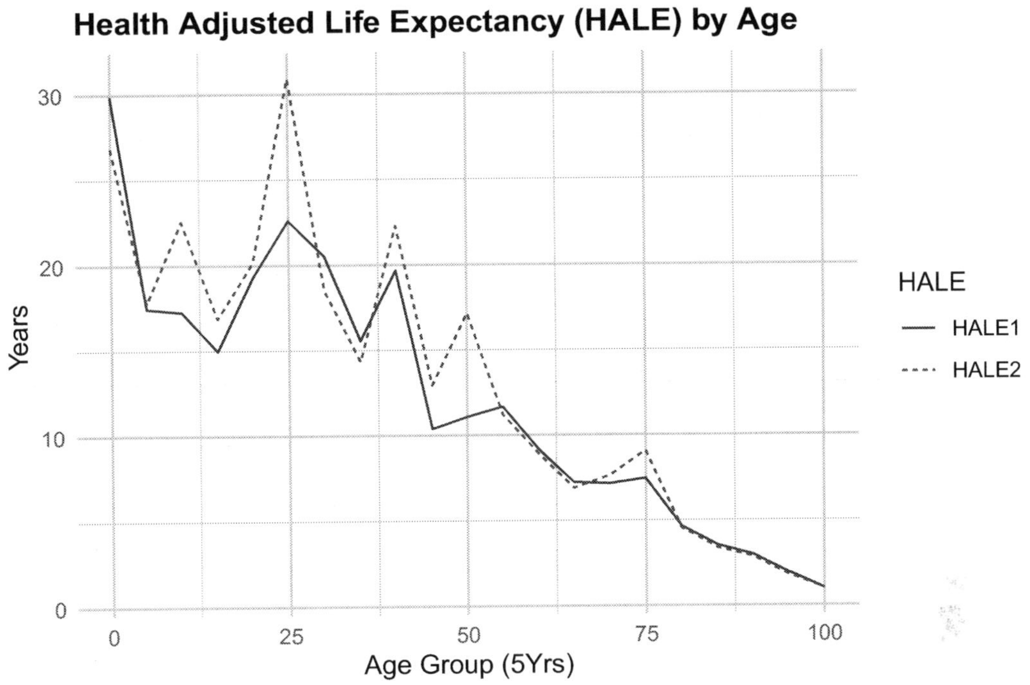

Figure 3.6 Health Adjusted Life Expectancy (HALE) by Age. The blue line represents the HALE for the simulated life table data, the dotted line represents the HALE for the adjusted life table data.

3.6 Summary

In this chapter, we have detailed the methods and calculations for evaluating the burden of disease using key health metrics: YLLs, YLDs, and DALYs. By understanding how to compute these metrics, we gain insights into the impact of diseases and injuries on populations, guiding public health decisions and interventions. We also introduced HALE, a metric that combines mortality and morbidity data to provide a comprehensive measure of population health. These metrics are invaluable tools for public health practitioners, policymakers, and researchers in their quest to improve global health outcomes.

As we confront new global health challenges like pandemics, ageing populations, and climate-related health risks, traditional metrics like DALYs and QALYs are evolving to meet new approaches to capture the complexity of health outcomes. The inclusion of well-being, resilience, and mental health is becoming increasingly essential to understanding the full impact of health conditions on individuals and populations.

In the next chapter (Chapter 4), we will delve deeper into the components and variations of these metrics, further enhancing our understanding of how to utilise them effectively in public health assessments.

4

Metrics Components

Learning Objectives

- Understand the construction and interpretation of life tables and life expectancy measures
- Analyse mortality levels and rates to assess population health dynamics
- Distinguish between incidence and prevalence and their relevance in disease monitoring
- Interpret disability weights and severity levels in the context of burden of disease estimation

In Chapter 3, we discussed the importance of health metrics in assessing the overall health status of a population and guiding the allocation of health resources. We have seen how to calculate key metrics by providing direct calculations of each of them, but haven't yet discussed the components that make up these metrics. In this chapter, we will investigate: **life expectancy**, **mortality rates**, **incidence and prevalence**, and **disability weights**. These components are crucial for understanding the burden of diseases and injury at both global and population levels.

4.1 Cause-Specific or Population-Wide

Health metrics are essential tools for evaluating the health status of a population and guiding public health interventions. They provide valuable insights into the burden of disease and injury, helping policymakers and public health officials make informed decisions about resource allocation and health policy. By combining these metrics, policymakers and public health officials can make informed decisions about how to improve the health outcomes of a population and reduce the burden of disease and injury.

> **What are the components of these health metrics, and how are they calculated?**

The evaluation of health metrics begins with the assessment of their components, which is crucial because results strongly depend on the types of **life tables**, **mortality rates**, and **disability weights** used in the analysis. Furthermore, it is important to consider whether the objective of the analyses is **cause-specific** or **population-wide**. This can significantly impact the granularity of the health metrics components, as in alignment with general principles in epidemiological research and health metrics analysis, discussed in the Global Burden of Disease (GBD) study methodologies.[1]

[1] Theo Vos et al., "Global Burden of 369 Diseases and Injuries in 204 Countries and Territories, 1990–2019: A Systematic Analysis for the Global Burden of Disease Study 2019," *The Lancet* 396, no. 10258 (October 2020): 1204–22, doi:10.1016/S0140-6736(20)30925-9.

DOI: 10.1201/9781032625935-4

Cause-specific metrics focus on disease intervention planning, such as assessing the burden of HIV or tuberculosis on specific populations. Population-wide metrics, on the other hand, are ideal for broader health policy decisions, like overall mortality rates or life expectancy, and provide a comprehensive view of the health landscape.

The results of health metrics calculations can vary significantly based on various factors, including geographic location, the type and severity of diseases or injuries, the specific causes of death or disability, and the age groups analysed (whether age-standardised or covering all ages). Additional variation arises from the chosen time points of analysis and whether the metrics are calculated across both sexes or specifically for males or females. Moreover, the disability weights applied can differ depending on the condition's severity, its impact on quality of life, and other contextual parameters, resulting in tailored calculations that reflect local health challenges more accurately.

In this chapter, practical examples and case studies are provided to illustrate the process of applying the components to the metrics. By understanding the structure of the components, you will be better equipped to analyse and interpret health data and make informed decisions about health policy and resource allocation.

4.2 Life Tables and Life Expectancy

The first component is the **life expectancy**, used for calculating the YLLs as in Equation 3.1. More specification about **life tables** used to calculate the **life expectancy** is in the Appendix A. As a key parameter in the calculation of health metrics, life expectancy is essential for estimating the number of years lost due to premature death.

The **standard life expectancy** is defined as the average number of years a person is expected to live based on current mortality rates, an important indicator of the overall health status of a population used to compare the health outcomes of different populations over time. It is calculated based on the **probability of survival** at each age, taking into account the **mortality rates** for that age group.

In life tables, the probability of survival and the mortality rates across different age groups are used for estimating the number of remaining expected life years. These tables provide crucial insights into the longevity patterns within a population, enabling researchers and policymakers to predict life expectancy trends and to assess public health strategies effectively.

Table 4.1 Extract of Global Health Observatory (GHO) Life Tables Components

age	lx	ndx	nLx	Tx	ex
40-44	92380	1320	458599	3530204	38
45-49	91060	1737	450958	3071605	34
50-54	89323	2547	440248	2620647	29

Where `lx` is the number of people alive at the beginning of the age, `ndx` is the number of people dying between age x and $x + 1$, `nLx` is the number of person-years lived between age x and $x + 1$, `Tx` is the total number of person-years lived by the cohort of persons alive at age x, and `ex` is the expected remaining lifetime at age x.

In the context of calculating Disability-Adjusted Life Years (DALYs), specifically for the component related to Years of Life Lost (YLLs), ex (the expected remaining lifetime at age x) is typically used rather than overall **life expectancy from birth** (le). This is because YLLs are calculated based on the difference between the age at death and the expected age at death, which is more accurately represented by the remaining life expectancy at a specific age.

To understand why the expected remaining lifetime at a specific age is used in the calculation of YLLs, consider the following example: if a person dies at age 50, the YLLs are calculated based on the difference between the expected remaining lifetime at age 50 and the actual age at death. This approach provides a more precise measure of the years of life lost due to premature death, as it accounts for the age-specific mortality rates and the probability of survival at that age.

While the life expectancy at birth provides an overall measure of the average number of years a person is expected to live, the expected remaining lifetime at a specific age is more relevant for calculating YLLs, as it reflects the impact of premature death on the remaining years of life for individuals at different ages.

4.2.1 Global Health Observatory Life Tables

The **Global Health Observatory (GHO) Life Tables** are essential tools provided by the World Health Organization (WHO) to support global health monitoring and assessment. They are part of the broader GHO data repository, which serves as WHO's gateway to health-related statistics for its 194 Member States. The GHO life tables provide data on life tables and life expectancy for different age groups. These tables are collected in the `{hmsidwR}` package and used to show how to derive key health metrics.

```
# install.packages("devtools")
devtools::install_github("Fgazzelloni/hmsidwR")
```

```
library(tidyverse)
library(hmsidwR)
```

The **`hmsidwR::gho_lifetables`** dataset contains five variables:

1. **indicator:** as shown in Table 3.1
2. **age group:** from <1 to 85+ in 5-year classes
3. **sex:** female, male, and both
4. **value:** indicators value
5. **year:** from 2000 to 2019

The life expectancy rates for each age group are calculated with consideration of the probability of survival based on key parameters such as age, and deaths probabilities for that age. More info about how to calculate the life expectancy can be found in the Appendix A section of this book.

Figure 4.1a shows the `ex - expectation of life at age x` represented for each age group while in Figure 4.1b ex is represented by averaging value across all age groups from 2000 to 2019.

By averaging across all age groups rather than plotting each line for each age group individually, we can visualise the overall trend in life expectancy over time. This provides a more comprehensive view of how life expectancy has changed across different time.

Table 4.2 Global Health Observatory Life Tables

```
gho_lifetables %>%
  filter(indicator == "ex", sex == "both") %>%
  select(-indicator, -sex) %>%
  head()
#> # A tibble: 6 x 3
#>     year age    value
#>    <dbl> <ord> <dbl>
#> 1  2000 <1      66.8
#> 2  2005 <1      68.4
#> 3  2010 <1      70.5
#> 4  2015 <1      72.3
#> 5  2019 <1      73.3
#> 6  2000 01-04  69.4
```

We can see a difference in the life expectancy values for different age groups, with the highest values for the youngest age groups and the lowest values for the oldest age groups. This reflects the impact of age on life expectancy, with younger individuals having a higher life expectancy than older individuals. The overall trend in life expectancy shows an increase over time, indicating improvements in health outcomes and longevity for the population. More on how to build these plots can be found in the Chapter 10 chapter of this book.

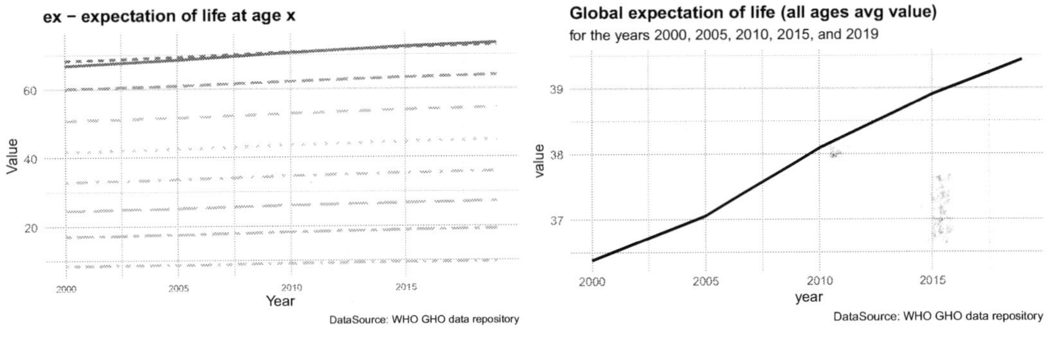

(a) ex - expectation of life at age x **(b)** GHO Life Tables

Figure 4.1 Global Health Observatory Life Tables - Expectation of Life

The mathematical formulation for calculating the expectation of life at age x is computed as:

$$e(x) = \frac{T(x)}{l(x)} \tag{4.1}$$

where $T(x)$ is the total number of person-years lived by the cohort of persons alive at age x, and $l(x)$ is the number of persons alive at age x.

It shows how *ex* is strongly related to the value of $T(x)$ and $l(x)$. The total number of person-years lived by the cohort of persons alive at age x ($T(x)$) typically referred to in demographic and actuarial studies, as a function to measure the cumulative amount of life that members of a cohort can expect to live beyond a certain age. Its changes over time indicate the effects of health policies, technological advancements, and socio-economic conditions on the longevity and health of populations.

4.2.1.1 Exercise

For example, at age 50, what is the life expectancy value if the total number of person-years lived by the cohort of persons alive at age 50 is 2,370,099 and the number of persons alive at age 50 is 89,867 ?[2]

4.3 Mortality Level and Rates

Another fundamental component of health metrics is the **mortality level** which indicates the number of deaths in a population. In the calculation of YLLs if the number of deaths are **cause-specific**, they are calculated for different diseases or injuries. If the number of deaths are **population-wide**, they are calculated for the entire population.

This component represents the count of deaths at each age or for specific diseases within a given time period. Data for this component is collected from vital registration systems, health surveys, hospital records, and epidemiological studies.

Here is a table containing the mortality rates for different age groups in two regions. The mortality rates are expressed as the number of deaths per 1,000 population in each age group. Data are used to illustrate the variation in mortality rates across age groups and regions, providing insights into the health risks faced by different populations.

Table 4.3 Example Mortality Rates by Age Group and Region

Age Group	Region A Mortality Rate (per 1,000)	Region B Mortality Rate (per 1,000)
0-1	40.5	30.0
1-5	5.2	4.0
5-10	1.8	1.5
10-15	0.9	1.0
15-20	1.2	1.3
20-30	1.5	1.8
30-40	2.0	2.2

4.3.1 Understanding Death Counts and Mortality Rates

While mortality rates themselves are not directly used in the formula for the calculation of YLLs, they are crucial for understanding the broader context of health risks and for estimating the death counts in populations where direct data on deaths might be incomplete or unreliable. In regions or for populations where vital registration data are incomplete, mortality rates derived from sample surveys or demographic models can be used to estimate the expected number of deaths.

[2]Answer: e(50) = T(50)/l(50) = 2,370,099/89,867 = 26.4 (see "Life Expectancy for CP, VS, TBI and SCI," n.d., https://www.lifeexpectancy.org/lifetable.shtml).

Table 4.4 Example Mortality Rates by Age Group and Region

Metric	Country X	Country Y
Total Population	5000000	20000000
Total Deaths	25000	40000
Mortality Rate (per 100,000)	500	200

An analysis of the mortality rates alongside YLLs provides a full picture of the health challenges faced by a population. While YLLs emphasise the impact of premature death, mortality rates help in understanding the probability and distribution of these deaths within the population.

The mortality rates can be calculated in different ways, depending on the specific nature of the analysis. In general, what is considered as the most common mortality rates is the **Crude Mortality Rate (CMR)**, which represents the number of deaths per 100,000 population.

$$CMR = \frac{\text{Number of deaths}}{\text{Total population}} * 100,000 \tag{4.2}$$

Other types of mortality rates include:

- **Age Specific Mortality Rate (ASMR)**: the number of deaths per 100,000 population in a specific age group

$$ASMR = \frac{\text{Number of deaths in a specific age group}}{\text{Total population in that age group}} * 100,000 \tag{4.3}$$

- **Cause-Specific Mortality Rate (CSMR)**: the number of deaths per 100,000 population due to a specific cause

$$CSMR = \frac{\text{Number of deaths due to a specific cause}}{\text{Total population}} * 100,000 \tag{4.4}$$

- **Infant Mortality Rate (IMR)**: the number of deaths per 1,000 live births in the first year of life

$$IMR = \frac{\text{Number of infant deaths}}{\text{Total number of live births}} * 1,000 \tag{4.5}$$

- **Maternal Mortality Rate (MMR)**: the number of maternal deaths per 100,000 live births

$$MMR = \frac{\text{Number of maternal deaths}}{\text{Total number of live births}} * 100,000 \tag{4.6}$$

These mortality rates are used to assess the impact of diseases or injuries on a population and to identify areas where improvements in health care are needed.

4.3.1.1 Example: Deaths Counts derived by Mortality Rates

Let's simulate **malaria** death counts in an African population with a **Case Fatality Rate (CFR)** ranging from 0.01% to 0.40%, and a case-incidence of 59.4 per 1000 population annually.[3] Calculate the number of expected malaria cases and the resulting deaths based on this rate for a simulated population of 100,000 individuals over a year:

[3] "World Malaria Report 2022," n.d., https://www.who.int/publications-detail-redirect/9789240064898.

- Define the Population: Assume a total population of 100,000.
- Set the Malaria Incidence Rate: 59.4 per 1000 population annually.
- Calculate Total Malaria Cases.
- Apply the Case Fatality Rate: Calculate estimated deaths using the CFR range.

```
# Define the total population
total_population <- 100000

# Define the incidence rate (cases per 1,000 population)
incidence_rate <- 59.4

# Calculate the total number of malaria cases per year
total_cases <- (incidence_rate / 1000) * total_population

# Case fatality rates (min and max)
cfr_min <- 0.0001 # 0.01%
cfr_max <- 0.004 # 0.40%

# Calculate estimated deaths for the minimum and maximum case fatality rates
deaths_min_cfr <- total_cases * cfr_min
deaths_max_cfr <- total_cases * cfr_max
```

```
#> [1] "Total population: 100000"
#> [1] "Malaria incidence rate per 1,000 population: 59.4"
#> [1] "Total estimated malaria cases per year: 5940"
#> [1] "Estimated deaths at minimum CFR (0.01%): 1"
#> [1] "Estimated deaths at maximum CFR (0.40%): 24"
```

In the simulation scenario, the incidence rate of 59.4 cases per 1,000 annually helps to understand how pervasive malaria is within the simulated population. By applying this rate to the entire population, we can estimate the total number of new cases per year. Combining this with the case fatality rate gives an estimate of the expected number of deaths, highlighting the impact of malaria on public health within that population.

4.4 Incidence and Prevalence

Incidence and prevalence are two fundamental concepts used in epidemiology to measure how often a disease occurs and how widespread it is within a population at a specific time.

- **Incidence** refers to the number of new cases of a disease that develop in a population during a specific time period. It provides information about the risk of contracting the disease and is usually expressed as a rate — for example, the number of new cases per 1,000 people per year.

The incidence rate, even identified as the cumulative incidence (risk) - r is considered as a measure of the probability the disease occurs in a specified period of time. It quantifies the risk of an individual in the population at risk developing the disease during the specified time period.

$$\text{Incidence rate} = \frac{\text{number of new cases at time t}}{\text{total population at risk}} * 1000 \quad (4.7)$$

- **Prevalence** measures the total number of cases of a disease in a population at a given time, including both new and existing cases. It is expressed as a proportion of the population and helps to provide a snapshot of how widespread the disease is.

The prevalence identifies the burden of disease at a specific time, rather than the probability of the disease to impact on the population, it expresses the probability of suffering from a disease, it is based on the total number of existing cases among the whole population.

$$\text{Prevalence} = \frac{\text{number of new + existing cases at time t}}{\text{total population}} \quad (4.8)$$

Like incidence, it can be multiplied by a factor of 10^n (where n is typically 1,000, 10,000, or 100,000) to express the prevalence per a standard number of people.

Table 4.5 Example Influenza Incidence and Prevalence Data

Metric	January	April	July	October	December
Incidence (new cases per 1,000 people)	5	3	1	2	6
Prevalence (existing cases per 1,000 people)	15	10	5	7	20

In summary, incidence measures the rate of new cases arising within a population over time, while prevalence measures the proportion of existing cases within the population at a specific point in time. These metrics are widely used in the literature and form the basis for many decisions in public health and clinical practice. They are discussed in foundational texts such as *"Epidemiology*: An Introduction" by Kenneth J. Rothman and in guidelines by health institutions like the Centers for Disease Control and Prevention (CDC) and the World Health Organization (WHO). Both metrics are crucial for understanding the dynamics and burden of diseases within populations.

4.4.1 Use of Prevalence in DALYs Calculation

In the context of the Global Burden of Diseases (GBD) study, the use of prevalence in the calculation of Disability-Adjusted Life Years (DALYs) is pivotal because DALYs aim to measure both the **current impact** of diseases and their **long-term effects** on populations as this metric combines years of life lost due to premature mortality (YLLs) with years lived with disability (YLDs). In particular, for YLDs calculations, prevalence rather than incidence is used for several reasons:

- **Direct Measurement of Burden**: Prevalence data directly reflect the current burden of disease in the population, including both new and ongoing cases. It provides a snapshot of all individuals affected by the disease at a given time, which is essential for calculating the total amount of health loss due to disabilities.
- **Incorporation of Disease Duration**: Using prevalence allows the calculation of YLDs to incorporate the duration of the disease until recovery or death. This is because prevalence captures both existing and new cases during the period of measurement.
- **Complexity of Disease Models**: Many chronic diseases or conditions with long duration are better captured through prevalence data. This approach simplifies the modelling by

Table 4.6 COVID-19 Cases and Recovered - simulate data

```
library(tidyverse, quietly = T)

population_size <- 100000 # Number of individuals
days <- 365 # Number of days

set.seed(123)
dates <- seq(as.Date("2019-01-01"),
             as.Date("2019-12-31"),
             by = "day")
```

avoiding the need for complex calculations that would otherwise be required to estimate the duration of each new case (from incidence data) and its progression over time.

The choice of prevalence over incidence in the calculation of YLDs thus reflects a pragmatic approach to capturing the current impact of diseases within a population, particularly for chronic diseases where ongoing management and sustained healthcare support are crucial.

4.4.1.1 Example: Calculating YLD for a Disease Using Prevalence

Suppose we want to calculate the **Years Lived with Disability (YLDs)** for a **chronic respiratory disease** in a population of 100,000 people. The prevalence rate of the disease is 2%, with a Disability Weight (DW) of 0.3 and an average duration of the disease is 5 years. The YLD is calculated using the formula:

1. Prevalent Cases = Population Size × Prevalence Rate

$$\text{Prevalent Cases} = 100,000 \times 0.02 = 2,000 \text{ cases}$$

2. YLD = Prevalent Cases × Disability Weight × Average Duration

$$\text{YLD} = 2,000 \times 0.3 \times 5 = 3,000$$

So, the YLD for chronic respiratory disease in this population over the average duration of the condition is 3,000 years. This YLD value would then be added to the YLL (Years of Life Lost) for the disease to calculate the total DALY.

4.4.1.2 Example: COVID-19 Incidence and Prevalence

Let's simulate some COVID-19 cases for a population of 100 000 individuals over 365 days. Consider an average infection time of 5 days or 1/5=0.2 (20%) rate of infection, and an average time of recovery of 20 days which corresponds to a recovery rate of 1/20=0.05 (5%)

Cases and recovered are simulated using a `Poisson distribution` with λ of 0.2 and 0.05, respectively. To model the count of rare events in a large population happening within a fixed interval of time or space, the Poisson distribution is particularly useful. It suits the initial spread of COVID-19 in many regions, and assumes that the events (new cases) occur independently of each other, which can be a reasonable approximation in the context of infection spread over short periods.

Table 4.7 COVID-19 Incidence and Prevalence - simulate data

```
covid_data <-
  transform(covid_data,
            Cum_Cases = cumsum(Cases),
            Cum_Recovered = cumsum(Recovered))

# Calculate daily incidence and prevalence per 100,000 population
covid_data <-
  transform(
    covid_data,
    Incidence = (Cum_Cases / population_size) * 1000,
    Prevalence = ((Cum_Cases - Cum_Recovered) / population_size) * 1000)
```

To apply the Poisson distribution, we use the `rpois()` function, which generates random numbers from a Poisson distribution with a specified rate parameter λ. The probability mass function of the Poisson distribution is given by:

$$P(X = k) = \frac{\lambda^k e^{-\lambda}}{k!} \tag{4.9}$$

where X is the random variable representing the number of events, k is the number of events, λ is the rate parameter, and e is the base of the natural logarithm.

```
cases <- rpois(length(dates), lambda = 0.2)
recovered <- rpois(length(dates), lambda = 0.05)
```

The simulated data are then combined into a data frame with the date, number of cases, and number of recovered individuals.

```
covid_data <- data.frame(
  Date = dates,
  Cases = cases,
  Recovered = recovered)
```

Let's have a look at the first few rows of the dataset:

```
#>         Date Cases Recovered
#> 1 2019-01-01     0         0
#> 2 2019-01-02     0         0
#> 3 2019-01-03     0         0
#> 4 2019-01-04     1         0
#> 5 2019-01-05     1         0
#> 6 2019-01-06     0         0
```

Calculate the cumulative incidence and prevalence over time:

```
#>         Date Cum_Cases Cum_Recovered Incidence Prevalence
#> 1 2019-01-01         0             0      0.00       0.00
#> 2 2019-01-02         0             0      0.00       0.00
#> 3 2019-01-03         0             0      0.00       0.00
#> 4 2019-01-04         1             0      0.01       0.01
#> 5 2019-01-05         2             0      0.02       0.02
#> 6 2019-01-06         2             0      0.02       0.02
```

```
total_cases <- sum(covid_data$Cases)
total_recoveries <- sum(covid_data$Recovered)
```

4.4.1.3 Incidence and Prevalence Rates for the Year

```
(incidence_rate <- total_cases / population_size)
#> [1] 0.00071
(prevalence_rate <- (total_cases - total_recoveries) / population_size)
#> [1] 0.00052
```

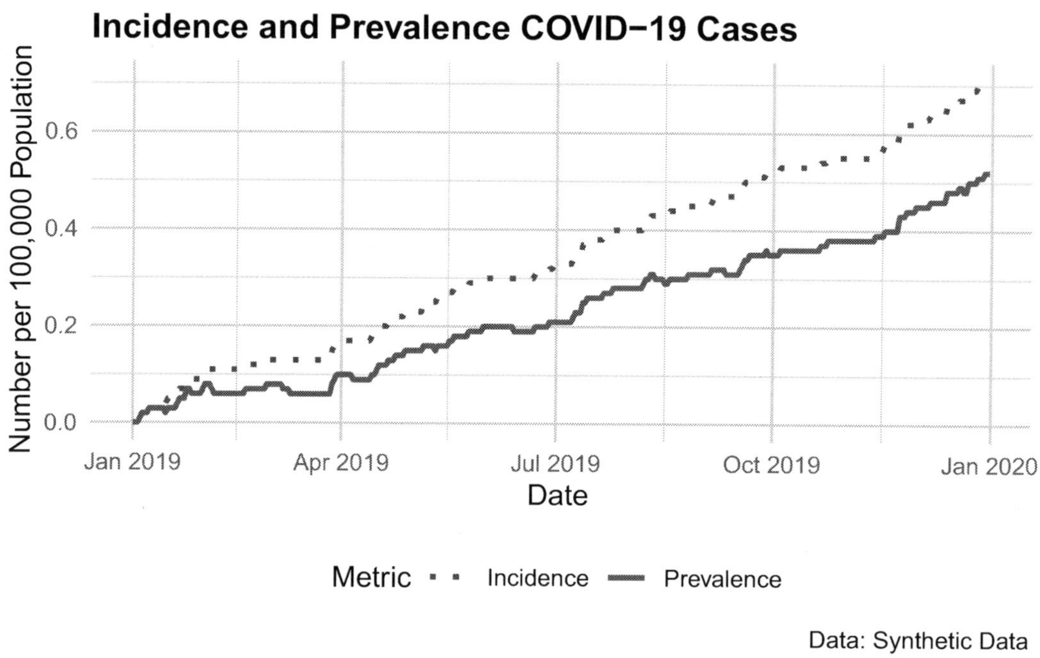

Figure 4.2 Incidence and Prevalence COVID-19 Cases - simulate data

4.5 Disability Weights and Severity Levels

The **disability weights** measure the **severity** of the health loss associated with specific health outcomes or diseases, ranging from 0 (no disability) to 1 (equivalent to death). These weights are used to calculate the number of years lived with a disability (YLDs) in the calculation of DALYs, and play a pivotal role between mortality and morbidity when estimating the Health Adjusted Life Expectancy (HALE).

The disability weights are crucial for understanding the impact of diseases and injuries on the health status of a population, if the disability weight of a specific disease is overestimated, the burden of the disease may be overestimated. Conversely, if the disability weight is underestimated, the burden of disease could result underestimated.[4]

The severity levels of a disease or injury are determined through a combination of clinical data, epidemiological studies, and expert input. These levels are crucial for understanding the burden of disease and for developing strategies in healthcare management and resource allocation. The severity levels can be assigned to be mild, moderate, or high, with respective probabilities reflecting the likelihood of each severity level occurring within the affected population.

Table 4.8 Example Disability Weights

Condition	Disability Weight
Mild Depression	0.15
Moderate Anxiety	0.30
Severe Stroke	0.75
Diabetes (without complications)	0.10
Advanced Dementia	0.85

For determining the disability weights, the severity levels are assigned based on the impact of the condition on an individual's quality of life. Higher weights are assigned to more severe conditions, reflecting the greater impact on an individual's health status, while lower weights are assigned to less severe conditions. Hence, the disability weights are calculated based on the severity of the condition and the impact on an individual's quality of life.

4.5.1 Methodology for Disability Weights

The disability weights can be derived or computed, depending on data availability. Often derived through large-scale population surveys, or expert panels through reviews of clinical descriptions and assessment scores based on understanding and professional experience. These methods involve trade-off exercises, such as **Time Trade Off (TTO)**[5] or **paired comparison** tasks.[6] Through surveys the respondents are asked to choose between different health states or to trade life years in different health states against a standard of full health. Expert panels would assess the severity of different health states based on clinical descriptions and their professional experience, rating the severity on a scale from 0 (no disability) to 1 (equivalent to death).

Computed disability weights methods can vary from applying techniques such as **Analytical Hierarchy Process (AHP)**[7] method used where health states are systematically compared in a pairwise fashion, and judgements about their relative severity are quantified. Or **Combining Results** from different methods and different populations to produce a set of

[4]Minsu Ock et al., "Disability Weights Measurement for 289 Causes of Disease Considering Disease Severity in Korea," *Journal of Korean Medical Science* 34, no. Suppl 1 (February 2019): e60, doi:10.3346/jkms.2019.34.e60.

[5]Anna K. Lugnér and Paul F. M. Krabbe, "An Overview of the Time Trade-Off Method: Concept, Foundation, and the Evaluation of Distorting Factors in Putting a Value on Health," *Expert Review of Pharmacoeconomics & Outcomes Research* 20, no. 4 (August 2020): 331–42, doi:10.1080/14737167.2020.1779062.

[6]Jürgen Rehm and Ulrich Frick, "Establishing Disability Weights from Pairwise Comparisons for a US Burden of Disease Study," *International Journal of Methods in Psychiatric Research* 22, no. 2 (May 2013): 144–54, doi:10.1002/mpr.1383.

[7]"Analytic Hierarchy Process," *Wikipedia*, March 2024, https://en.wikipedia.org/w/index.php?title=Analytic_hierarchy_process&oldid=1214553274.

Table 4.9 Disability Weights

```
disability_weights %>%
  filter(year == 2019) %>%
  select(specification, severity, dw) %>%
  head()
#> # A tibble: 6 x 3
#>   specification                    severity    dw
#>   <chr>                            <chr>    <dbl>
#> 1 Infectious disease, acute episode mild     0.006
#> 2 Infectious disease, acute episode moderate 0.051
#> 3 Infectious disease, acute episode mild     0.006
#> 4 Infectious disease, acute episode mild     0.006
#> 5 Infectious disease, acute episode mild     0.006
#> 6 Infectious disease, acute episode mild     0.006
```

disability weights that reflect a consensus view. Statistical models might be used to aggregate these results and ensure that they are consistent across different scales.

The Global Burden of Disease (GBD) study led by the Institute for Health Metrics and Evaluation (IHME) is one of the most comprehensive efforts to estimate disability weights for a wide range of health conditions. The GBD study periodically updates and refines disability weights based on extensive global surveys and expert consultations. In the 2010 iteration, for instance, IHME used community surveys across multiple countries, including Bangladesh, Indonesia, Peru, and Tanzania, and an online survey to gather feedback on how people perceive the severity of different health states. Respondents were asked to rank or rate hypothetical health conditions, which provided data for calculating standardised disability weights.

4.5.1.1 Disability Weights Data

Here is an example of a table containing the disability weights for twelve combinations of different conditions such as Infectious disease, Non-communicable diseases, and other health conditions.

Data are from the results of a systematic analysis of Global burden of 369 diseases and injuries in 204 countries and territories, 1990–2019.[8] The table can be downloaded from the {hmsidwR} package, and contains the first two cause-specific disability weights for the year 2019, as well as the severity level of the condition set as to be mild, moderate, severe, and combined for selected communicable, and Non-communicable diseases. To access the data:

```
library(hmsidwR)

disability_weights <- hmsidwR::disweights
```

The table here shows the first 6 rows of the disability weights for cause1, severity, and disability weights for the year 2019 for 204 countries and territories.

If we focus on the first cause of disability for infectious disease, we can see that the disability weight varies along with the severity level. This indicates that the condition associated with a moderate level of severity has a disability weight of 0.057. This is set to reflect the impact

[8] Vos et al., "Global Burden of 369 Diseases and Injuries in 204 Countries and Territories, 1990–2019".

Table 4.10 Severity and Disability Weights

```
library(hmsidwR)
disability_weights <- hmsidwR::disweights

disability_weights %>%
  filter(year == 2019,
         cause1 == "Infectious disease") %>%
  group_by(severity) %>%
  summarize(dw = mean(dw))
#> # A tibble: 4 x 2
#>   severity      dw
#>   <chr>      <dbl>
#> 1 mean      0.219
#> 2 mild      0.0148
#> 3 moderate 0.0572
#> 4 severe   0.162
```

of the severity condition on an individual's quality of life.

4.6 Summary of the DALYs' Components

4.6.1 YLLs Components

The components of YLLs include several factors that contribute to the calculation of premature death due to a disease or injury. These components are:

- **Age at death**: The age at which a person died due to a disease or injury is a crucial component of YLL. The earlier the age at death, the greater the impact on potential years of life lost.
- **Life expectancy**: The expected age at death in a population without the disease or injury is an important component of YLL. This value is used to compare the actual age at death with the expected age at death and determine the number of years of life lost.
- **Standard life expectancy**: To make comparisons across populations and over time, YLL is often expressed relative to a standard life expectancy, typically set at an age of 70 years.
- **Population size**: The size of the population affected by a disease or injury is another important component of YLL. A larger population will have a greater impact on overall YLL, regardless of the age at death.
- **Cause of death**: The cause of death is also considered when calculating YLL, as different causes may have different impacts on potential years of life lost.

4.6.2 YLDs Components

The estimation of YLDs requires certain epidemiological parameters such as prevalence, incidence, case-fatality rate, relative risk, odds ratio, hazard ratio, mean, incidence ratio, severity, duration and remission.

In particular, we are interested in the major factors that contribute to the calculation of the number of years lived with a disability due to a disease or injury. These components are:

- **Prevalence and Incidence**: The prevalence of a condition is the number of cases of a particular disease or injury present in a population at a given time. This is an important component of YLD as it determines the number of people who are affected by a disease or injury and the overall impact on the population. The incidence is the impact of new cases on a population in a specified time period, and it is calculated by considering the number of new cases affected by a condition divided by the size of a population. Both incidence and prevalence can be used in the calculation.

- **Disability weight**: The disability weight reflects the severity of the disability caused by a disease or injury. It is used to quantify the impact of a condition on quality of life, with higher weights assigned to more severe conditions.

  Prior to 2010, the calculation of YLDs included elements of discounting and age weighting, with discount rates that typically ranged from 3% to 4% per year. Considering the future years of healthy life valued less than present years, the practice aimed to reflect the economic theory of time preference, where immediate benefits are preferred over future benefits.

  However, due to its complexity and ethical implications, this approach has been criticised. By 2010, the World Health Organization (WHO) and other health organisations began to consider simplifying the methodology. The focus shifted to only the disability weights used to quantify the severity of different health conditions, leaving aside the element of discounting

- **Age**: The age of the person affected by a disease or injury is also considered when calculating YLD. Conditions that occur at an earlier age will have a greater impact on the number of years lived with disability.

- **Population size**: The size of the population affected by a disease or injury is another important component of YLD. A larger population will have a greater impact on overall YLD, regardless of the age of the affected individuals.

- **Duration of disability**: The duration of disability is also considered when calculating YLD. Conditions that last for a longer period of time will have a greater impact on the number of years lived with disability.

4.6.3 DALYs Components

Both YLLs and YLDs are components of the DALYs and are used to provide a comprehensive assessment of the impact of disease and injury on a population. By combining YLLs and YLDs, the DALYs take into account both premature death and the impact of disease or injury on quality of life, providing a more comprehensive view of the overall burden of disease.

DALYs are especially useful in guiding the allocation of health resources as they provide a common numerator, allowing for the expression of utility in terms of dollar/DALY.

For example, in Gambia, the provision of the pneumococcal conjugate vaccine costs $670 per DALY saved. This number can then be compared to other treatments for other diseases, to determine whether investing resources in preventing or treating a different disease would be more efficient in terms of overall health.[9]

[9]"Disability-Adjusted Life Year," December 8, 2023, https://en.wikipedia.org/w/index.php?title=Disability-adjusted_life_year&oldid=1188922629.

Table 4.11 Germany lungcancer

```
hmsidwR::germany_lungc %>%
  select(age, sex, prevalence, dx) %>%
  head()
#> # A tibble: 6 x 4
#>   age   sex    prevalence    dx
#>   <chr> <chr>       <dbl> <dbl>
#> 1 10-14 male         0.08 0.322
#> 2 10-14 female       0.18 0.457
#> 3 10-14 both         0.13 0.779
#> 4 15-19 male         0.48 1.27
#> 5 15-19 female       0.9  1.56
#> 6 15-19 both         0.68 2.83
```

4.7 Case Study: Germany Lung Cancer Study

For this case study, we used data from the GBD study for Germany, related to the number of deaths due to lung-cancer in 2019. Data are available in the `{hmsidwR}` package and, and includes the upper and lower bounds of the estimates and the 5-yrs age group for both sexes. We do not have information for the 0-4, 5-9 and 85+ age groups.

Here we can see the first 6 rows of the data, that we are going to use to calculate the YLLs, the YLDs and finally the DALYs.

Joining `germany_lungc` with the GHO life tables (`gho_lifetables`) we can build a new dataset with all information needed for calculating the YLLs for the lung cancer deaths in Germany in 2019.

```
gelung_YLL <- germany_lungc %>%
  filter(sex == "both") %>%
  left_join(gho_lifetables %>%
    filter(year == 2019, indicator == "ex") %>%
    select(-indicator, -year) %>%
    rename(life_expectancy = value)) %>%
  group_by(age) %>%
  reframe(dx, life_expectancy, YLL = dx * life_expectancy)


gelung_YLL %>%
  head()
#> # A tibble: 6 x 4
#>   age        dx life_expectancy   YLL
#>   <chr>   <dbl>           <dbl> <dbl>
#> 1 10-14   0.779            66.4  51.7
#> 2 15-19   2.83             61.6  174.
#> 3 20-24   6.15             56.8  349.
#> 4 25-29  13.5              52.1  704.
#> 5 30-34  43.0              47.4 2041.
#> 6 35-39 105.               42.8 4502.
```

Table 4.12 Lung cancer - Disability Weights

```
lung_dw <- hmsidwR::disweights %>%
  filter(year == 2019,
         str_detect(sequela, "lung")) %>%
  select(sequela, dw)
```

Now to calculate the YLDs due to lung-cancer we need to consider not fatal disability status. This can appear in conjunction with other conditions, or morbidities, that are not fatal but are acting together with the lung-cancer.[10] The disability weights are available from GBD study[11] are the same as those found in the `disweights` dataset.

So, 0.451 is the disability weight for the metastatic phase of lung, or lung cancer. We can use this value together with the prevalence of the disease to show how to calculate the YLDs for the lung cancer deaths in Germany in 2019. The number of lung cancer cases in Germany in 2019 is 34,000, and the prevalence of the disease is 0.0004 for all ages and sex. While considering 5-yrs age groups with a common disability weight of 0.451. Total YLDs can be calculated as the sum of the product of the prevalence and the disability weight for each age group.

```
prev_germany_lungc <- germany_lungc %>%
  filter(sex == "both") %>%
  select(age, prevalence)

prev_germany_lungc %>% head()
#> # A tibble: 6 x 2
#>   age   prevalence
#>   <chr>      <dbl>
#> 1 10-14       0.13
#> 2 15-19       0.68
#> 3 20-24       0.98
#> 4 25-29       1.66
#> 5 30-34       3.85
#> 6 35-39       9.24
```

```
gelung_YLL %>%
  select(age, YLL) %>%
  left_join(gelung_YLD %>% select(age, YLD)) %>%
  mutate(DALY = YLL + YLD)
#> # A tibble: 16 x 4
#>    age      YLL      YLD    DALY
#>    <chr>  <dbl>    <dbl>   <dbl>
#>  1 10-14   51.7   0.0586    51.7
#>  2 15-19  174.    0.307    175.
#>  3 20-24  349.    0.442    350.
#>  4 25-29  704.    0.749    705.
#>  5 30-34 2041.    1.74    2043.
```

[10] Michael Porst et al., "The Burden of Disease in Germany at the National and Regional Level," *Deutsches Ärzteblatt International* 119, no. 46 (November 2022): 785–92, doi:10.3238/arztebl.m2022.0314.

[11] *Ihmeuw/Ihme-Modeling* (Institute for Health Metrics; Evaluation, 2024), https://github.com/ihmeuw/ihme-modeling.

Table 4.13 Lung Cancer Cases in Germany 2019

```
gelung_YLD <- prev_germany_lungc %>%
  mutate(dw = 0.451, YLD = prevalence * dw)

gelung_YLD %>%
  head()
#> # A tibble: 6 x 4
#>   age   prevalence    dw    YLD
#>   <chr>      <dbl> <dbl>  <dbl>
#> 1 10-14       0.13 0.451 0.0586
#> 2 15-19       0.68 0.451 0.307
#> 3 20-24       0.98 0.451 0.442
#> 4 25-29       1.66 0.451 0.749
#> 5 30-34       3.85 0.451 1.74
#> 6 35-39       9.24 0.451 4.17
```

```
#>  6 35-39    4502.    4.17     4506.
#>  7 40-44   10814.   10.0     10824.
#>  8 45-49   28982.   28.3     29010.
#>  9 50-54   73451.   58.7     73510.
#> 10 55-59  121449.  101.     121550.
#> 11 60-64  137749.  139.     137888.
#> 12 65-69  135861.  164.     136025.
#> 13 70-74  108057.  169.     108226.
#> 14 75-79   95872.  136.      96007.
#> 15 80-84   66681.  112.      66793.
#> 16 85+     35158.   77.1     35235.
```

```
(YLLs <- sum(gelung_YLL$YLL))
#> [1] 821896.1
(YLDs <- sum(gelung_YLD$YLD))
#> [1] 1000.589
(DALYs <- YLLs + YLDs)
#> [1] 822896.6
```

Per 1000 population, the YLLs, YLDs, and DALYs for lung cancer deaths in Germany in 2019 are 821, 1, and 822, respectively. These metrics provide a comprehensive view of the impact of lung cancer on the health status of the population, combining the years of life lost due to premature death with the years lived with disability.

```
DALYs / 1000 # DALYs per 1000 population
#> [1] 822.8966
```

The value of the metrics changes when different disability weights are adopted. It is noteworthy that the value for the Years Lived with Disabilities (YLDs) is often quite small compared to the contribution made by the Years of Life Lost (YLLs) in the calculation of Disability-Adjusted Life Years (DALYs). This disparity highlights how mortality frequently dominates the overall disease burden in many health evaluations, underscoring the critical impact of premature death on public health metrics.

For instance, consider the disability weights for lung cancer as calculated in a study tailored to the Korean population.[12] These weights are subdivided into four groups corresponding to the stages of the disease, from 1 to 4. Each stage reflects increasing severity and a corresponding increase in the disability weight. Such gradations are crucial for accurately reflecting the progression of the disease and its escalating impact on patients' lives. This differentiation allows health policymakers and researchers to fine-tune interventions and allocate resources more effectively, targeting the stages that contribute most significantly to health deterioration.

Cause of Disease	Disability Weights	lower	upper
Trachea, bronchus and lung cancers (stage 1)	0.600	0.542	0.656
Trachea, bronchus and lung cancers (stage 2)	0.738	0.686	0.785
Trachea, bronchus and lung cancers (stage 3)	0.758	0.710	0.801
Trachea, bronchus and lung cancers (stage 4)	0.906	0.873	0.932

In conclusion, disability weights have a fundamental role in influencing the overall calculations of DALYs, as they reflect the severity of health conditions and their impact on quality of life. Assigning appropriate weights to different diseases and injuries might be challenging, but it is essential for accurately assessing the burden of disease and guiding health policy decisions. The case study on lung cancer in Germany illustrates how the combination of YLLs and YLDs provides a comprehensive view of the health impact of a specific condition, helping to inform public health strategies and resource allocation.

[12] Ock et al., "Disability Weights Measurement for 289 Causes of Disease Considering Disease Severity in Korea".

5

Causes and Risks

Learning Objectives

- Identify major causes of disease and associated risk factors using health data
- Formulate clear and focused research questions for health outcomes analysis
- Gain an introductory understanding of causal inference concepts and their application in public health research

"...fear is the most pervasive emotion of modern society..."[1]

What qualifies as a risk is subject to dynamic social change[2] , as well as the perception of risk has evolved over time, influenced by factors such as media coverage and sociopolitical dynamics.

Historically, major risks included starvation, infections, and violent conflicts, while modern risks are often associated with lifestyle choices and chronic diseases such as obesity, cardiovascular disease, and cancer. Despite advancements in healthcare and increasing life expectancy in post-industrial countries, the focus often shifts to perceived threats like terrorism, global pandemics such as COVID-19, and environmental catastrophes. This shift is reflected in the increasing combination of quantitative analyses and public health interventions, tracking changes in risk-related discourse and identifying key risk topics over time.

Furthermore, tools like topic modelling and sentiment analysis help identify how the public perceives various risks and how these perceptions evolve over time.

In the field of public health, the latest GBD results reveal significant insights into the causes and risks associated with health metrics and infectious diseases. The primary risks identified include behavioural, environmental, occupational, and metabolic factors.

5.1 Conditions and Injuries

Conditions and injuries associated with the burden of disease and injury vary according to specific causes and risks. In this book causes and risk factors include:

- **Lifestyle choices**: Poor diet, physical inactivity, tobacco use, and excessive alcohol consumption are major risk factors for many chronic diseases and injuries, including heart disease, stroke, cancer, and liver disease.

[1] Joanna Bourke, *Fear: A Cultural History* (Catapult, 2007).
[2] Ying Li, Thomas Hills, and Ralph Hertwig, "A Brief History of Risk," *Cognition* 203 (October 2020): 104344, doi:10.1016/j.cognition.2020.104344.

DOI: 10.1201/9781032625935-5

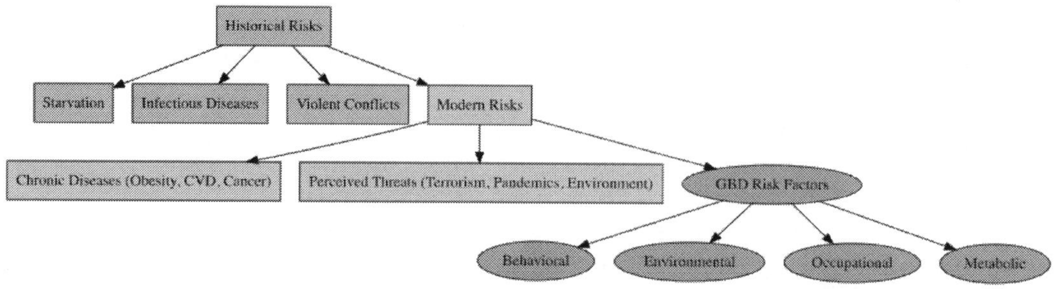

Figure 5.1 FlowChart of Historical vs. Modern Risks: this flowchart illustrates how risk perception has evolved over time, shifting from historical to modern risks. It integrates key risk factors identified in the Global Burden of Disease (GBD) study.

- **Environmental factors**: Exposure to pollutants, such as air pollution and toxic chemicals, can increase the risk of certain diseases and injuries.
- **Infections**: Many diseases, such as tuberculosis, HIV/AIDS, and malaria, are caused by infectious agents.
- **Poverty**: People living in poverty are often more susceptible to health problems due to limited access to healthcare, healthy food, and safe living conditions.
- **Ageing**: As people get older, they are at an increased risk of many health problems, including chronic diseases and disabilities.
- **Genetics**: Some diseases and injuries are caused by genetic factors, such as a genetic predisposition to certain cancers.
- **Injuries**: Injuries, such as falls, road traffic accidents, and violence, can also contribute to the burden of diseases and injuries.

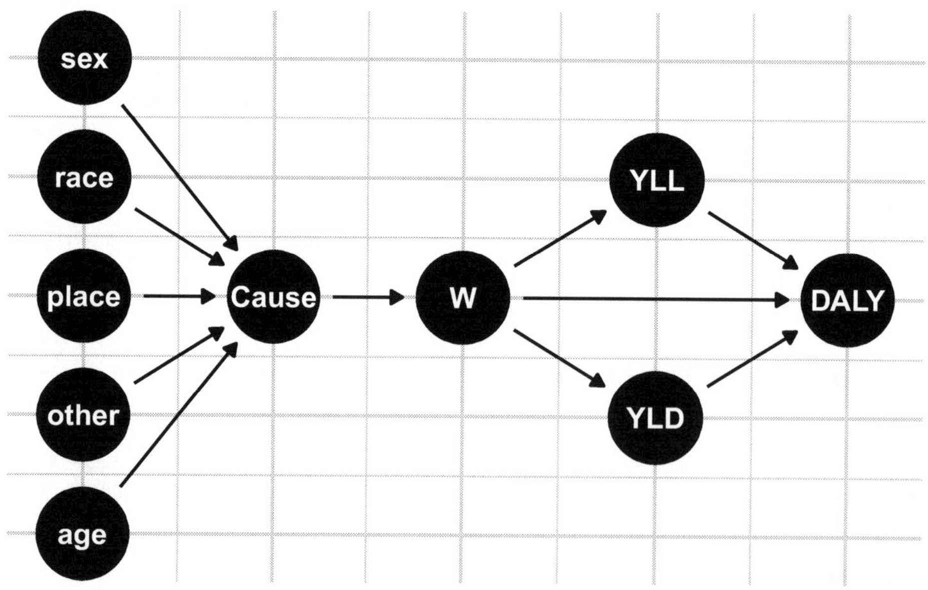

Figure 5.2 Causal relationships leading to fueling DALYs value. Weights (W), Years Lived with Disability (YLD), and Years of Life Lost (YLL) are the main components of the DALY metric.

A particular health condition can have multiple causes (co-morbidities) and risk factors. For instance, a poverty status and the lack of access to healthcare facilities, is proven to be increasing the risk of infectious diseases, while poor diet and physical inactivity can increase the risk of chronic diseases. Acting in favour of addressing the *underlying causes and risk factors* for diseases and injuries is crucial for prompt public health interventions and can help reduce the overall burden of disease.

5.2 Risk Measures

In health metrics, *risk* refers to the likelihood that an individual will experience a specific health outcome, such as illness or injury, due to certain behaviours, exposures, or conditions. Risk factors are variables that increase the probability of developing a particular health condition or experiencing an adverse health outcome; they are measurable probabilities influenced by factors like lifestyle (e.g., smoking or diet), environmental exposures (e.g., air pollution), or underlying health conditions.

To provide a comprehensive framework for assessing the burden of different risk factors on population health and guide effective public health strategies to mitigate these risks, key measures are used to assess risks and their impact on health outcomes:

- Risk-specific exposures
- Relative risks (RRs)
- Theoretical Minimum-Risk Exposure Levels (TMRELs)
- Population Attributable Fractions (PAFs)

5.2.1 Risk-Specific Exposures

The quantification of risks and causes involves the evaluation of a set of behavioural, environmental and occupational, and metabolic risks. Pairs of risk-outcome are investigated based on observations and statistical evidence. Convincing evidence consists of plausible associations between exposure and disease in terms of size, duration and effects. Common examples of risk exposures in health metrics include: smoking, physical inactivity, high blood pressure (hypertension), and others.

Risk combinations can be **additive** (the occurrence of a least one event, A or B), **multiplicative** (the occurrence of both of two events, A and B) or just **interactive,** acting to influence other pairs, this action is generally identified as possible **confounding**, to be distinguished by factors in the causal pathway between exposure and outcome.

To have an idea of the impact of different risk factors on a cause of illness, the **Socio-demographic Index (SDI)** provides insights into the potential magnitude of social, cultural and demographic factors looking at the risk exposures and possible paths for policy interventions. The life expectancy level is closely correlated to the level of the SDI indicator as it is based on average income per person, educational attainment, and total fertility rate (TFR). Higher SDI values typically indicate better socio-economic conditions, including improved access to healthcare, education, and sanitation, which can mitigate various health risks. Conversely, lower SDI values are associated with higher risk exposure due to limited access to healthcare, poorer living conditions, and other socio-economic challenges. An application of the SDI index on time series is on Chapter 9.

One more element to take into consideration is the **Comparative Risk Assessment (CRA)**[3] divided into attributable and avoidable burden. Considering as the objective the potential reduction of future disease burden, four types of **minimum risk exposure** distributions are identified:

- Theoretical
- Plausible
- Feasible
- Cost-effective

The following provide a high level overview on quantifying attributable burden by using the theoretical minimum risk.

5.2.2 Relative Risks (RRs)

The relative risk (or Risk Ratio) is a measure of the strength of the association between an exposure and an outcome. It compares the likelihood of a particular health outcome, occurring in individuals exposed to a specific risk factor, to the likelihood in those who are not exposed. This metric helps quantify how much a risk factor, like smoking or high blood pressure, increases the probability of an adverse health effect.

To calculate the risk-outcome pairs, such as mortality and morbidity, the attributable burden of a risk is decomposed to identify the impact on disease burden across factors like location, age, sex, and specific causes of disease.[4] This decomposition considers the combined effect of all risk exposures, which are categorised into metabolic, behavioural, and environmental risk factors. Each category contributes distinctly to the overall health outcome, enabling a nuanced understanding of how multiple exposures collectively influence disease burden and health outcomes.

The relative risk is the ratio between the proportions of exposed and unexposed groups.

$$RR = \frac{p_0}{p_1} \tag{5.1}$$

where p_1 and p_0 are the proportions of exposed and unexposed groups respectively. Or, in terms of population, these group would approx the values of the real population:

$$RR = \frac{p_1}{p_0} = \frac{d_1/n_1}{d_0/n_0} \tag{5.2}$$

where d_1/n_1 and d_0/n_0 are the proportion of the population with and without the disease.

For example, let's say we are studying the association between smoking (exposure) and lung cancer (outcome). We want to calculate the relative risk of lung cancer among smokers compared to non-smokers. If the relative risk is 2, it means that smokers are twice as likely to develop lung cancer compared to non-smokers.

[3]Stanaway et al., "Global, Regional, and National Comparative Risk Assessment of 84 Behavioural, Environmental and Occupational, and Metabolic Risks or Clusters of Risks for 195 Countries and Territories, 1990–2017".

[4]Christopher J. L. Murray et al., "Global Burden of 87 Risk Factors in 204 Countries and Territories, 1990–2019: A Systematic Analysis for the Global Burden of Disease Study 2019," *The Lancet* 396, no. 10258 (October 17, 2020): 1223–49, doi:10.1016/S0140-6736(20)30752-2.

```
exposed <- c(50, 10)
unexposed <- c(20, 5)

# Calculate the relative risk
relative_risk <- function(exposed, unexposed) {
  (exposed[1] / sum(exposed)) / (unexposed[1] / sum(unexposed))
  }

relative_risk(exposed, unexposed)
#> [1] 1.041667
```

In this case, a relative risk of 1.04 indicates that the exposed group is 1.04 times more likely to develop the outcome compared to the unexposed group.

A second example is to calculate the relative risk based on the number of events and person-time at risk for exposed and unexposed groups. Let's consider the following scenario:

```
d1 <- 50 # Number of events in the exposed group
n1 <- 10 # Person-time at risk in the exposed group
d0 <- 20 # Number of events in the unexposed group
n0 <- 5 # Person-time at risk in the unexposed group

# Calculate the relative risk
relative_risk_d <- (d1 / n1) / (d0 / n0)

# Print the relative risk
relative_risk_d
#> [1] 1.25
```

In this case, the relative risk based on the number of events and person-time at risk is 1.25, indicating that the exposed group has a 1.25 times higher risk of developing the outcome compared to the unexposed group.

In summary, the relative risk can be calculated using two different formulas:

- The first formula, $RR = p_1/p_0$, calculates the relative risk directly using the proportions of events p_1 in the exposed group compared to the unexposed group p_0 . This formula provides a more simplified view of the relative risk based solely on event proportions.
- The second formula, $RR = \frac{d_1/n_1}{d_0/n_0}$, considers both the **number of events** $(d1, d0)$ and **person-time at risk** $(n1, n0)$ for each group. This formula takes into account the **incidence rate** in addition to **event proportions**, providing a more specific understanding of the relative risk by incorporating information about the **duration of exposure**.

5.2.3 Relative Risks and Network Analysis

In some cases, relative risks can be modelled using **network analysis**, a specialised approach within statistical modelling which extends the concept of mixed effects to compare multiple treatments while accounting for various factors and dependencies. The relationship between variables, represented by nodes and edges, considers the potential interactions or dependencies between different risk factors and outcomes. This approach is generally favourable when exploring complex relationships among multiple variables.

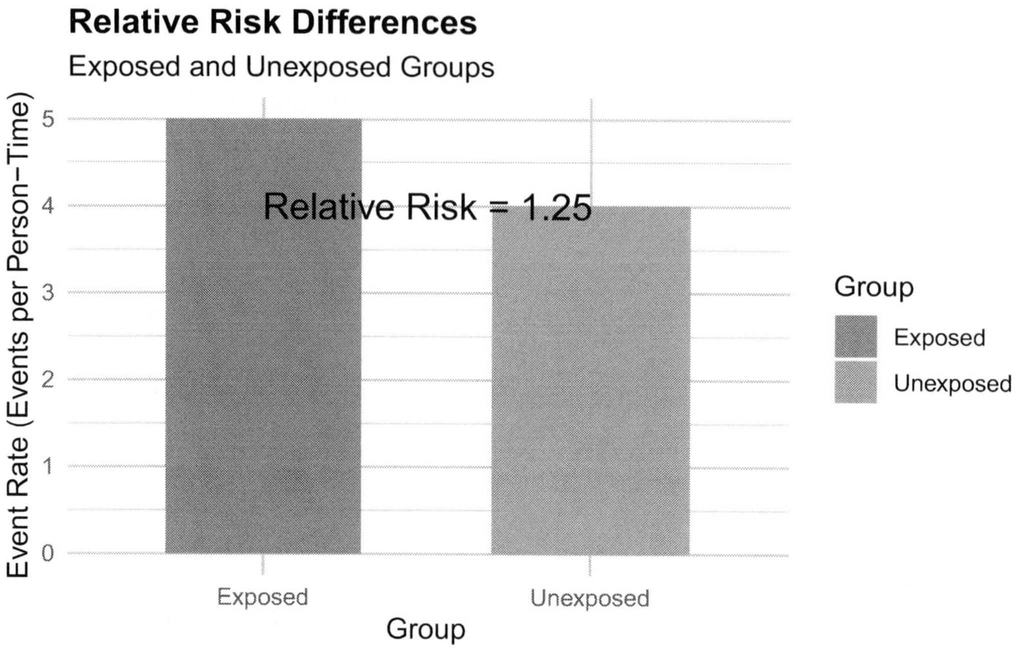

Figure 5.3 Bar chart showing the relative risk of outcome between exposed and unexposed groups. The relative risk is calculated based on the number of events and person-time at risk for each group.

To represent the network we can use a **Directed Acyclic Graph (DAG)** for drawing causal relationships between variables, such as the relationship between health risks and diseases.

This is an example of a **Network graph** representing the causal pathways between different variables, such as smoking, physical inactivity, high blood pressure, lung cancer, heart disease, and stroke. By visualising the relationships between these variables, we can identify the direct and indirect effects of risk factors on health outcomes.

The following code shows one more example of a network graph that would be helpful to identify the relationship between outcome (O), exposure (E) and different risk factors made with the `{ggdag}` package and the `dagify()` function.

```
# Load the library
library(ggdag)
set.seed(555)
# Define the DAG structure
dag <- dagify(
  y ~ x,
  x ~ c1 + c2 + c3,
  c1 ~ c2 + c3,
  c1 ~ c3)

# Plot the DAG
ggdag(dag) + theme_dag_grid()
```

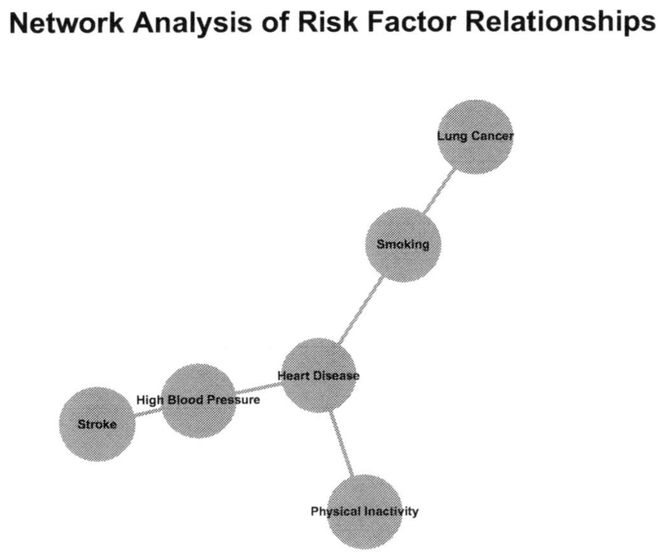

Figure 5.4 Directed Acyclic Graph (DAG) - Network Analysis of Risk Factor Relationships.

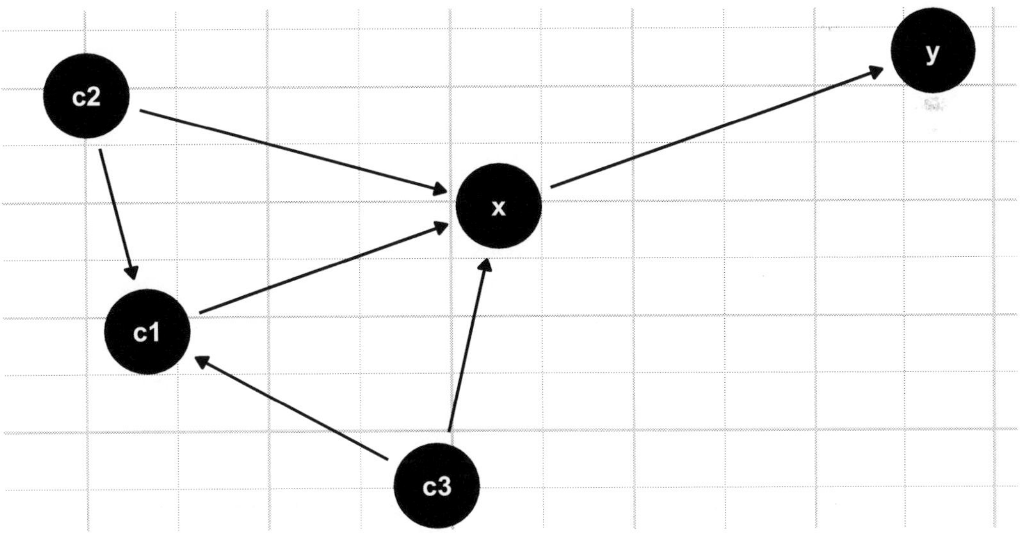

Figure 5.5 DAG between outcome (O), exposure (E) and different risk factors.

5.2.3.1 Simulation of Risk Exposure

The simulation of the risk exposure can be done replicating a logistic regression model with a DAG structure. We can use the `{dagitty}` package, and the `simulateLogistic()` function. The model estimates the probability of an outcome (O), given exposure (E) to different risk factors, such as C1, C2, and C3 (confounders). The relative risk is calculated based on the estimated probabilities of the outcome given exposure and no exposure to the risk factors.

```
# Load necessary libraries
library(dagitty)
library(tidyverse)

# Create DAG structure
dag <- dagitty("dag { E -> O
                      C1 -> O
                      C2 -> O
                      C3 -> O }")

dat <- dag %>% tidy_dagitty()
# Generate data
set.seed(123)
n <- 1000
data <- simulateLogistic(dag)

head(data)
#>    C1 C2 C3  E  O
#> 1  1 -1  1  1 -1
#> 2 -1 -1 -1  1  1
#> 3  1  1  1  1  1
#> 4  1  1 -1 -1 -1
#> 5  1  1 -1 -1 -1
#> 6 -1 -1 -1  1  1
```

```
# Fit logistic regression model
model <- glm(O ~ E + C1 + C2 + C3,
             data = data,
             family = "binomial")

# Extract estimated probabilities
pr_outcome_exp <- predict(model, type = "response")
pr_outcome_no_exp <- predict(model,
                             newdata = data.frame(E = "1",
                                                  C1 = data$C1,
                                                  C2 = data$C2,
                                                  C3 = data$C3),
                             type = "response")

# Calculate relative risk
relative_risk <- pr_outcome_exp / pr_outcome_no_exp
```

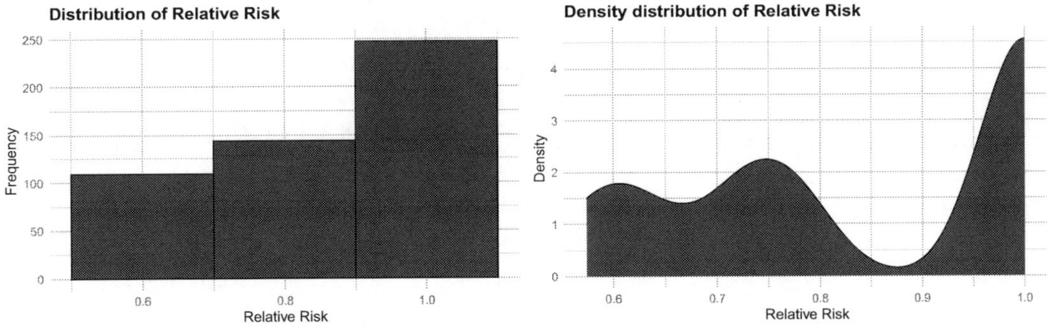

(a) Histogram of Relative Risk **(b)** Density distribution of Relative Risk

Figure 5.6 Histogram and density distribution of Relative Risk.

5.2.4 Theoretical Minimum-Risk Exposure Levels (TMRELs)

Risk factors associated with a particular health condition are considered based on the **Theoretical minimum risk exposure levels (TMRELs)** and as a function of the risk exposure or **relative risk (RR)** value. Not all the variables that are thought to be risk factors increasing causes for a particular health condition are always the driving cause of the condition, for this reason a minimum level of risk exposure is established for the risk to be considered involved as effective in the outcome.

Moreover, disease attributable to a particular risk factor or combination of risk factors need to be ascertained by investigating the risk-outcome relationship. Risk factors can also act indirectly on the outcome via intermediate risks, such as the association of low fruit consumption and heart disease influenced by systolic blood pressure which acts as mediator between the two.

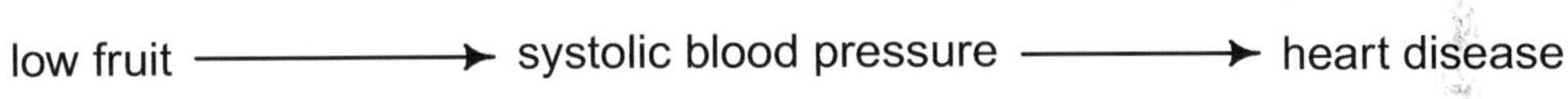

Figure 5.7 DAG: Risk-Outcome leading to heart disease. The relationship between low fruit consumption, systolic blood pressure, and heart disease.

Examples of risk factors with established **Theoretical Minimum Risk Exposure Levels (TMRELs)** include particulate matter air pollution, high systolic blood pressure, and smoking. For systolic blood pressure, the TMREL is typically set around 110/70 mmHg. Research has shown that maintaining blood pressure near this level is associated with the lowest risk for cardiovascular disease and stroke. Similarly, for particulate matter air pollution, the TMREL is set at the lowest level of exposure that is feasible and achievable, typically based on World Health Organization (WHO) guidelines. For smoking, the TMREL is set at zero, as any level of smoking is associated with increased health risks.

In terms of **Disability-Adjusted Life Years (DALYs)**, the overall level is significantly influenced by behavioural, environmental, and occupational risks. Behavioural risks, such as smoking and physical inactivity, and environmental exposures, like air pollution, contribute heavily to DALYs by increasing both mortality and disability rates within affected populations. Occupational risks further add to the burden, particularly in regions where workplace safety standards are lower, underscoring the need for targeted interventions across different population groups.

5.2.5 Population Attributable Fractions (PAFs)

The **Population Attributable Fraction (PAF)** is a measure used to quantify the proportion of disease incidence in a population that can be attributed to a specific risk factor. It represents the proportion of risk that would be reduced in a given year if the exposure to a risk factor in the past were reduced to an ideal exposure scenario.

PAF is calculated based on the prevalence of the risk factor in the population and the relative risk associated with that risk factor. The formula for calculating PAF is as follows:

$$PAF = \frac{P_e \times (RR - 1)}{1 + P_e \times (RR - 1)} \tag{5.3}$$

Where:

- P_e is the prevalence of the risk factor in the population.
- RR is the relative risk associated with the risk factor, representing the increased risk of disease among individuals exposed to the risk factor compared to those who are not exposed.

The PAF ranges from 0% to 100%. A PAF of 0% indicates that the risk factor has no impact on the incidence of the disease, while a PAF of 100% indicates that all cases of the disease in the population can be attributed to the risk factor.

PAF is useful for public health interventions as it provides insight into the potential impact of reducing or eliminating a specific risk factor on the incidence of disease in the population. By targeting interventions to reduce exposure to the risk factor, public health efforts can effectively reduce the burden of disease in the population and improve overall health outcomes.

5.3 Causal Inference

Causality concerns the relationship between two variables, where one variable (*the cause*) directly influences the other (*the effect*). For example, regular exercise improves cardiovascular health, or adequate sleep supports cognitive function. However, causality is distinct from correlation, which indicates a statistical association without implying a direct influence. For instance, a correlation between television watching and obesity does not imply a causal link. Establishing causality requires systematically evaluating alternative explanations and accounting for confounding factors that could affect both the cause and effect.

Causal inference is essential for understanding the underlying causes of a condition or phenomenon, even if these causes are not immediately apparent. It often requires a structured data analysis to uncover hidden causal relationships within the observed data.

Performing causal inference requires setting up an experiment, where there are **treatment** and **outcome** elements. The *treatment* is the intervention applied to the data. For example, to confirm the statement that *regular exercise leads to improved cardiovascular health*, an intervention may be designed to introduce another variable, such as regular fruit consumption, and observe its combined effect with exercise on cardiovascular health.

In this investigation, the primary factors are exercise and fruit intake. The goal is to examine whether their combination improves cardiovascular health. Once the intervention is analysed

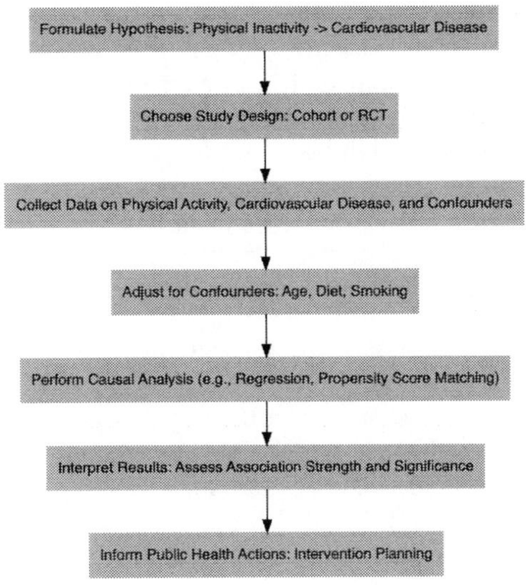

Figure 5.8 Causal Inference Flowchart. The flowchart outlines the steps involved in performing causal inference, from formulating a hypothesis to informing public health actions.

by measuring changes in cardiovascular health (the response variable), the next step is to apply a control procedure, often using a **counterfactual** scenario. This approach helps assess what might have happened in the absence of the treatment, providing a benchmark to confirm the treatment's true effect.

5.4 Summarising the Relationship between Risk and Outcome

The relationship between risk and outcome in epidemiology is central to understanding the causes of disease and guiding preventive strategies. This relationship involves assessing how exposure to certain risk factors affects the likelihood of developing specific health outcomes. Epidemiological studies quantify the strength of this association through measures like **Relative Risk (RR)** and **Population Attributable Fraction (PAF)**.

Relative Risk (RR) compares the risk of developing a health outcome among individuals exposed to a risk factor with those who are not exposed. An RR greater than 1 indicates an increased risk associated with the exposure. For example, if smokers have a relative risk of 15 for lung cancer compared to non-smokers, this suggests a strong association between smoking and lung cancer.

Population Attributable Fraction (PAF) estimates the proportion of disease incidence in a population that can be attributed to a specific risk factor, helping quantify the potential impact of reducing or eliminating that exposure on the overall disease burden. For example, if smoking accounts for 30% of lung cancer cases in a population, the PAF for smoking-related lung cancer is 0.30.

To establish causality, epidemiologists must demonstrate consistent associations, dose-response relationships (where increased exposure heightens risk), temporal precedence (exposure precedes outcome), and rule out alternative explanations. Ultimately, understanding these risk-outcome relationships enables evidence-based public health decisions, informing preventive strategies, interventions, and policies to improve population health.

Table 5.1 Table showing risk measures, definitions, and examples.

Risk Measure	Definition	Example
Relative Risk (RR)	Measures the likelihood of an outcome occurring in an exposed group relative to a non-exposed group.	Smokers have a 15x higher relative risk (RR = 15) of lung cancer compared to non-smokers.
Population Attributable Fraction (PAF)	Estimates the proportion of disease cases that could be prevented if a specific risk factor were eliminated.	If smoking accounts for 30% of lung cancer cases, then the PAF for smoking is 0.30.
Theoretical Minimum Risk Exposure Level (TMREL)	Represents the ideal level of exposure to a risk factor that minimises adverse health effects.	The TMREL for PM2.5 (air pollution) is set around 2.4 $\mu g/m^3$, as exposure below this level is associated with minimal health risk.

In conclusion, the study of risk and outcome has evolved beyond traditional epidemiological methods to embrace advanced techniques like transfer learning. This interdisciplinary approach enables the application of insights from epidemiology to other fields and viceversa, deepening our understanding of the complex relationships between risk factors and health outcomes. Machine learning and data-driven techniques help identifying patterns, and develop predictive models that extend beyond conventional frameworks, offering fresh perspectives on population health and guiding targeted interventions.

Part II

Machine Learning

6

Introduction to Machine Learning

> **"Human beings are not just passive victims of disease. They are active participants in the biological confrontation between man and microbe."**

This chapter will walk you through a basic construction of a machine learning model, providing a simple explanation of how to model fast-growing phenomena, such as in the case of the spread of infectious diseases. Then in the following chapters of this second section you will dive deep into different techniques for modelling starting from feature engineering to making predictions.

6.1 Deterministic and Stochastic Modelling

The spread of a virus can be seen as a **random process**, since the number of individuals who are infected at any given time can change randomly. The exact number of individuals who will be infected in the future cannot be determined with certainty, as it depends on various factors such as the contagiousness of the virus, the behaviour of individuals, and the efficacy of mitigation measures.

A **deterministic model**, on the other hand, could be used to model the spread of a virus under certain conditions, such as a fixed number of individuals, constant contagiousness, and no mitigation measures. This type of model can be used to make predictions about the spread of a virus under certain assumptions, but it will not account for the randomness and uncertainty associated with real-world scenarios. In general, a **stochastic process**, or random process[1] is the type of model which attempts to replicate uncertain outcomes, using probabilities. On the other hand, in a **deterministic system** the outcome is obtained from a given input, and for this reason it is reproducible.

Most models used to study the spread of a virus are a **combination of both deterministic and stochastic models**. For example, the SIR (Susceptible-Infected-Recovered) model is a deterministic model that describes the dynamics of the spread of a virus, but it also includes stochastic elements such as random interactions between individuals.

6.2 Machine Learning Models

What a machine learning model is and how it differs from statistical models (deterministic and stochastic) is all a matter of parameter calibration. Understanding the differences

[1] Robert P. Dobrow, *Introduction to Stochastic Processes with R* (John Wiley & Sons, 2016).

DOI: 10.1201/9781032625935-6

between deterministic and stochastic models is crucial for effectively applying machine learning techniques, as it informs the selection of the appropriate modelling approach based on the data characteristics and analysis goals. Machine learning models learn from data to automatically adjust their parameters, optimising them to minimise errors or maximise performance on a given task. Compared to traditional statistical models, they are more flexible and adaptable to complex data patterns.

Machine Learning (ML) techniques are identified as subfields of the **Artificial Intelligence (AI)** technology, acting by learning relationships in the data. Learning from experience (E), ML computes tasks (T) to improve performance (P). The origins of ML, dating back to the late 1950s, only flourished in the 1990s with the aim of minimising loss on unseen samples.[2]

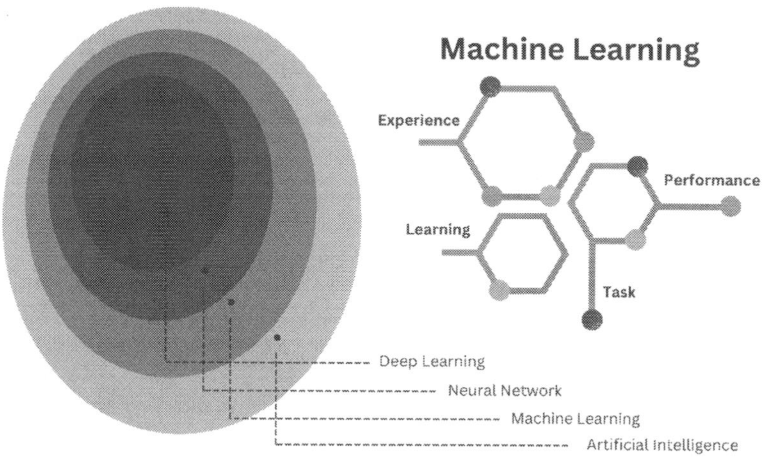

Figure 6.1 Machine Learning Cycle

The **Machine Learning Cycle** is a continuous process that involves the following steps: data collection, data preprocessing, model selection, model training, model evaluation, and model deployment. The cycle is iterative, with each step informing the next, and the process is repeated until the desired performance is achieved. The goal of the Machine Learning cycle is to develop models that can make accurate predictions or decisions based on data.

The emergence of infections is an ongoing evolution and adaptation.[3] In the late 1970s, Dr. René Dubos believed that '*the relationship between humans and microbes is dynamic and influenced by various factors, including environmental conditions, human behaviour, and microbial adaptation*'. The importance of understanding the complex interactions between hosts and pathogens in the emergence and spread of infectious diseases is described as dynamic interplay between organisms and their environment, a **process of continuous adaptation and interaction**. Organisms continuously respond to changes in their surroundings to maintain balance and survival. This is analogous to what happens inside a machine learning model environment. It involves continuous parameter learning and adjustment achieved

[2]"Machine Learning," *Wikipedia*, April 2024, https://en.wikipedia.org/w/index.php?title=Machine_learning&oldid=1220758567.

[3]Lyle D. Broemeling, *Bayesian Analysis of Infectious Diseases: COVID-19 and Beyond* (New York: Chapman; Hall/CRC, 2021), doi:10.1201/9781003125983.

through a technique called tuning or parameter calibration, resulting in a range of possible alternative scenarios and simulations of the observed data.

6.2.1 Empirically Driven Models

To locate machine learning models within the models framework, we can think about the scope of the analysis, which in this case is predicting the future and preventing undesired outcomes.

In particular, these types of models are subdivided in:

1. **Mechanistic Model**: For example the SIR model is a **classic compartmental model** used to simulate the spread of infectious diseases. It divides the population into three compartments: susceptible (S), infectious (I), and recovered (R). The equations describe the rate of change of each compartment over time, where β represents the transmission rate and γ represents the recovery rate.

$$\text{SIR model} \begin{cases} \frac{dS}{dt} &= -\beta \cdot S \cdot I \\ \frac{dI}{dt} &= \beta \cdot S \cdot I - \gamma \cdot I \\ \frac{dR}{dt} &= \gamma \cdot I \end{cases} \tag{6.1}$$

2. **Empirically Driven Model**: Empirically driven models do not have explicit mathematical equations like mechanistic models. Instead, they **learn patterns** and relationships directly from data. An example of an empirically driven model is **Random Forest** which is a machine learning algorithm that builds multiple decision trees and combines their predictions to make accurate predictions. It works by splitting the data into subsets and building a decision tree for each subset. The final prediction is made by aggregating the predictions of all decision trees. Unlike mechanistic models, Random Forest does not rely on explicit equations or known relationships but instead learns patterns from the input data.

Machine learning models fall under the category of **empirically driven models**. Unlike **mechanistic models**, which are based on explicit equations and known relationships between variables (such as the differential equations used in infectious disease modelling), machine learning models derive patterns and relationships directly from data without explicit knowledge of the underlying mechanisms. Therefore, while both mechanistic and empirically driven models are used for prediction, they operate on different principles:

> **Mechanistic models rely on known relationships and equations, while machine learning models learn patterns from data.**[4]

Before delving deep into machine learning techniques for analysing health data and metrics, it's essential to proceed step by step in building a modelling framework. This approach begins with a thorough understanding of the modelling procedures.

[4] Ruth E. Baker et al., "Mechanistic Models Versus Machine Learning, a Fight Worth Fighting for the Biological Community?" *Biology Letters* 14, no. 5 (May 16, 2018): 20170660, doi:10.1098/rsbl.2017.0660.

6.2.2 Learning Methods

There are a variety of models available, and the decision on which model to use depends on the type of **learning method** either **supervised** or **unsupervised**. Supervised learning is applied when data are labelled, meaning that the dataset includes both the independent (predictors) and dependent (outcome) variables. It is the classical approach to machine learning, where the model learns to predict the outcome variable based on the input variables. Unsupervised learning, on the other hand, only includes the input variables, so there is no a direct objective, or a "response" variable to focus on. The model learns to find patterns and relationships in the data without explicit labels, making it useful for clustering and dimensionality reduction.

The **nature of the data** is also fundamental, including whether the outcome is continuous or discrete, and whether the number of predictors exceeds the number of observations. Models can range from non-linear to multilevel, and they can involve more complex combinations. A major distinction is made between **regression** and **classification** based on whether the outcome variable is continuous.

Machine learning models are all types of models that can be all of the above but allow for: **learning from data through model parameters auto-calibration**. Learning from data is a process where an algorithm adjusts its parameters to minimise the errors in predictions. Each algorithm has its method of learning.

6.2.3 Parameters and Hyper-Parameters

In machine learning and statistical modelling, parameters and hyperparameters are two distinct concepts, each playing a crucial role in building and tuning models.

Parameters are the **internal** coefficients or weights that the model learns from the training data. These values are adjusted during the training process to minimise the loss function and improve the model's accuracy. For instance, in a linear regression model, parameters include the **slope coefficients** and the **intercept** (Equation 6.3). Parameters are optimised during the training phase using optimization algorithms that perform selection, mutation, and crossover of the **coefficients**. The goal is to find the set of parameters that best fit the training data.

Hyperparameters are the **external** settings of the model that can be redefined by the practitioner, or optimised using techniques such as grid search, random search, or more advanced methods like Bayesian optimization. This process involves evaluating model performance with different hyperparameter settings. Examples of hyperparameters are the sample size, the number of trees on a random forest model, the learning rate, the regularisation setting (λ) in ridge and lasso regression, and so on.

More will be explained below, but it's important to understand that creating a model might involve high-level calculations. This means progressing beyond a basic equation to include parameter selection and hyperparameter optimization. In particular, in the study of infectious diseases, the focus is on how variables will evolve over time. For this reason, selecting the appropriate model requires an understanding of the underlying patterns and dynamics of growth.

6.3 The Steps of Building a Model

The process of constructing a model that would be able to explain the relationships between dependent and independent variables in a given system is intended as model development. At the heart of this process is the application of a model function to estimate coefficients that minimise the difference between the model's predictions and the observed data.

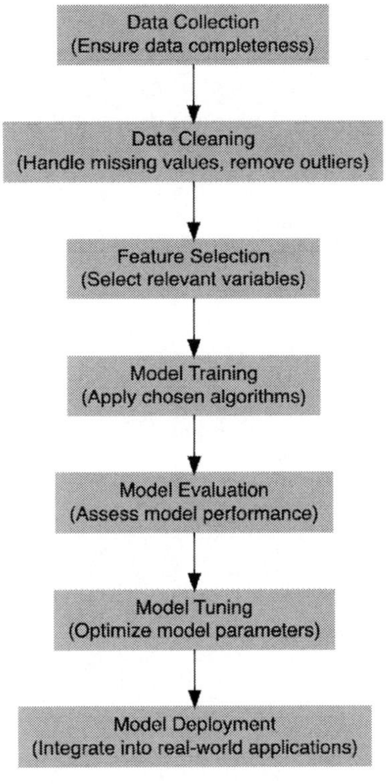

Figure 6.2 Model Building Process

Let's break this down further: Suppose we have a response variable, denoted as y, which represents the number of deaths or infections in our dataset. Additionally, we have some other variables called predictors $x_1, x_2, ...$, which are factors that may influence the level of y. These predictors are selected based on the type of analyses, and could include factors such as demographics, secondary health outcomes (morbidity), population density, temperature, vaccination rates, etc. The goal of model development is to create a mathematical function that captures the relationship between the response variable y (or dependent variable) responding to changes in predictor variables x_i (or independent variables) within the study.

This function, often referred to as the model equation or model function, is typically represented as:

$$y = f(x_1, x_2, ...) + \epsilon \tag{6.2}$$

Here, f represents the relationship between the predictors and the response, and *epsilon* represents the error term, which captures the difference between the observed values of y and the values predicted by the model. To estimate the coefficients of the model function, we employ statistical techniques such as **linear regression** for continuous response variables, **logistic regression** for binary response variables, and various **machine learning algorithms** that include tuning parameters to handle more complex dataset and model specifications. These techniques analyse the relationship between the predictors and the response in the dataset and determine the optimal coefficients that minimise the difference between the observed (y) values and the values predicted by the model $(\hat{y})$.

Once the model coefficients are estimated, we can use the model function to predict future values of y for new values of predictor variables x_i. This allows us to simulate the effect of different scenarios or make predictions about future outcomes based on the relationships identified in the data. Overall, the model development process is a crucial step in the modelling framework, as it sets the foundation for understanding and analysing the relationships between variables in a given system. It enables us to extract insights from the data, make predictions, and inform decision-making in various fields, including epidemiology, public health, economics, and environmental science.

6.3.1 Example: Cholera

The first dataset used is from the `{HistData}` package `HistData::CholeraDeaths1849`, made of 730 observations and 6 variables, with 2 causes of deaths: cholera and diarrhoea. For this example we select just the deaths due to cholera within 12 months in 1849. Let's have a look at the first 6 rows of the dataset:

```
library(tidyverse)
library(HistData)

cholera <- HistData::CholeraDeaths1849 %>%
  filter(cause_of_death == "Cholera") %>%
  select(date, deaths)

cholera %>% head()
#> # A tibble: 6 x 2
#>   date       deaths
#>   <date>      <dbl>
#> 1 1849-01-01     13
#> 2 1849-01-02     19
#> 3 1849-01-03     28
#> 4 1849-01-04     24
#> 5 1849-01-05     23
#> 6 1849-01-06     39
```

The response variable is `y = deaths` due to cholera, and the only predictor we are considering on this first step is `x = date` in days from 1849-01-01 to 1849-12-31. Let's visualise our data by using the `{ggplot2}` package with `geom_line()` as layer.

```
cholera %>%
  ggplot(aes(x = date, y = deaths)) +
  geom_line() +
  labs(
```

```
  title = "Deaths due to Cholera in London (1849)",
  x = "Date", y = "N. deaths")
```

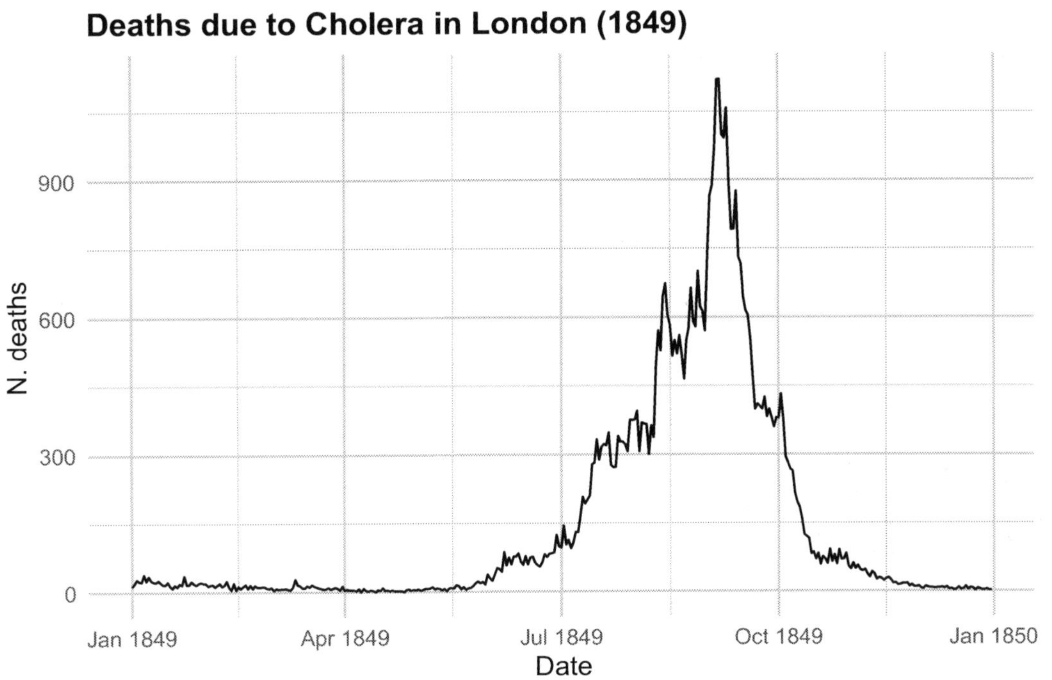

Figure 6.3 Deaths due to Cholera in London (1849)

Now let's observe in mathematical terms what happens when we start investigating the relationship between the response and the predictor, to explain the behaviour of the variables.

The following mathematical formulation represent our observed data, where β_0 and β_1 are the parameters, respectively the intercept and the slope allowing the computation of the equivalence between y and x [5].

$$y = \beta_0 + \beta_1 x \tag{6.3}$$

When a model is attempted, the values of the slope (β_0) and the intercept (β_1) are estimated[6] in order to be able to replicate the values (y) of the response by applying x to our model function.

$$\hat{y} = \hat{\beta}_0 + \hat{\beta}_1 x \tag{6.4}$$

where $\hat{\beta}_0$ is the estimate value of the intercept, and $\hat{\beta}_1$ the estimated value of the slope. So, the estimated data will approximate the observed data, with some margin of error (ϵ):

$$y \sim \hat{y} + \epsilon \tag{6.5}$$

[5] We can compare this formulation to a general $Y = a + mx$ linear function. In our case a would be the intercept and m the slope of the line that will summarise the information between y and x.

[6] The hat ($\hat{}$) on top of the variables indicates the values are estimated.

The difference between y and $\hat{y}$ is the error we make when applying a model.

$$y - \hat{y} = \epsilon \tag{6.6}$$

Reducing the error (ϵ) as much as possible can lead to better fit of the model.

While the case of having just one predictor influencing our response variable might be useful for educational purposes, as illustrated in the data above, scenarios involving more than one predictor are more realistic and lead to increased complexity in the model function. This situation typically results in a multivariate linear model, often referred to as **multiple linear regression**.

$$y = \beta_0 + \beta_1 x_1 + \beta_2 x_2 + ... + \beta_n x_n \tag{6.7}$$

In this case more than one predictor is used to investigate the varying effects of the response variable. A compact form of the model function with more than one predictor can be stated as:

$$y = \beta_0 + \sum_{i=1}^{p} \beta_i x_i = \beta_0 + \beta X \tag{6.8}$$

In this notation, the capital X takes the form of a matrix containing various x_i: $X = (x_1, x_2, x_3, ..., x_p)$, the predictors, and the $\beta = (\beta_1, \beta_2, \beta_3, ..., \beta_p)$ are the coefficient to be estimated.

> Valuable insights into the trends and drivers of cholera mortality can be gained in order to inform public health interventions and policies aimed at reducing the burden of this disease.

If we were to investigate this spread as we hadn't seen before and looked at some point in time, let's say in between June and August 1849 we could have thought that the trend was linear and growing in time. And actually is until some point, as we know what happened next. In the first plot the model line (blue line) is obtained with the `geom_smooth()` function with the specification `method = "lm"` . In the second plot we have used all data up to August, and we can clearly see the infections spread smoothly to finally explode shaping an elbow curve. The `geom_smooth()` selected the best function that suits the data with a **locally estimated scatterplot smoothing**, or **LOESS**, which is a nonparametric method for smoothing a series of data in which no assumptions are made about the underlying structure of the data.

```
cholera %>%
  filter(date >= "1849-06-01" & date <= "1849-08-01") %>%
  ggplot(aes(x = date, y = deaths)) +
  geom_point() +
  geom_smooth(method = "lm", se = F) +
  labs(
    title = "Deaths due to Cholera in London (June to August 1849)",
    subtitle = "Linear Model",
    x = "Date", y = "N. deaths")

cholera %>%
  filter(date <= "1849-08-01") %>%
  ggplot(aes(x = date, y = deaths)) +
  geom_point() +
  geom_smooth(se = F) +
```

```
  labs(
    title = "Deaths due to Cholera in London (January to August 1849)",
    subtitle = "method LOESS",
    x = "Date", y = "N. deaths")
```

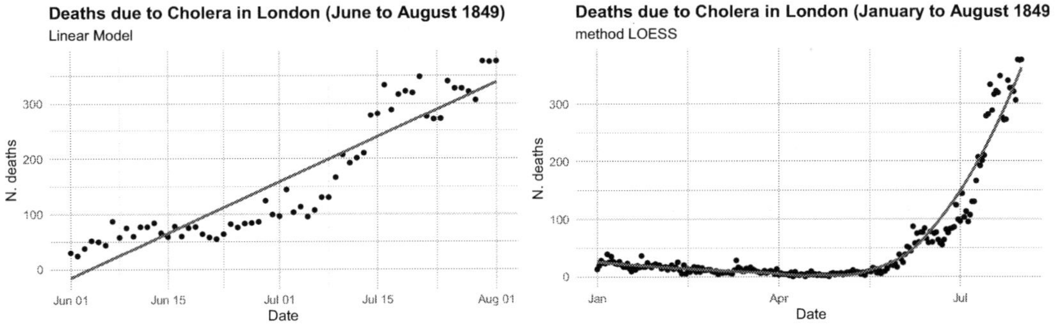

(a) Deaths due to Cholera in London (June to August 1849)

(b) Deaths due to Cholera in London (January to August 1849)

Figure 6.4 Deaths due to Cholera in London (1849)

In the case of `CholeraDeaths1849`, and in the context of infectious diseases, the trend typically starts at a certain point, then increases to reach a peak—the highest level of infection spread—before eventually decreasing back to the initial level. This pattern is inherently **non-linear**.

To visualise both linear and non-linear trends we can use a `geom_smooth()` function[7], with `method = "lm"` for linear model and `method = "gam"` for applying a **general additive model**.

```
ggplot(cholera, aes(x = date, y = deaths)) +
  geom_line() +
  geom_smooth(method = "lm", se = F) +
  geom_smooth(method = "gam",
              color = "darkred", se = F)
```

6.3.1.1 GAM - Generalised Additive Model

The purpose of creating a model is to identify underlying patterns within a series of observations. This requires the model to interpolate given observations in order to represent the overall pattern accurately. For instance, in the visualisation above, the blue line made with the `geom_smooth()` function, when specified with `method = "lm"`, helps us visualise the direction of a linear pattern in the data. However, it's evident that the data points form a bell-shaped curve as distribution of deaths over time, indicating a non-linear relationship between date and cholera deaths. In the second layer we used `method= "gam"`, **Generalised Additive Models (GAMs)** flexible extensions of linear models, the most suitable choice for this data used to model non-linear relationships between the response and predictor variables. They are particularly useful when the relationship between the variables is complex and cannot be adequately captured by linear models.

$$g(\mu) = \beta_0 + f(x) \tag{6.9}$$

[7]More about data visualisations techniques are in chapter Chapter 10.

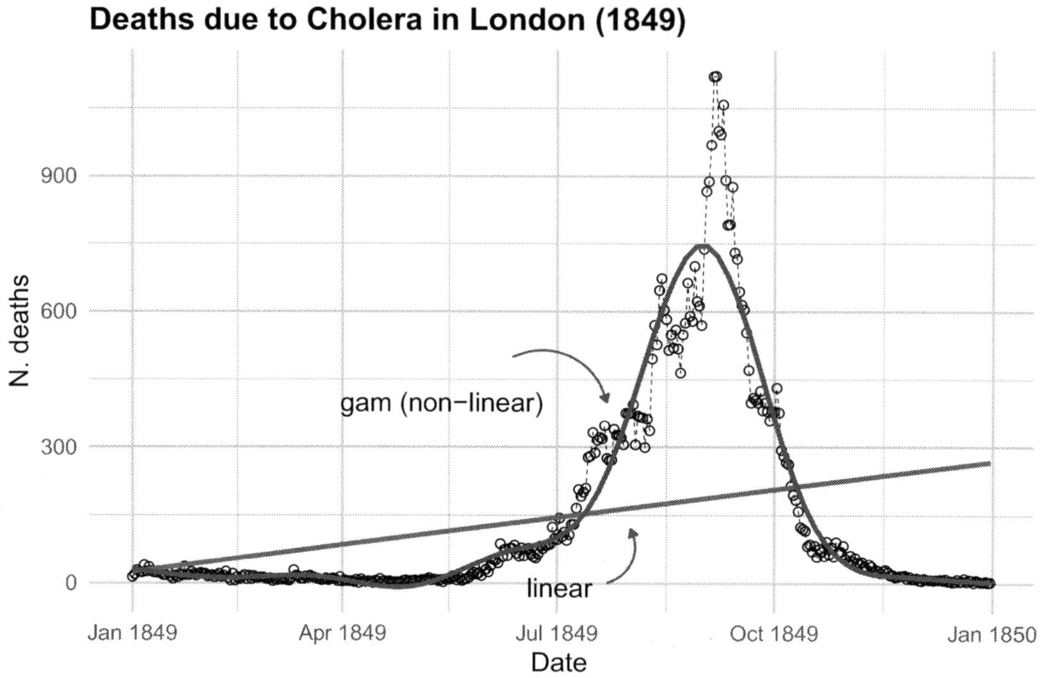

Figure 6.5 Deaths due to Cholera in London (1849)-GAM

where: $g()$ is a link function, μ is the expected value of the response variable, β_0 is the intercept term, $f()$ represents the smooth functions of the predictor variable. In case of more than one predictor: $g(\mu) = \beta_0 + f_1(x_{i1} + f_2(x_{i2} + f_3(x_{i3} + ...)$ there will be $p = 1, .., j$ number of $f()$ smooth functions as many as the number of predictors.

What is happening here is a transformation of the predictors through the application of a function: $x \sim f(x)$. The smooth functions are estimated using non-parametric techniques such as splines (polynomial transformations) or kernel functions. These smooth functions allow for flexible modelling of the relationship between the predictor variables and the response variable, capturing non-linearities and complex patterns in the data. The link function $g()$ is typically chosen based on the distributional characteristics of the response variable, to represent the data mean trend.

```
# Load the mgcv package
library(mgcv)

# use the days instead of the full date
cholera$days <- row_number(cholera)

# Fit a GAM using the gam() function
gam_model <- gam(deaths ~ s(days), data = cholera)

# Print the summary of the GAM model
summary(gam_model)
#>
#> Family: gaussian
```

```
#> Link function: identity
#>
#> Formula:
#> deaths ~ s(days)
#>
#> Parametric coefficients:
#>             Estimate Std. Error t value Pr(>|t|)
#> (Intercept)  146.008      3.583   40.74   <2e-16 ***
#> ---
#> Signif. codes:  0 '***' 0.001 '**' 0.01 '*' 0.05 '.' 0.1 ' ' 1
#>
#> Approximate significance of smooth terms:
#>           edf Ref.df   F p-value
#> s(days) 8.969      9 431  <2e-16 ***
#> ---
#> Signif. codes:  0 '***' 0.001 '**' 0.01 '*' 0.05 '.' 0.1 ' ' 1
#>
#> R-sq.(adj) =  0.914   Deviance explained = 91.6%
#> GCV = 4818.7  Scale est. = 4687      n = 365
```

The smooth term for days is significant, as indicated by the approximate significance test. The effective degrees of freedom (edf) for the smooth term are 8.969, suggesting a moderately flexible relationship between deaths and time. The adjusted R-squared value is 0.914, indicating that the model explains approximately 91.4% of the variance in the response variable (deaths). The deviance explained is 91.6%, suggesting that the model fits the data well.

Overall, the model suggests that there is a positive relationship between increasing time and the number of deaths due to cholera, with the number of deaths increasing over time to reach a peak and then eventually slow down to zero. However, it's essential to consider the context of the data and potential confounding variables before drawing conclusions about causality or making predictions based solely on this model. Other important factors influencing the spread are social behaviour and vaccination. We will talk more about infectious diseases spread in section 4 Chapter 14.

6.3.2 Example: Epidemic X

6.3.2.1 SEIR Model

In this example we simulate data of an epidemic to build a SEIR (susceptible, exposed, infected, recovered) model, a case a little more complicated than just making a SIR (susceptible, infected, recovered) model (Equation 6.1). More about the compartmental models will be shown in Chapter 8, Chapter 14 and in Chapter 15.

So, let's start looking at how our simple linear equation $y = \beta_0 + \beta_1 x$ can be changed to become a differential equation. A differential equation describes how a quantity changes with respect to another quantity, in particular time in this case. So, we are interested in the variation of y within time.

$$y' = \frac{dy}{dt} = \frac{y_1 - y_0}{t_1 - t_0} \tag{6.10}$$

And this is explained by the variation of the predictors in time, the calculation is a derivative. Recall that the derivative of a constant is 0, in our case β_0 is the constant.

$$\frac{dy}{dt} = \frac{d(\beta_0 + \beta_1 x)}{dt} = \beta_1 \frac{dx}{dt} \tag{6.11}$$

This equation describes how y changes with respect to time t, taking into account the rate of change of x with respect to time t, and the constant slope β_1 of the line.

$$y' = \beta_1 \frac{dx}{dt} \tag{6.12}$$

The Equation 6.12 will be used in the model to describe how individuals move between compartments over time.

For this example we use a package named {deSolve} which solves differential equations.

```
# Load required packages
library(deSolve) # For solving differential equations
```

We define a function for making the SEIR model, and its parameters. β is the transmission rate, σ the rate of latent individuals becoming infectious, and γ the rate of recovery.

```
SEIR <- function(time, state, parameters) {
  # variables need to be in a list
  with(as.list(c(state, parameters)), {
    # Parameters
    beta <- parameters[1] # Transmission rate
    sigma <- parameters[2] # Rate of latent individuals becoming infectious
    gamma <- parameters[3] # Rate of recovery

    # SEIR equations
    dS <- -beta * S * I / N
    dE <- beta * S * I / N - sigma * E
    dI <- sigma * E - gamma * I
    dR <- gamma * I

    # Return derivatives
    return(list(c(dS, dE, dI, dR)))
  })
}
```

Then simulate starting parameters by assigning a value to them.

```
N <- 1000 # Total population size
beta <- 0.3 # Transmission rate
sigma <- 0.1 # Rate of latent individuals becoming infectious
gamma <- 0.05 # Rate of recovery
```

Set an initial state and a time vector, let's say 100 days.

```
initial_state <- c(S = N - 1, E = 1, I = 0, R = 0)

# Time vector
times <- seq(0, 100, by = 1)
```

Here we use the `ode()` function from the `{deSolve}` package for solving the differential equations in the the SEIR model function that we created above.

```
output <- deSolve::ode(y = initial_state,
                       times = times,
                       func = SEIR,
                       parms = c(beta = beta,
                                 sigma = sigma,
                                 gamma = gamma))
```

The output is class "deSolve", "matrix" :

```
class(output)
#> [1] "deSolve" "matrix"
```

So, it needs to be converted to be a dataframe of time, susceptible, exposed, infected and recovered. All simulated values in 100 days of an epidemic.

```
simulated_data <- as.data.frame(output)

head(simulated_data)
#>   time        S         E          I           R
#> 1    0 999.0000 1.0000000 0.00000000 0.000000000
#> 2    1 998.9857 0.9186614 0.09324728 0.002384628
#> 3    2 998.9452 0.8699953 0.17567358 0.009145043
#> 4    3 998.8812 0.8483181 0.25070051 0.019828923
#> 5    4 998.7954 0.8493639 0.32110087 0.034138118
#> 6    5 998.6890 0.8699856 0.38915443 0.051899977
```

This plot shows the simulated data of the SEIR model, with the number of susceptible, exposed, infectious, and recovered individuals over time. The number of susceptible individuals decreases over time as they become exposed and infected, while the number of exposed and infectious individuals increases before eventually decreasing as individuals recover from the infection.

```
# Plot simulated data
ggplot(simulated_data, aes(x = time)) +
  geom_line(aes(y = S, color = "Susceptible")) +
  geom_line(aes(y = E, color = "Exposed")) +
  geom_line(aes(y = I, color = "Infectious")) +
  geom_line(aes(y = R, color = "Recovered")) +
  labs(title = "Simulation of SEIR Model",
       x = "Time", y = "Population") +
  scale_color_manual(values = c(
    "Susceptible" = "navy", "Exposed" = "orange",
    "Infectious" = "brown", "Recovered" = "darkgreen"))
```

6.3.2.2 Random Forest

The next step is to calibrate this model by applying a machine learning algorithm. A `random forest` model is a type of model that uses an algorithm called **ensemble learning** to build multiple decision trees and combine their predictions to make accurate predictions. It works by splitting the data into subsets and building a decision tree for each subset. The final prediction is made by aggregating the predictions of all decision trees. Unlike mechanistic

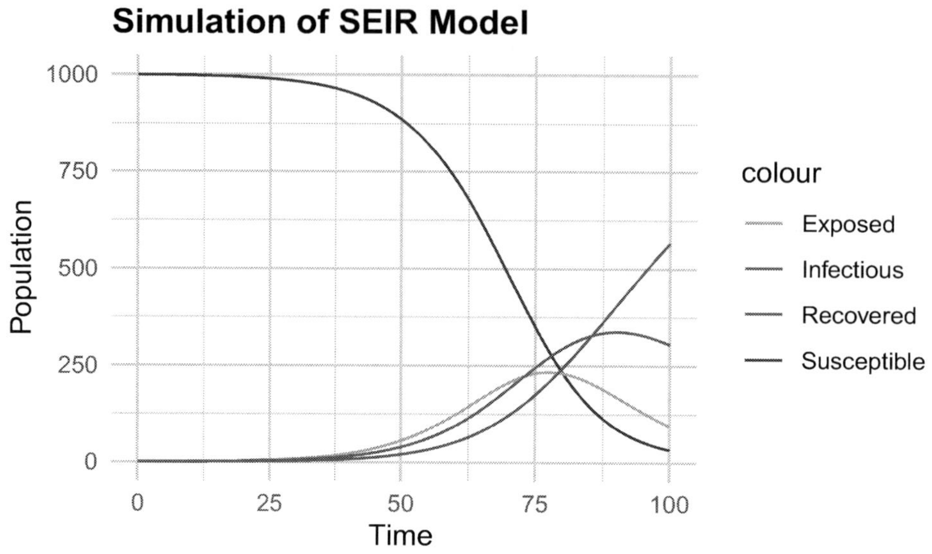

Figure 6.6 Simulation of SEIR Model: Susceptible, Exposed, Infectious, and Recovered individuals over Time interact with each other determining the scenario of the Epidemic. With the increase of the number of exposed and infectious individuals, the number of susceptible individuals decreases over time. The number of exposed and infectious individuals increases before eventually decreasing as individuals recover from the infection.

models, Random Forest does not rely on explicit equations or known relationships but instead learns patterns from the input data.

The `randomForest()` function from the `{randomForest}` package is used to predict the number of new infections in the simulated data, and train the model to which some normally distributed noise is added to the simulated data.

```
simulated_data <- cbind(simulated_data,
                        noise = rnorm(nrow(simulated_data),
                                      mean = 0,
                                      sd = 5))
```

Simulated data are split into **training** and **testing** sets to train the model and evaluate its performance. What this means is that the model is trained on a subset of the data (the training set) and then tested on the remaining data (the testing set) to assess its predictive performance.

```
# Load required packages
library(randomForest)

# Split the data into training and testing sets
set.seed(123)
train_index <- sample(nrow(simulated_data),
                      0.8 * nrow(simulated_data))
train_data <- simulated_data[train_index, ]
test_data <- simulated_data[-train_index, ]
```

```
# Train the Random Forest model - non machine learning yet!
rf_model <- randomForest(
  formula = I ~ .,
  data = round(train_data)
)
# Plot the tree
reprtree:::plot.getTree(rf_model, k = 3, depth = 4, cex = 0.8)
```

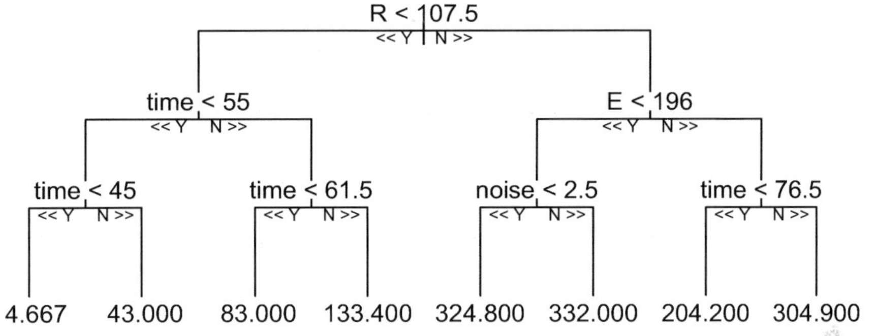

Figure 6.7 Tree of Random Forest Model for Epidemic X: The model splits the sample by determining the most probable number of infected individuals, using multiple decision trees to enhance accuracy. Each tree in the forest evaluates different features and criteria to make predictions, combining their outputs to form a consensus estimate. This approach helps to reduce overfitting and improve the robustness of the model in predicting the spread and impact of the epidemic.

It can be seen that the Random Forest model is trained on the simulated data, and the decision tree is built grouping the data into different categories, in this case the model uses the input variables (S, E, R, noise) with `depth = 4` to set the limit of the number of splits in the tree. Things can change with a different set of parameters, such as the number of trees, the number of variables to consider at each split, and the minimum number of data points required to split a node.

To predict the number of new infections based on the input variables, the `predict()` function is used on the test set, and the Root Mean Squared Error (RMSE) is then calculated to evaluate the model's performance. It quantifies how much the predicted values deviate from the actual values. The smaller the RMSE, the closer the predicted values are to the actual values, indicating a better predictive model performance. Conversely, a higher RMSE indicates a greater error between predicted and actual values.

```
# Make predictions on the test set
predictions <- predict(rf_model, newdata = test_data)

# Calculate Root Mean Squared Error (RMSE)
(rmse <- sqrt(mean((test_data$I - predictions)^2, na.rm = T)))
#> [1] 5.4194
```

This means that the model's predictions deviate from the actual values by an average of 8.66 new infections. This value can be used to assess the model's performance and identify areas for improvement.

```
cbind(test_data, pred = predictions) %>%
  ggplot(aes(I, pred)) +
  geom_point() +
  geom_abline() +
  labs(
    title = "Prediction of Infections for Epidemic X",
    subtitle = "Simulate Data",
    x = "Infections", y = "Predicted values")

cbind(test_data, pred = predictions) %>%
  ggplot(aes(x = time)) +
  geom_point(aes(y = I)) +
  geom_line(aes(y = pred), color = "navy") +
  labs(
    title = "Prediction of Infections for Epidemic X",
    subtitle = "Simulate Data",
    x = "Time (Day)", y = "Obeserved vs Estimated values")
```

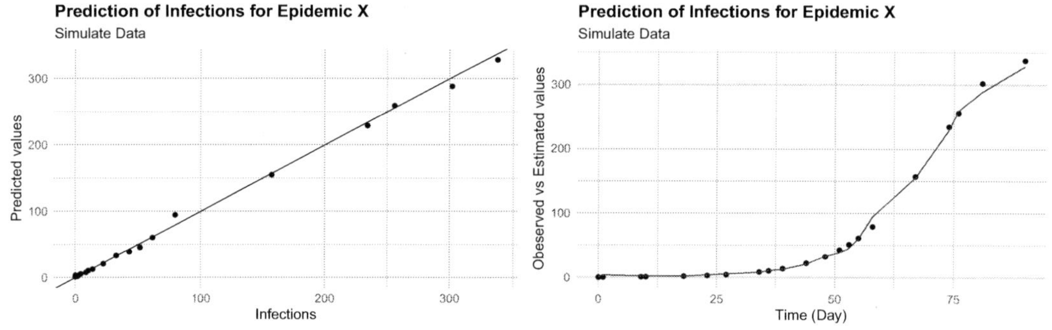

(a) Prediction of Infections for Epidemic X **(b)** Observed vs Estimated values

Figure 6.8 Prediction of Infections for Epidemic X: The model predicts the number of new infections based on the input variables, using the Random Forest algorithm to enhance accuracy. The plot shows the relationship between the observed and predicted values, with the line representing the ideal prediction where the observed and predicted values are equal. The Root Mean Squared Error (RMSE) is calculated to evaluate the model's performance, with a lower RMSE indicating a better predictive model.

6.3.2.3 Optimization with Tidymodels

Random Forest model is a powerful machine learning algorithm that can be tuned to improve its performance. The **tuning process** involves selecting the optimal values for the hyperparameters of the model, such as in the case of a random forest model, the number of trees, the number of variables to consider at each split, and the minimum number of data points required to split a node. These hyperparameters can significantly impact the model's performance, and tuning them can help improve the model's accuracy and generalisation to new data.

For this task we use the `{tidymodels}` package, a collection of packages for modelling and machine learning using the tidyverse principles. The `{tidymodels}` package provides a consistent interface for modelling tasks, making it easier to build, tune, and evaluate machine learning models.

```
library(tidymodels)
library(dials)
tidymodels_prefer()

# Spending data
set.seed(1231) # Set seed for reproducibility

# Split the data into training and testing sets
split <- initial_split(simulated_data, prop = 0.8)
train_data <- training(split)
test_data <- testing(split)

# Create a resampling scheme: 5-fold cross-validation
cv_folds <- vfold_cv(train_data, v = 5)

# Create a recipe for data preprocessing
data_recipe <- recipe(I ~ ., data = train_data) %>%
  step_nzv(all_predictors()) %>%
  step_normalize(all_numeric())

# Define the Random Forest model
rf_ranger_model <-
  # tuning parameters - Machine Learning Application
  rand_forest(trees = tune(),
              min_n = tune()) %>%
  set_engine("ranger") %>%
  set_mode("regression")
```

Automate tuning parameters is performed, in this case, using a Bayesian Optimization with the `tune_bayes()` function to specify the grid of hyperparameters to search over. You can specify the number of iterations and initial random points to start the optimization. The `tune_bayes()` function uses the `bayes_opt()` function from the `{tune}` package to perform the optimization.

```
# Bayesian optimization
set.seed(123)
bayes_results <- tune_bayes(rf_ranger_model,
                            data_recipe,
                            resamples = cv_folds,
                            metrics = metric_set(rmse, rsq),
                            # Number of initial random points
                            initial = 5,
                            # Total iterations including initial points
                            iter = 20,
                            param_info = parameters(rf_ranger_model))
```

Examine the results of the Bayesian optimization to identify the optimal hyperparameters for the Random Forest model. The `show_best()` function displays the best hyperparameters based on the optimization results.

```
# Summarise the tuning results
show_best(bayes_results, metric = "rmse")
#> # A tibble: 5 x 9
#>   trees min_n .metric .estimator   mean     n std_err .config .iter
#>   <int> <int> <chr>   <chr>       <dbl> <int>   <dbl> <chr>   <int>
#> 1  1873     2 rmse    standard   0.0352     5 0.00844 Iter14     14
#> 2  1801     2 rmse    standard   0.0353     5 0.00855 Iter9       9
#> 3  1839     2 rmse    standard   0.0354     5 0.00832 Iter11     11
#> 4  1883     2 rmse    standard   0.0356     5 0.00831 Iter16     16
#> 5  1709     2 rmse    standard   0.0356     5 0.00863 Iter10     10
```

Extract the best parameters:

```
best_bayes <- select_best(bayes_results, metric = "rmse")

best_bayes
#> # A tibble: 1 x 3
#>   trees min_n .config
#>   <int> <int> <chr>
#> 1  1873     2 Iter14
```

Finally, we can use the best hyperparameters to train the Random Forest model on the training data and evaluate its performance on the test data. The `fit()` function fits the model using the best hyperparameters, and the `predict()` function makes predictions on the test data. We can then calculate the Root Mean Squared Error (RMSE) to evaluate the model's performance.

```
# Final model with best parameters
final_bayes_model <- finalize_model(rf_ranger_model,
                                    best_bayes)
final_fit <- fit(final_bayes_model,
                 formula = I ~ .,
                 data = train_data)

# Predict and evaluate on test data
predictions <- predict(final_fit, new_data = test_data)
augumented <- augment(final_fit, new_data = test_data)
eval_metrics <- metrics(estimate = .pred,
                        truth = I,
                        data = augumented)

eval_metrics
#> # A tibble: 3 x 3
#>   .metric .estimator .estimate
#>   <chr>   <chr>          <dbl>
#> 1 rmse    standard       4.25
#> 2 rsq     standard       0.999
#> 3 mae     standard       2.34
```

```
# Calculate Root Mean Squared Error (RMSE)
err <- (test_data$I - predictions$.pred)^2
rmse <- sqrt(mean(err, na.rm = T))
```

```
paste("RMSE:", rmse)
#> [1] "RMSE: 4.25017352277781"
```

```
augumented %>%
  ggplot(aes(I, .pred)) +
  geom_point() +
  geom_abline() +
  labs(
    title = "Prediction of Infections for Epidemic X",
    subtitle = "Simulate Data",
    x = "Infections", y = "Predicted values")

augumented %>%
  ggplot(aes(x = time)) +
  geom_point(aes(y = I)) +
  geom_line(aes(y = .pred), color = "navy") +
  labs(
    title = "Prediction of Infections for Epidemic X",
    subtitle = "Simulate Data",
    x = "Time (Day)", y = "Obesrved vs Estimated values")
```

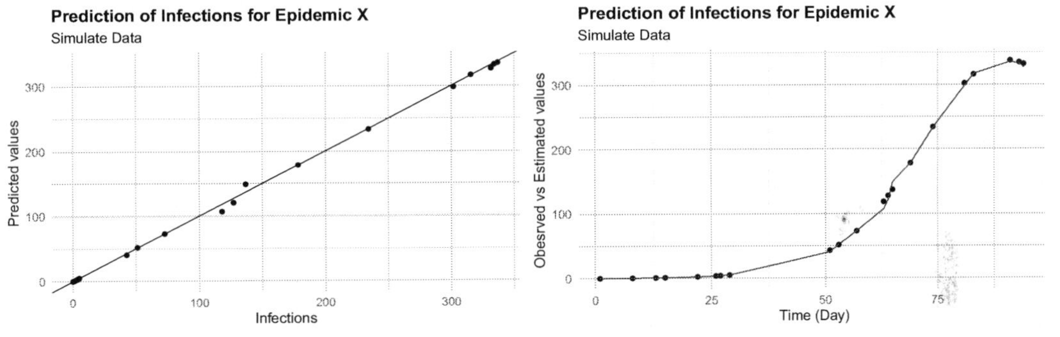

(a) Prediction of Infections for Epidemic X **(b)** Observed vs Estimated values

Figure 6.9 Prediction of Infections for Epidemic X

6.3.3 Example: Epidemic Y

6.3.3.1 INLA: An Empirical Bayes Approach to GAMs

In this example is a simulation of an epidemic in 100 days based on temperature level and number of cases simulated with a random poisson distribution.

The model used is the **INLA - integrated nested Laplace approximation**[8] model, an excellent choice for applications requiring repeated model fitting. The INLA approach is particularly useful for fitting complex models, such as Generalised additive models (GAMs), which involve non-linear relationships between predictors and the response variable.

[8] "Approximate Bayesian Inference for Latent Gaussian Models by Using Integrated Nested Laplace Approximations - Rue - 2009 - Journal of the Royal Statistical Society: Series b (Statistical Methodology) - Wiley Online Library," n.d., https://rss.onlinelibrary.wiley.com/doi/full/10.1111/j.1467-9868.2008.00700.x.

$$y_i = \beta_0 + \sum_{j=1}^{n} f_j(x_{i,j}) + \epsilon_i \tag{6.13}$$

$$f_j(x_{i,j}) = \sum_{k=1}^{p} \beta_{j,k} B_{j,k}(x_{i,j}) \tag{6.14}$$

where y_i represent the response vector of observations, $f_j(x_{i,j})$ the smooth function of the predictors (random effects), $B_{j,k}$ basis function such as splines, β_0 and β_j the intercept and the coefficients respectively. While ϵ_i is the error term with a Gaussian distribution:

$$\epsilon_i \sim Norm(0, \sigma^2) \tag{6.15}$$

Used as:

```
INLA::inla(y ~ x1 + x2 + ... + xn, data = data)
```

It is also a valid alternative to **Markov Chain Monte Carlo (MCMC)** methods used to compute the joint posterior distribution of the model parameters[9] - (Appendix B). Due to the deterministic nature of its approximations, the use of a **Laplacian approximation** to estimate the individual posterior marginals of the model parameters, allows for faster computation, and more efficient estimation of the posterior distribution, making it a popular choice for Bayesian inference in large-scale applications. However, it's worth noting that for very complex models or those with multi-modal posteriors, MCMC might still be preferred due to its flexibility and ability to characterise the entire posterior distribution.

In INLA, each of GAMs components are treated as random effects with specific prior distributions (typically Gaussian). The smoothness of these effects is controlled by hyperparameters, which INLA estimates from the data. The model is then fitted using the `{INLA}` package, which provides a fast and efficient way to estimate the posterior distribution of the model parameters.

Let's assume new `epidemic_data` with columns `day`, `cases`, and `temperature`. To model the number of cases as a function of time and temperature, considering a non-linear effect of time using a **random walk model** (`model = "rw2"`) and a linear effect of temperature:

```
install.packages("INLA",
  repos = c(getOption("repos"),
    INLA = "https://inla.r-inla-download.org/R/stable"),
  dep = TRUE)
```

```
library(INLA)
```

```
# Sample data creation
set.seed(123)
epidemic_data <- data.frame(
  day = 1:100,
  temperature = rnorm(100, mean = 20, sd = 5),
  cases = rpois(100,
```

[9] W. R. Gilks, S. Richardson, and David Spiegelhalter, eds., *Markov Chain Monte Carlo in Practice* (Chapman; Hall/CRC, 1995), doi:10.1201/b14835.

```
                  lambda = 10 + sin(1:100 / 20) * 10 + rnorm(100,
                                                              sd = 5)))

# Define the model formula
formula <- cases ~ f(day, model = "rw2") + temperature

# Fit the model using INLA
result <- inla(formula,
               family = "poisson",
               data = epidemic_data)
```

```
# Summary of the results
result$summary.fixed
```

The model summary shows the estimated coefficients for the fixed effects of the model, including the intercept and the effect of temperature. The estimated coefficients represent the average effect of each predictor on the response variable, accounting for the non-linear effect of time and the linear effect of temperature. The summary also includes the standard errors and 95% credible intervals for each coefficient, providing a measure of uncertainty around the estimates.

```
result$summary.hyperpar %>% t()
#>              Precision for day
#> mean                 23176.059
#> sd                   14734.793
#> 0.025quant            4473.788
#> 0.5quant             19952.248
#> 0.975quant           60407.981
#> mode                 13533.496
```

```
# Extracting the fitted values and the effect of time
time_effect <- result$summary.random$day
fitted_values <- result$summary.fitted.values

# Creating a data frame for plotting
plot_data <- data.frame(Day = epidemic_data$day,
                        FittedCases = fitted_values$mean,
                        Lower = fitted_values$`0.025quant`,
                        Upper = fitted_values$`0.975quant`)

# Plotting the results
ggplot(plot_data, aes(x = Day)) +
  geom_ribbon(aes(ymin = Lower, ymax = Upper),
              fill = "lightblue",
              alpha = 0.4) +
  geom_line(aes(y = FittedCases),
            color = "blue") +
  labs(title = "Fitted GAM for Epidemic Y",
       x = "Day", y = "Fitted number of cases")
```

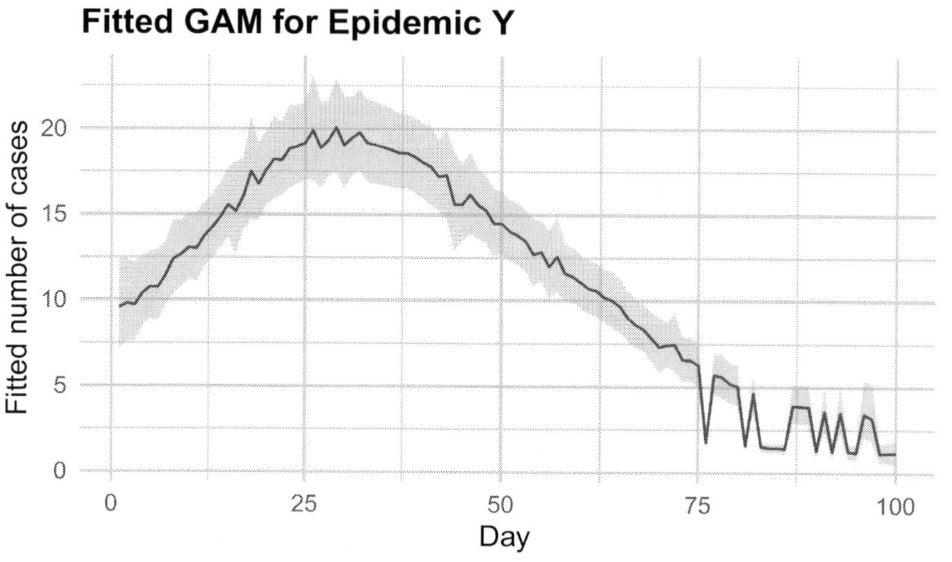

Figure 6.10 Fitted GAM for Epidemic Y: The plot shows the fitted values of the GAM model for Epidemic Y, with the shaded area representing the 95% credible interval around the mean estimate. The blue line represents the mean estimate of the number of cases over time, capturing the non-linear trend in the data.

The `inla()` function allows a model specification, in this case a `Poisson` is used and a formula. The non-linear effect is a second-order random walk `model = "rw2"`, a statistical modelling approach used to represent a type of prior commonly used in Bayesian modelling for time series or spatial data where you expect smoothness and some degree of continuity between adjacent observations. In particular, GAMs are used to capture non-linear trends by fitting smooth, flexible functions to the data. These functions can be represented through various basis functions, and a second-order random walk is one such basis function. The random walk model assumes that the values of the response variable are correlated with their neighbours, creating a smooth, continuous effect over time.

6.4 Measures of Machine Learning Models

To evaluate the performance of machine learning models, the loss function and the evaluation metrics are used to assess how well the model generalizes to new, unseen data. The loss function quantifies the discrepancy between the predicted outcomes and the actual values, providing a measure of the model's performance. The evaluation metrics, such as accuracy, precision, recall, and F1 score, provide additional insights into the model's performance and can help identify areas for improvement.

6.4.1 Loss Functions

The **loss function** is a method for evaluating how well a machine learning algorithm model features a dataset. The **cost function** is the average of all loss function values.

The accuracy of predictive models is checked with **loss functions**, which measure the discrepancy between the predicted outcomes and the actual values. This adjustment of the model learning process is performed through iterative adjustments of the model parameters with the objective to improve the model's performance.

Models are trained to a specific loss function that guides the optimization process and quantifies the model performance.

6.4.1.1 Regression Loss Functions

Regression loss functions are for regression tasks where the prediction involves continuous numbers, and include:

- **Mean Squared Error (MSE):** MSE calculates the average of the squares of the errors, i.e., the average squared difference between the estimated values and the actual value. This loss function is sensitive to outliers as it squares the errors before averaging them.

$$MSE = \frac{1}{n}\sum_{i=1}^{n}(\hat{Y_i} - Y_i)^2 \tag{6.16}$$

- **Mean Absolute Error (MAE):** MAE measures the average magnitude of the errors in a set of predictions, without considering their direction (i.e., it averages the absolute differences between predictions and actual outcomes). Unlike MSE, MAE is not overly sensitive to outliers, making it suitable for datasets with anomalies.

$$MAE = \frac{1}{n}\sum_{i=1}^{n}|\hat{Y_i} - Y_i| \tag{6.17}$$

- **Mean Squared Logarithmic Error (MSLE):** MSLE is useful when targeting a regression model to predict exponential growth. By taking the log of the predictions and actual values, MSLE transforms the target variable to reduce the skew of the distribution, which can lead to more stable predictions across a range of values.

$$MSLE = \frac{1}{n}\sum_{i=1}^{n}(log(\hat{Y_i} + 1) - log(Y_i + 1))^2 \tag{6.18}$$

6.4.1.2 Classification Loss Functions

Classification loss functions are for classification tasks, where the output is categorical, typical loss functions include:

- **Binary Cross-Entropy:** Also known as log loss, this function measures the performance of a classification model whose output is a probability value between 0 and 1. It is particularly useful for binary classification tasks.

$$L = -\frac{1}{m}\sum_{i=1}^{m}(y_i * log(\hat{y_i}) + (1 - y)log(1 - \hat{y})) \tag{6.19}$$

- **Hinge Loss:** Often used with Support Vector Machines (SVMs), hinge loss evaluates the margin of classification errors, providing a penalty for miss-classified points to improve model accuracy.

$$L = max(0, 1 - y * f(x)) \tag{6.20}$$

Choosing the right loss function: The selection of a suitable loss function depends on the specific characteristics of the data and the model application. For instance, if predicting precise values is crucial and the data range is wide, MSE might be appropriate. Conversely, for models where the prediction scale is logarithmic or the data contains many outliers, MSLE or MAE could be more effective.

The choice of a loss function is not merely a technical decision but a strategic one, affecting how a model learns and performs on unseen data. Each loss function has its strengths and trade-offs, making it vital for practitioners to understand their implications thoroughly. Understanding these measures and how they influence model training and predictions can greatly enhance the effectiveness of machine learning applications.

6.4.2 Evaluation Metrics

While loss functions are used during the training process to guide the optimization of the model parameters, **evaluation metrics** measure how well the model's predictions align with the actual outcomes, providing a signal to adjust the model.

6.4.2.1 Regression Evaluation Metrics

For regression tasks, the following metrics are commonly used to assess the model's predictive performance:

- **Root Mean Squared Error (RMSE):** A measure of the average deviation between predicted and actual values, calculated as the square root of the average of the squared differences between predicted and actual values. It is commonly used in regression tasks to assess the model's predictive accuracy.

$$RMSE = \sqrt{\frac{1}{n}\sum_{i=1}^{n}(Y_i - \hat{Y}_i)^2} \tag{6.21}$$

- **R-squared (R2):** A statistical measure of how well the model fits the data, indicating the proportion of variance in the dependent variable that is explained by the independent variables. It ranges from 0 to 1, with higher values indicating a better fit.

$$R^2 = 1 - \frac{SS_{residual}}{SS_{total}} \tag{6.22}$$

- **Adjusted R-squared:** A modified version of R-squared that adjusts for the number of predictors in the model, providing a more accurate measure of the model's goodness of fit. It penalises the addition of unnecessary predictors that do not improve the model's performance.

$$AdjustedR^2 = 1 - \frac{(1 - R^2)(n - 1)}{n - k - 1} \tag{6.23}$$

6.4.2.2 Classification Evaluation Metrics

For classification tasks, the following metrics are commonly used to evaluate the model's performance:

- **Accuracy:** The proportion of correctly classified instances out of the total instances in the dataset. It is a simple and intuitive measure of a model's performance, but it may not be suitable for imbalanced datasets.

$$Accuracy = \frac{TP + TN}{TP + TN + FP + FN} \tag{6.24}$$

- **Precision:** The proportion of true positive predictions out of all positive predictions made by the model. It is a measure of the model's ability to avoid false positives.

$$Precision = \frac{TP}{TP + FP} \tag{6.25}$$

- **Recall (Sensitivity):** The proportion of true positive predictions out of all actual positive instances in the dataset. It is a measure of the model's ability to identify all positive instances.

$$Recall = \frac{TP}{TP + FN} \tag{6.26}$$

- **Confusion Matrix:** A table that summarises the performance of a classification model, showing the number of true positive (TP), true negative (TN), false positive (FP), and false negative (FN) predictions. It is used to calculate metrics such as accuracy, precision, recall, and specificity.
- **F1 Score:** The harmonic mean of precision and recall, providing a balanced measure of a model's performance. It is particularly useful when dealing with imbalanced datasets.

$$F1 = 2 \times \frac{Precision \times Recall}{Precision + Recall} \tag{6.27}$$

- **Receiver Operating Characteristic (ROC) Curve:** A graphical representation of the trade-off between true positive rate (sensitivity) and false positive rate (1-specificity) across different threshold values. It is used to evaluate the performance of binary classification models.

$$TPR = \frac{TP}{TP + FN}; \; FPR = \frac{FP}{FP + TN} \tag{6.28}$$

- **Area Under the Curve (AUC):** The area under the ROC curve, which provides a single value to summarise the model's performance. An AUC of 0.5 indicates a random classifier, while an AUC of 1.0 indicates a perfect classifier.

$$AUC = \int_0^1 TPR(FPR)dFPR \tag{6.29}$$

These are only a few of the most common loss functions and evaluation metrics able to provide insights into the model's performance to generalize to new data and make accurate predictions.

6.4.3 Public Health Loss Functions

> "The public may be less interested in environmental quality than in economic prosperity."
> Dubos

In the field of public health the measures of cost like mortality and morbidity are used to evaluate the outcome of health and well-being of a population.

The most common analyses methods are:[10]

- Cost-utility, using quality-adjusted life years (QALYs)
- Cost-effectiveness, for specific outcomes, such as life expectancy or medical outcomes.

[10] Marja Hult et al., "Cost-Effectiveness Calculators for Health, Well-Being and Safety Promotion: A Systematic Review," *The European Journal of Public Health* 31, no. 5 (May 10, 2021): 997–1003, doi:10.1093/eurpub/ckab068.

As mentioned in the history of health metrics (Chapter 2), the cost-utility framework has been employed for calculating QALYs. Over time, this measure has been criticised for potentially discriminating against certain disabilities in the population by assigning costs that were perceived as either too high or too low, and for failing to capture the full spectrum of human health conditions.

Moreover, comprehensive tools that assess the impacts through cost-effectiveness measures to estimate the effectiveness of health interventions should also include a measure of disability. The measure of DALYs (Disability-Adjusted Life Years), developed in 1993, took major consideration of the disability status in evaluating the well-being of a population. It was further enhanced by incorporating a layer based on disability weights.

In summary, the measures for a cost-effectiveness intervention involve a careful calibration of following components: mortality, morbidity, and disability.

7

Techniques for Machine Learning Applications

Learning Objectives

- Apply feature engineering techniques to prepare data for modelling
- Evaluate and select the most appropriate machine learning model based on data characteristics
- Understand the fundamentals of key machine learning algorithms and their applications

Selecting the most suitable machine learning model involves understanding **the goals of the analysis**, the **nature of the data**, and the **statistical and machine learning methods** that best suit the tasks. In Chapter 6, we learned about what machine learning models are, provided examples for building a model framework, and selected common metrics for model performance calibration and evaluation.

In this chapter, we focus on the strategies for selecting appropriate models by leveraging the strengths of different techniques, specifically for health metrics and for infectious diseases. We will explore various considerations involved in addressing potential biases, and discuss actions to prevent them.

7.1 Goals of the Analysis and Nature of Data

The identification of the primary **goal of the analysis** is fundamental. Whether it involves trend analysis, investigating the relationships between response and predictor variables, or strictly forecasting to predict future outcomes, the strategy for model selection varies accordingly.

Health Metrics Data:

- **Composite Measures:** Health metrics like DALYs are composite measures that include both mortality and morbidity data, often requiring sophisticated regression models capable of handling continuous variables and multiple predictors. By examining the components of DALYs (e.g., Years of Life Lost (YLLs) and Years Lived with Disability (YLDs)), we can identify the key drivers such as mortality rates, disease prevalence, and risk factors.

- **Regression Models:** Regression models, including **linear regression**, **Ridge regression**, and **Lasso regression**, are commonly used to handle these continuous variables and address challenges like correlation and multicollinearity with appropriate techniques such as regularisation.

DOI: 10.1201/9781032625935-7

Infectious Disease Data:

- **Categorical and Continuous Data:** Infectious disease data can be categorical (e.g., disease presence or absence) or continuous (e.g., incidence rates). Classification models are suitable for categorical outcomes, while regression models are appropriate for continuous data.
- **Disease Dynamics:** Understanding the dynamics of infectious diseases, such as transmission rates, incubation periods, and immunity, informs the selection of models. Common models include compartmental models (e.g., SIR, SEIR) and agent-based models.

Common considerations for health metrics and infectious diseases data type:

- **Seasonality and Trends:** The data may exhibit seasonality or trends, necessitating the use of time series analysis models like **ARIMA** or seasonal decomposition to capture these patterns.
- **Simulation Models:** These models can predict the impact of interventions on DALYs and infectious diseases, estimating the effectiveness of different interventions and guiding policy decisions. Examples of these types of models are: **SIR** models, and **Agent-based models**. In addition, **confidence intervals** and **sensitivity analyses** help assess the uncertainty associated with these predictions.
- **Bayesian Models:** These models can estimate parameters and make predictions based on prior knowledge and observed data, incorporating uncertainty and variability.
- **Predictive modelling:** Such as **decision trees**, **support vector machines (SVM)**, and **Long Short-Term Memory (LSTM) neural networks**, can predict disease outbreaks, identify high-risk populations, and optimise resource allocation.

7.2 Statistical and Machine Learning Methods

The choice of model depends on the type of data, the relationships between variables, and the goals of the analysis. Once we have these factors well identified, we are a step forward in restricting the range of applicable models.

The next step involves conducting a thorough **exploratory data analysis (EDA)**. This initial exploration helps to uncover the underlying structure of the data, the relationships between variables, and the way the response variable—which may also be referred to as the outcome variable—depends on predictors. This phase is critical as it informs the necessity of subsequent data adjustments and transformations.

The importance of data preparation and exploratory data analysis in machine learning are the building blocks in the preparation of machine learning digestible data. **Feature engineering** is a technique that involves creating new features from existing ones based on domain knowledge or transformation of data to improve the model's ability to discern patterns. For example, creating features like **moving averages** or differences between consecutive days can reveal trends and cycles that are not immediately apparent from raw data.

Another example is the **standardisation** process, which is crucial when dealing with variables measured in different units. It involves rescaling the features so they have a mean of zero and a standard deviation of one. This process is particularly important when variables span several orders of magnitude; without standardisation, a model might incorrectly interpret the scale of a feature as a proxy for importance.

Furthermore, the application of transformations, such as **logarithmic** scaling or the application of **spline** functions can help in managing skewed data or enhancing model ability to capture non-linear relationships, which result particularly useful in complex data modelling. In addition, tailored adjustments, and more sophisticated manipulations have been implemented over time to allow estimation of missing values in order to obtain customised, flexible, and more homogeneous data. For more information on feature engineering, see[1] useful for effective machine learning strategy application, covering various techniques and appropriate use cases, focusing on practical understanding and implementation.

7.3 Model Selection Strategies

In developing predictive models for health metrics and infectious diseases, selecting the appropriate model is critical to ensure accurate and reliable forecasts. Here are outlined sample strategies employed in the model selection process, we introduce the **Rabies** dataset used for our discussion and demonstrate the selection of a suitable model for analysing its impact. Rabies, although nearly 100% fatal once symptoms appear, presents a unique challenge due to the relative rarity of cases and limited availability of comprehensive data. This scarcity complicates efforts to model the disease accurately and develop effective public health strategies.

To address these challenges, we explore advanced modelling techniques that can enhance the robustness of our analyses despite data limitations, which involves evaluating multiple models based on their performance and selecting the best-fitting models to achieve the most accurate predictions.

7.4 Example: Rabies

The **rabies** dataset from the `{hmsidwR}` package contains information on death rates and disability-adjusted life years (DALYs) per 100,000 inhabitants due to rabies and all causes of mortality in Asia and for the Global region from 1990 to 2019. Rabies ([2]) is a fatal viral infection, and it is also classified as an infectious disease that can infect all mammals causing acute encephalitis. Caused by the rabies virus, which belongs to the Lyssavirus genus, it is transmitted to humans through the bite of an infected animal such as bats, raccoons, skunks, foxes, and obviously dogs, which are the main source of human rabies deaths.[3] Rabies defined as **neglected tropical disease (NTD)** predominantly affects already marginalised, poor and vulnerable populations. Although effective human vaccines and immunoglobulins exist for rabies, these are often not readily available or accessible to everyone.[4]

[1] Brandon Butcher and Brian J. Smith, *The American Statistician* 74, no. 3 (July 2020): 308–9, doi:10.1080/00031305.2020.1790217.

[2] CDC, "About Rabies," May 14, 2024, https://www.cdc.gov/rabies/about/index.html.

[3] Katie Hampson et al., "Estimating the Global Burden of Endemic Canine Rabies," *PLOS Neglected Tropical Diseases* 9, no. 4 (April 2015): e0003709, doi:10.1371/journal.pntd.0003709.

[4] "Rabies," n.d., https://www.who.int/news-room/fact-sheets/detail/rabies.

In this example we consider the number of DALYs per 100,000 inhabitants due to rabies in Asia and the Global region, as our response variable, the dataset is made available in the `{hmsidwR}` package. It is composed of 240 observations and 7 variables: `measure`, `location`, `cause`, `year`, `val`, `upper`, `lower`.

```
library(tidyverse)
hmsidwR::rabies %>%
  filter(year >= 1990 & year <= 2019) %>%
  select(-upper, -lower) %>%
  head()
#> # A tibble: 6 x 5
#>   measure location cause       year    val
#>   <chr>   <chr>    <chr>      <dbl>  <dbl>
#> 1 Deaths  Global   All causes  1990 1107.
#> 2 Deaths  Asia     Rabies      1990    0.599
#> 3 Deaths  Global   All causes  1994 1095.
#> 4 Deaths  Global   All causes  1992 1090.
#> 5 Deaths  Asia     Rabies      1992    0.575
#> 6 Deaths  Asia     Rabies      1994    0.554
```

Selecting only the `cause == Rabies` , the first thing to notice is that deaths rates and DALYs are on different units, rates and years respectively.

```
library(tidyverse)
rabies <- hmsidwR::rabies %>%
  filter(year >= 1990 & year <= 2019) %>%
  select(-upper, -lower) %>%
  pivot_wider(names_from = measure, values_from = val) %>%
  filter(cause == "Rabies") %>%
  rename(dx_rabies = Deaths, dalys_rabies = DALYs) %>%
  select(-cause)

rabies %>% head()
#> # A tibble: 6 x 4
#>   location  year dx_rabies dalys_rabies
#>   <chr>    <dbl>     <dbl>        <dbl>
#> 1 Asia      1990     0.599         33.1
#> 2 Asia      1992     0.575         31.9
#> 3 Asia      1994     0.554         30.7
#> 4 Asia      1991     0.585         32.3
#> 5 Asia      1995     0.551         30.5
#> 6 Asia      1997     0.502         27.9
```

It can be seen that the number of deaths due to rabies is much lower than the number of DALYs. This difference in scale can affect the model's ability to learn from the data. To address this issue, we can scale and centre the numeric variables to make them more comparable.

```
p1 <- rabies %>%
  ggplot(aes(x = year, group = location, linetype = location)) +
  geom_line(aes(y = dx_rabies),
            linewidth = 1) +
  geom_line(aes(y = dalys_rabies))
```

```
p2 <- rabies %>%
  # apply a scale transformation to the numeric variables
  mutate(year = as.integer(year),
         across(where(is.double), scale)) %>%
  ggplot(aes(x = year, group = location, linetype = location)) +
  geom_line(aes(y = dx_rabies),
            linewidth = 1) +
  geom_line(aes(y = dalys_rabies))
```

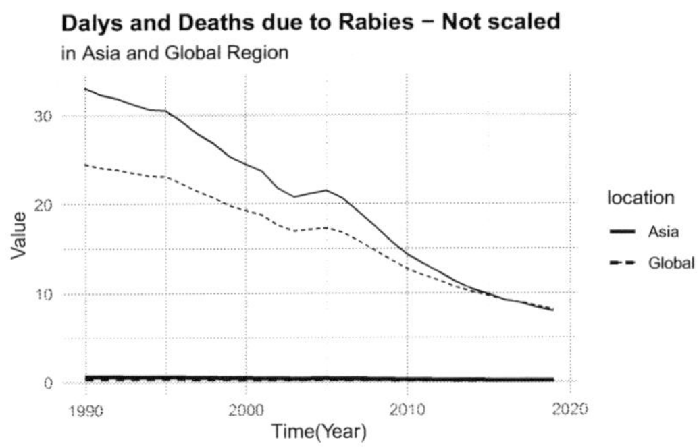

(a) Not scaled

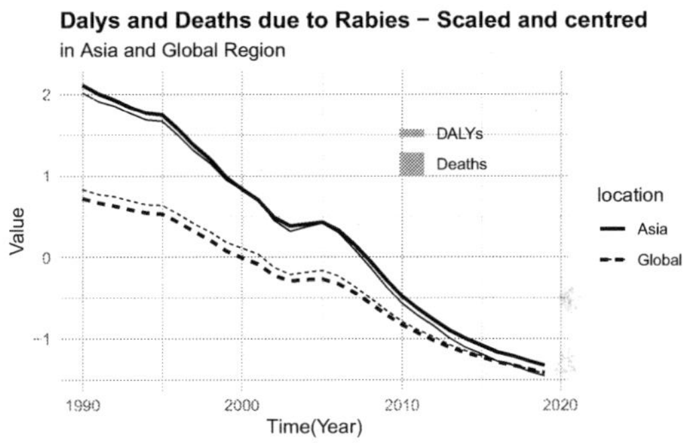

(b) Scaled and centred

Figure 7.1 Not Scaled and Scaled and Centred

Creating new features from existing ones provide additional predictive power. Then, combine the cause vector in a way to obtain two vectors for death rates due to rabies and all causes, scale and centre the numeric variables to obtain homogeneous data to use in the model.

```
all_causes <- hmsidwR::rabies %>%
  filter(year >= 1990 & year <= 2019) %>%
  select(-upper, -lower) %>%
  pivot_wider(names_from = measure, values_from = val) %>%
  filter(!cause == "Rabies") %>%
  rename(dx_allcauses = Deaths, dalys_allcauses = DALYs) %>%
  select(-cause)

dat <- rabies %>%
  full_join(all_causes, by = c("location", "year"))

dat %>% head()
#> # A tibble: 6 x 6
#>   location  year dx_rabies dalys_rabies dx_allcauses dalys_allcauses
#>   <chr>    <dbl>     <dbl>        <dbl>        <dbl>           <dbl>
#> 1 Asia      1990     0.599         33.1        1179.          50897.
#> 2 Asia      1992     0.575         31.9        1151.          49532.
#> 3 Asia      1994     0.554         30.7        1120.          48084.
#> 4 Asia      1991     0.585         32.3        1166.          50412.
#> 5 Asia      1995     0.551         30.5        1116.          47766.
#> 6 Asia      1997     0.502         27.9        1072.          46164.
```

To be able to visualise the magnitude of difference between death rates and DALYs for both rabies and all causes, it is necessary to scale or standardise the data as shown above.

```
p3 <- dat %>%
  select(-year, -location) %>%
  scale() %>%
  cbind(dat %>% select(year, location)) %>%
  ggplot(aes(x = year,
             group = location,
             linetype = location)) +
  geom_line(aes(y = dx_rabies),
            linewidth = 1) +
  geom_line(aes(y = dx_allcauses))

p4 <- dat %>%
  select(-year, -location) %>%
  scale() %>%
  cbind(dat %>% select(year, location)) %>%
  ggplot(aes(x = year,
             group = location,
             linetype = location)) +
  geom_line(aes(y = dalys_rabies),
            linewidth = 1) +
  geom_line(aes(y = dalys_allcauses))
```

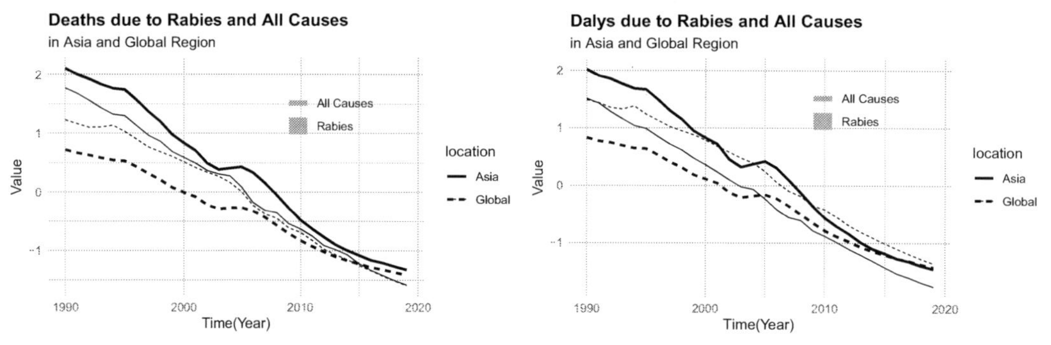

(a) Deaths due to Rabies and All Causes **(b)** Dalys due to Rabies and All Causes

Figure 7.2 Scaled and centred

For this task, we will use the `{tidymodels}` meta-package, as it provides a consistent interface for modelling and machine learning tasks. In particular, we define and execute modelling workflows, to create tailored data pre-processing tasks on various modelling specifications, and evaluate the performance using resampling techniques, to eventually select the best model. A more detailed explanation of the `{tidymodels}` framework can be found in the book.[5]

[5]Max Kuhn Silge and Julia, *Tidy Modeling with r*, n.d., https://www.tmwr.org/.

7.4.1 Training Data and Resampling

Splitting data into training and test allows the model to train a subsection of the data and then test its performance on the remaining part of the data, the test set. In this case, we will use the `initial_split()` function to split the data into training and test sets. The proportion assigned to trains can vary but it is usually assigned to be 80%, also a stratification option can be set.

```
library(tidymodels)

set.seed(11012024)
split <- initial_split(dat, prop = 0.8, strata = location)
training <- training(split)
test <- testing(split)
```

After that, it is important to create a set of folds, which means a set of subgroups of the original data by grouping following specific directions based on the type of **resampling technique**. Resampling techniques are used to evaluate the model's performance and estimate its generalisation error. There are various types of resampling techniques, it depends on the specific characteristics of your dataset, and the goals of your analysis. Some of the most common resampling techniques include:

- **k-Fold Cross-Validation** for general model evaluation and hyperparameter tuning.
- **Bootstrap Resampling** to estimate the variability of your model and for smaller datasets.
- **Time Series Cross-Validation** for time-dependent data to preserve temporal structure.
- **Spatial Resampling** for spatially correlated data to account for spatial dependencies.
- **Stratified Resampling** when dealing with imbalanced datasets to ensure proper representation of all classes.

In this case, we will use **k-Fold Cross-Validation** to evaluate the model's performance. The `vfold_cv()` function creates a set of folds for cross-validation, which is used to train and test the model on different subsets of the data.

```
set.seed(11102024)
folds <- vfold_cv(training, v = 10)
```

7.4.2 Data Preprocessing and Featuring Engineering

As already seen in the exploratory phase, preprocessing data is a crucial step in machine learning. This process can include techniques for handling missing values, standardisation of the data, encoding categorical variables, and removing highly correlated variables.

In this case, we will use the `{recipes}` package to create a recipe, with a set of preprocessing steps. The `recipe()` function allows us to define a model formula and use various `step_<functions>()` for manipulating data. We are going to set up 3 recipes, the first is a basic one which includes all variables and does not perform any data transformation.

```
rec <- recipe(dalys_rabies ~ ., data = training)
```

The second recipe includes some key steps to transform the data into a way specific models would be able to understand and learn from it. Models such as k-nearest neighbours, or support vector machines, that rely on distance metrics, can be sensitive to differences in feature scales.

For instance, non-standardised year data can dominate the model's decision-making process, leading to biased results. By scaling and centring the data, we ensure that all features contribute equally to the model's predictions.

We can create more complex recipes with more steps, but for this example, we will use a step for encoding the location variable (Asia, Global) into a numeric vector, and a second step to normalise (or standardise) all predictors.

```
rec1 <- recipe(dalys_rabies ~ ., data = training) %>%
  # convert nominal variables to dummy variables
  step_dummy(all_nominal_predictors()) %>%
  # scale the numeric variables
  step_normalize(all_numeric_predictors())
```

Once the recipe is created, we can apply it to the data using the `prep()` function, which estimates the necessary parameters for the transformations and applies them to the data. Then, to check the results we can use the `juice()` function to extract the processed data.

```
rec1 %>%
  prep() %>%
  juice() %>%
  select(1, 2, 5) %>%
  head()
#> # A tibble: 6 x 3
#>     year dx_rabies dalys_rabies
#>    <dbl>     <dbl>        <dbl>
#> 1 -1.61       2.12         33.1
#> 2 -1.17       1.79         30.7
#> 3 -1.50       2.02         32.3
#> 4 -1.06       1.76         30.5
#> 5 -0.847      1.40         27.9
#> 6 -0.738      1.23         26.8
```

Trained data can be also tested on new data, in this case we test them on the `test` set with the `bake()` function.

```
rec1 %>%
  prep() %>%
  bake(new_data = test) %>%
  select(1, 2, 5) %>%
  head()
#> # A tibble: 6 x 3
#>     year dx_rabies dalys_rabies
#>    <dbl>     <dbl>        <dbl>
#> 1 -1.39     1.94           31.9
#> 2 -0.521    0.870          24.5
#> 3 -0.412    0.743          23.7
#> 4  0.131    0.375          20.7
#> 5 -0.738    0.255          20.7
#> 6 -0.521    0.0443         19.3
```

DALYs often aggregate various health impacts, and can have highly skewed distributions. This skewness arises due to several factors: the presence of outliers, the nature of the health condition being measured, and the distribution of the data itself. To handle the skewness of the data, we can apply:

- Log Transformation: $log(DALYs + 1)$
- Sqrt Transformation: $\sqrt{DALYs}$
- Yeo-Johnson Transformation, a generalisation of the Box-Cox transformation that can handle both positive and negative values: $((DALYs + 1)^p - 1)/p$.

Let's apply the **Yeo-Johnson transformations** to the response variable (`dalys_rabies`) and see how the density distribution changes with different values of λ. This is a step that can be tuned with a machine learning algorithm.

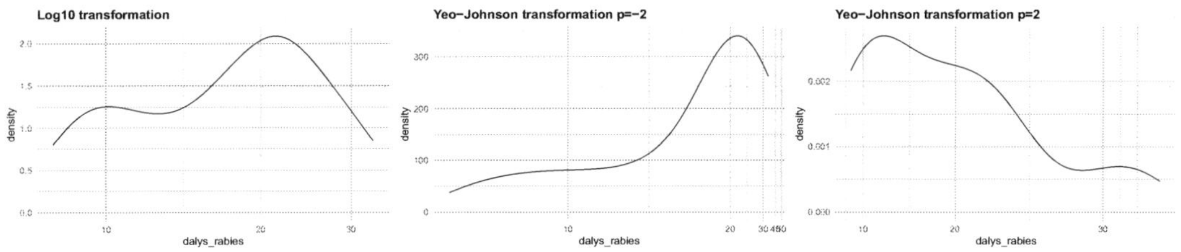

(a) Log10 **(b)** Yeo-Johnson p=-2 **(c)** Log10

Figure 7.3 Response variable transformation

Let's now create a third recipe with the `step_YeoJohnson()` function.

```
rec2 <- rec1 %>%
  # apply Yeo-Johnson transformation to the response variable
  step_YeoJohnson(dalys_rabies)

rec2 %>%
  prep() %>%
  juice() %>%
  select(1, 2, 5) %>%
  head()
#> # A tibble: 6 x 3
#>     year dx_rabies dalys_rabies
#>    <dbl>     <dbl>        <dbl>
#> 1 -1.61       2.12         5.97
#> 2 -1.17       1.79         5.78
#> 3 -1.50       2.02         5.91
#> 4 -1.06       1.76         5.77
#> 5 -0.847      1.40         5.54
#> 6 -0.738      1.23         5.44
```

7.4.3 Correlation, Multicollinearity, and Overfitting

To be noted is that we haven't applied any **correlation** selection step on this data. Filtering out highly correlated predictors, such as those with a correlation greater than 80% to avoid multicollinearity, would lead to excluding crucial variables. On the other hand, including all possible covariates in a model often yields implausible signs on covariates or unstable coefficients, as well as overfitting.[6]

[6]Kyle J. Foreman et al., "Modeling Causes of Death: An Integrated Approach Using CODEm," *Population Health Metrics* 10, no. 1 (January 2012): 1, doi:10.1186/1478-7954-10-1.

When multiple predictors are correlated, but all are crucial for the analysis (e.g., deaths due to rabies, total deaths, and total DALYs for all causes), applying a correlation step that filters out correlated variables can be problematic. One way to overcome bias arising from it is using regularisation techniques like **Ridge Regression** or **Lasso Regression** is often the best approach to handle multicollinearity without removing any predictors. Alternatively, **Principal Components Analysis (PCA)** can reduce dimensionality while retaining most of the variance. These methods ensure all important predictors are included in the model without the adverse effects of multicollinearity.

7.4.4 Model Specification

The next step is to outline the model specification. There are various type of models that can be used. We start with a **random forest**. This choice is typically done due to the algorithm's features, which is able to create **multiple bootstrap samples** (random samples with replacement) from the original dataset. Each bootstrap sample is used to train a separate decision tree.

7.4.5 Model 1: Random Forest

Rabies death rates may exhibit complex relationships with predictor variables. Random forests are capable of capturing non-linear relationships between predictors and the target variable.

Also, it handles multicollinearity, missing data, provides variables importance and is an ensemble learning method, which means they combine the predictions of multiple individual decision trees to produce a more accurate and stable prediction.

In our simplified case this type of model will do random samples with replacement of data. In `{tidymodels}` we can select different types of engines, in the case of random forest we could use random forest, ranger, and others. The difference between these engines derives from the specific type of calculation used to make the estimation. The Ranger engine is notably faster than random forest, so let's use that for this example.

```
rf_mod <- rand_forest(mtry = tune(),
                      trees = tune(),
                      min_n = tune(),
                      mode = "regression",
                      engine = "ranger")

wkf <- workflow(preprocessor = rec,
                spec = rf_mod)

rf_res <- tune_grid(object = wkf,
                    resamples = folds,
                    grid = 5,
                    control = control_grid(save_pred = TRUE))

show_best(rf_res, metric = "rmse") %>%
  select(-n, -std_err)
#> # A tibble: 5 x 7
#>    mtry trees min_n .metric .estimator  mean .config
#>   <int> <int> <int> <chr>   <chr>      <dbl> <chr>
```

```
#> 1     4  1794     7 rmse    standard   0.692 Preprocessor1_Model1
#> 2     5    85    17 rmse    standard   1.38  Preprocessor1_Model5
#> 3     1   446    16 rmse    standard   2.15  Preprocessor1_Model4
#> 4     3  1338    34 rmse    standard   2.79  Preprocessor1_Model2
#> 5     2  1151    31 rmse    standard   2.91  Preprocessor1_Model3
```

```
rf_res_tuned <- select_best(rf_res, metric = "rmse")

rf_res_tuned
#> # A tibble: 1 x 4
#>    mtry trees min_n .config
#>   <int> <int> <int> <chr>
#> 1     4  1794     7 Preprocessor1_Model1
```

```
rf_fit <- wkf %>%
  finalize_workflow(select_best(rf_res,
                                metric = "rmse")) %>%
  fit(training)

rf_fit %>%
  predict(new_data = test) %>%
  bind_cols(test) %>%
  rmse(truth = dalys_rabies, estimate = .pred)
#> # A tibble: 1 x 3
#>   .metric .estimator .estimate
#>   <chr>   <chr>          <dbl>
#> 1 rmse    standard       0.506
```

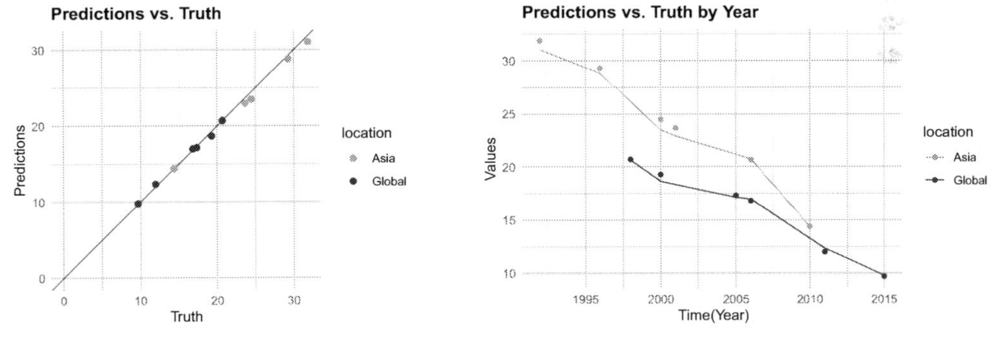

(a) Predictions vs. Truth   **(b)** Predictions vs. Truth by Year

Figure 7.4 Predictions vs. Truth

7.4.6 Model 2: Generalised Linear Model (GLM)

Generalised Linear Models (GLMs) involve statistical estimation rather than the iterative parameter tuning, common in many machine learning techniques. However, adding a machine learning feature through parameter calibration can be done using techniques such as cross-validation and grid search to find the best model settings.

To introduce a machine learning feature with parameter calibration into our modelling of the rabies data, we can use a technique like cross-validation combined with a **regularisation method** or an algorithm that supports parameter tuning. Here, we can employ a model from the `glmnet` package, which fits a generalised linear model via **penalised maximum likelihood**. The regularisation path is computed for the lasso or elastic-net penalty at a grid of values for the regularisation parameter lambda.

Adding Machine Learning Features with `{glmnet}` and Cross-Validation

```
if (!require(glmnet)) install.packages("glmnet")
library(glmnet)
```

For `glmnet`, we need to input matrices rather than data frames, and create matrices for the independent variables (predictors) and the dependent variable (response).

```
predictors <- model.matrix(dalys_rabies ~ .,
                           data = dat)[, -1] # Remove intercept
response <- dat$dalys_rabies
```

Use cross-validation to find the optimal lambda value, which controls the strength of the regularisation:

```
# Set seed for reproducibility
set.seed(123)

# Fit the model with cross-validation
cv_model <- cv.glmnet(predictors,
                      response,
                      family = "gaussian")
cv_model
#>
#> Call:  cv.glmnet(x = predictors, y = response, family = "gaussian")
#>
#> Measure: Mean-Squared Error
#>
#>      Lambda Index Measure      SE Nonzero
#> min 0.09043    48 0.05662 0.01147       2
#> 1se 0.13120    44 0.06564 0.01192       2
```

Extracting the best model, we can see that λ is 0.165.

```
# Get the best lambda value
best_lambda <- cv_model$lambda.min
paste("Best Lambda:", best_lambda)
#> [1] "Best Lambda: 0.0904304071218807"
```

And plot the lambda selection with the `plot()` function.

```
# Plot the lambda selection
plot(cv_model)
```

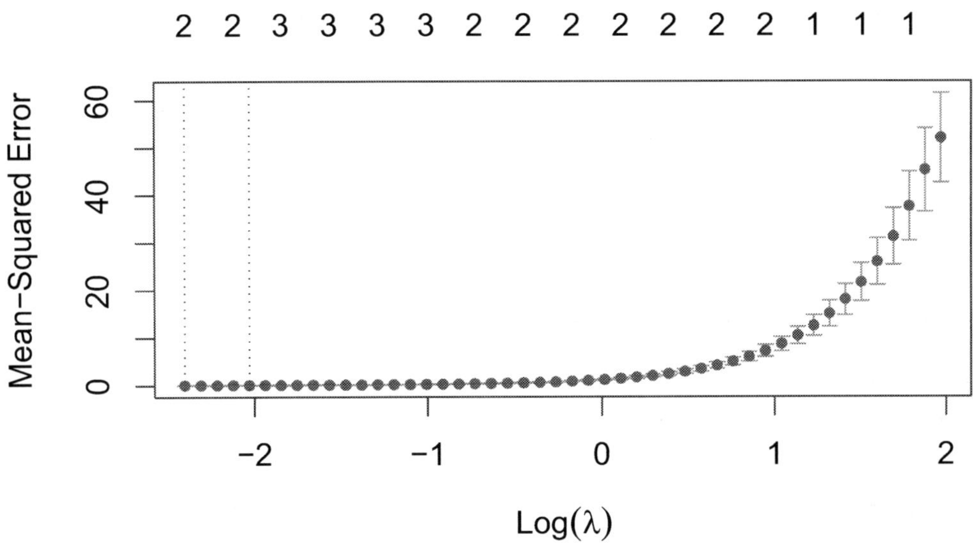

Figure 7.5 Cross-Validation Optimal Lambda

Then, fitting the final model with the selected best lambda, we can predict and evaluate the model.

```
final_model <- glmnet(predictors,
                      response,
                      family = "gaussian",
                      lambda = best_lambda)

# Predict using the final model
predictions <- predict(final_model,
                       # values of the penalty parameter lambda
                       s = best_lambda,
                       # matrix of new values for x
                       newx = predictors
                       )

# Calculate Mean Squared Error
rmse <- sqrt(mean((response - predictions)^2))
paste("Root Mean Squared Error:", rmse)
#> [1] "Root Mean Squared Error: 0.224854043214572"
```

By incorporating `glmnet` and using lambda selection via cross-validation, we introduce a **machine learning feature—parameter calibration** into our analysis. This approach not only helps in minimising overfitting but also enhances model performance by selecting the most effective regularisation parameter. The cross-validation process used here is crucial for confirming that our model's parameters are optimally tuned for the given data, embodying a key aspect of machine learning methodologies.

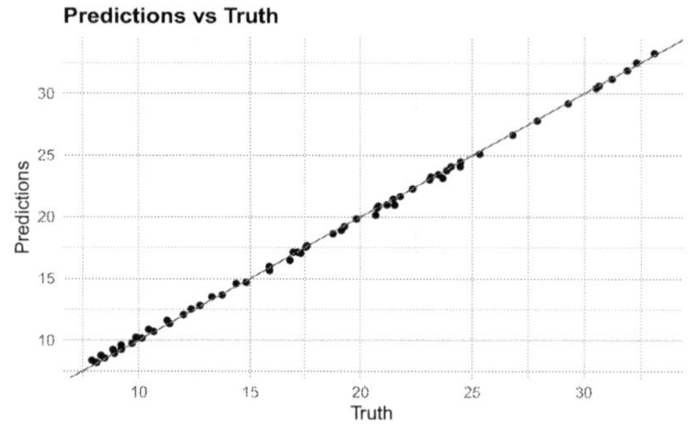

(a) Predictions vs. Truth

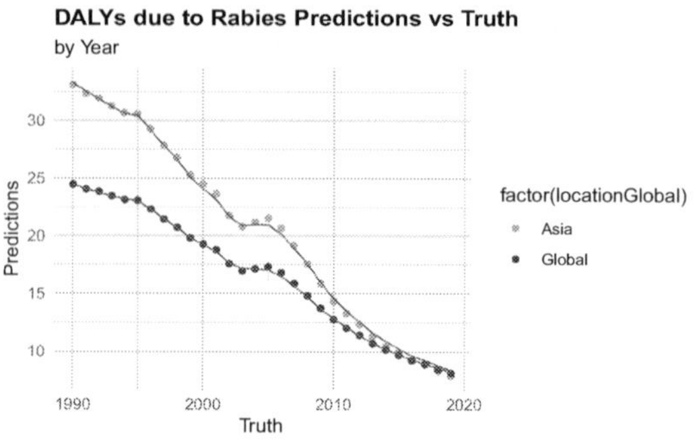

(b) Predictions vs. Truth by Year

Figure 7.6 Predictions vs. Truth

7.4.7 Testing Multiple Models

In the example above, we used two models to predict DALYs due to rabies, a random forest with `{tidymodels}` and a generalised linear model with `{glmnet}` with a Root Mean-Square Error of 0.448 and 0.257 respectively. The Random Forest model has a higher RMSE, which means it has a higher prediction error compared to the GLM model. However, we haven't applied any of the preprocessing steps, and there are many other models that could be used to predict DALYs such as:

1. **Support Vector Machines (SVM)**: SVMs are a powerful machine learning algorithm that can be used for both classification and regression tasks. They work by finding the hyperplane that best separates the data into different classes or groups.
2. **Extreme Gradient Boosting (XGBoost)**: Known for its high performance in various prediction tasks, XGBoost can handle missing values and is effective for large datasets.
3. **K-Nearest Neighbours (KNN)** models are a type of instance-based learning algorithm that stores all available cases and classifies new cases based on a similarity measure.
4. **Long Short-Term Memory (LSTM) Networks**: For temporal or sequential health data, LSTM networks can capture dependencies over time, making them suitable for time-series prediction of disease progression and outcomes.

Each of these models has its own strengths and weaknesses, and the choice of model will depend on the specific characteristics of the data and the goals of the analysis. By testing multiple models and comparing their performance, we can identify the best model for the given data and task.

Let's use the `{parsnip}` package and the `workflow_set()` function to fit a set of models to the rabies data. We will fit a **Support Vector Machine (SVM)**, and a **K-Nearest neighbours (KNN) model** to the data and compare their performance.

```
linear_reg_spec <-
  linear_reg(penalty = tune(),
             mixture = tune()) %>%
```

```
  set_engine("glmnet")

svm_p_spec <-
  svm_poly(cost = tune(),
           degree = tune()) %>%
  set_engine("kernlab") %>%
  set_mode("regression")

knn_spec <-
  nearest_neighbor(neighbor = tune(),
                   dist_power = tune(),
                   weight_func = tune()) %>%
  set_engine("kknn") %>%
  set_mode("regression")
```

```
library(rules)
library(baguette)
# Combine workflows into a workflow set
workflow_set <- workflow_set(preproc = list(scaled = rec1,
                                            yeo_johnson = rec2),
                             models = list(linear_reg = linear_reg_spec,
                                           svm = svm_p_spec,
                                           knn = knn_spec))

grid_ctrl <-control_grid(save_pred = TRUE,
                         parallel_over = "everything",
                         save_workflow = TRUE)

# Fit and evaluate the models with hyperparameter tuning
grid_results <- workflow_set %>%
  workflow_map(seed = 1503,
               resamples = folds,
               grid = 5,
               control = grid_ctrl)
```

```
# Show the results
grid_results %>%
  collect_metrics() %>%
  arrange(mean) %>%
  select(1, 5, 7, 9) %>%
  head()
#> # A tibble: 6 x 4
#>   wflow_id               .metric  mean std_err
#>   <chr>                  <chr>   <dbl>   <dbl>
#> 1 yeo_johnson_svm        rmse    0.148  0.0168
#> 2 yeo_johnson_knn        rmse    0.150  0.0331
#> 3 yeo_johnson_knn        rmse    0.173  0.0271
#> 4 yeo_johnson_svm        rmse    0.175  0.0177
#> 5 yeo_johnson_linear_reg rmse    0.178  0.0239
#> 6 yeo_johnson_linear_reg rmse    0.179  0.0243
```

```
autoplot(grid_results,
         rank_metric = "rmse",
         metric = "rmse",
         select_best = TRUE) +
  geom_text(aes(y = mean - 0.1,
                label = wflow_id),
            angle = 90,
            hjust = 1,
            color = "black",
            size = 3.5) +
  lims(y = c(-1.5, 0.9)) +
  theme(legend.position = "none")
```

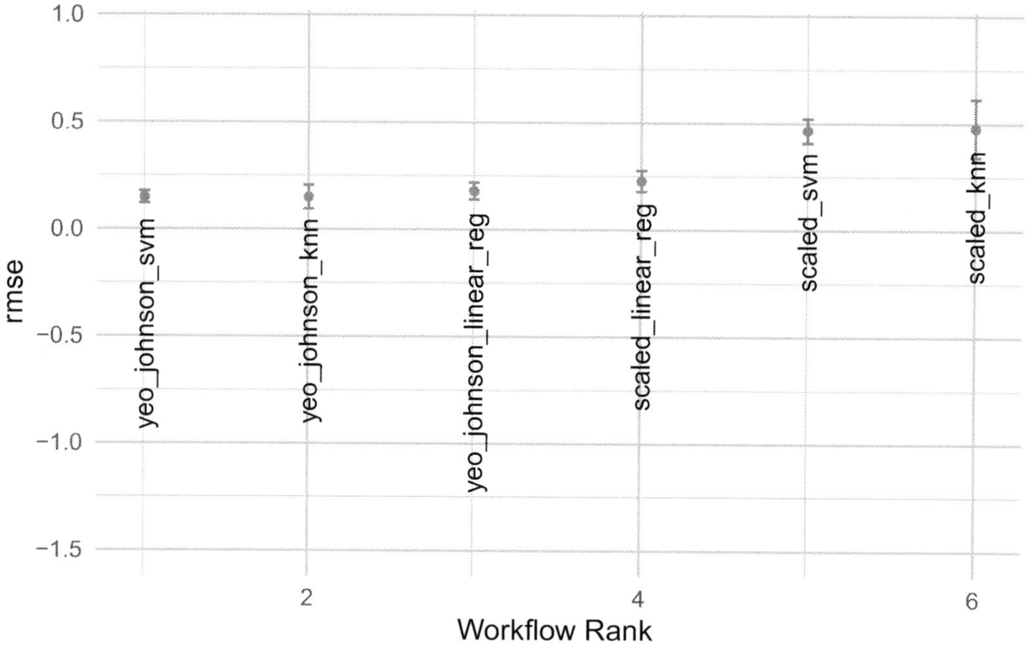

Figure 7.7 Model Performance

7.5 Summary

The integration of machine learning techniques into public health data analysis can significantly enhance the predictive power and robustness of models. By leveraging the capabilities of machine learning algorithms, we can extract valuable insights from complex health data, enabling more informed decision-making and policy formulation in public health contexts. The examples provided in this chapter illustrate the application of machine learning techniques to health metrics data, demonstrating the importance of feature engineering, model selection, and parameter calibration in enhancing the predictive accuracy and relevance of models. By following best practices in machine learning, public health researchers and practitioners can harness the power of data-driven insights to address critical health challenges and improve population health outcomes.

Best Practices for Machine Learning in Public Health:

- Conduct exploratory data analysis to understand the underlying structure of the data and relationships between variables.
- Apply feature engineering techniques to create new variables and enhance the model's predictive power.
- Select machine learning models that are contextually appropriate and robust for public health data analysis. Such as Random Forest, Generalised Linear Models, and others.
- Use parameter calibration techniques such as cross-validation, regularisation, monte carlo, and grid search to optimise model performance.
- Evaluate model performance using appropriate metrics and visualisation tools to assess predictive accuracy and relevance.

The integration of machine learning methodologies into public health data analysis represents a significant opportunity to advance the field of public health and enhance our understanding of health metrics and disease dynamics.

8

Essential R Packages for Machine Learning

Learning Objectives

- Gain an overview of essential R packages for modelling and data analysis
- Apply various modelling frameworks using appropriate R tools
- Learn how to discover and evaluate new R packages for specific analytical tasks

This chapter provides an overview of the most suitable R-packages for machine learning. It also discusses the combination of packages and functions to achieve the desired results. Additionally, it explores how to find new R-packages and evaluate their suitability for a given task.

8.1 Inside and Outside of the Library Boxes

When it comes to R, the possibilities are endless. With over 15,000 packages available on CRAN (Comprehensive R Archive Network) and countless others on GitHub and other repositories, the universe of available packages is vast. How to untangle among all of them? Which one to choose? Sometimes, it is rather favourable to start by working out of the library boxes, which means using functions provided in the built-in packages inside a fresh R installation.

However, the vast majority of the time, the best way to start is by using the packages that are already available in the R ecosystem. These packages are designed to make your life easier by providing pre-built functions for common tasks. They can help you save time and effort by automating repetitive tasks and streamlining complex analyses.

Life has become easier with the advent of wrapping functions and the reduction of lines of code through the use of functions found in packages. In the past, data analysis and modelling required extensive coding, often involving repetitive tasks and lengthy scripts. As a result, users can achieve sophisticated results more efficiently, without the need to write lengthy and intricate scripts from scratch. This shift has not only simplified the process of data analysis and modelling but has also democratised access to advanced statistical techniques, making them more accessible to a broader audience.

DOI: 10.1201/9781032625935-8

8.2 Essential R Packages for Machine Learning

Some of the most used modelling packages that are particularly useful for machine learning modelling of the spread of infectious diseases and evaluating DALYs variation due to infectious disease include:

8.2.1 Meta-Packages

1. `{tidymodels}`:[1] This framework provides a collection of packages for modelling and machine learning tasks, including {tidyr}, {dplyr}, and ggplot2. It offers a consistent and tidy workflow for data preprocessing, model building, evaluation, and visualisation.
2. `{caret}`:[2] The caret framework (short for **C**lassification **A**nd **RE**gression **T**raining) provides a unified interface for training and evaluating machine learning models. It supports a wide range of algorithms and offers convenient functions for hyperparameter tuning and model selection.
3. `{mlr3}`:[3] This is a modern and extensible framework for machine learning. It provides a unified interface for modelling tasks, making it easy to train and evaluate a wide range of machine learning algorithms.

8.2.2 Engines

Engines are the actual implementations of machine learning algorithms. They perform the computations necessary to train and evaluate models. Engines can be integrated into various meta-packages/frameworks to leverage their specific algorithms and computational efficiencies. Each engine might have its own set of parameters and functionalities, which can be accessed through the high-level interfaces provided by meta-packages.

1. `{randomForest}`: For random forest models.
2. `{xgboost}`: An optimised distributed gradient boosting library designed to be highly efficient, flexible, and portable. It implements machine learning algorithms under the gradient boosting framework.
3. `{glmnet}`: For lasso and ridge regression. Provides efficient procedures for fitting generalised linear models via penalised maximum likelihood.
4. `{nnet}`: For neural networks.
5. `{kernlab}`: For kernel-based machine learning methods.
6. `{e1071}`: For support vector machines and other functions.
7. `{lme4}`: For linear and generalised linear mixed-effects models.
8. `{mgcv}`: For generalised additive models.
9. `{rpart}`: For recursive partitioning and regression trees.
10. `{h2o}`: A powerful machine learning framework that can be efficiently integrated with `{tidymodels}`. `{h2o}` offers a range of machine learning algorithms, including linear models, tree-based models, and ensemble methods, with efficient handling of large datasets and support for parallel computing.

[1]Silge and Julia, *Tidy Modeling with r*.
[2]Max Kuhn, *The Caret Package*, n.d., https://topepo.github.io/caret/.
[3]"Mlr-Org," n.d., https://mlr-org.com/.

11. {keras3}, the R interface to Keras, is a deep learning technique which provides high-level **neural networks** API written in Python. Designed to enable fast experimentation with deep learning models on top of {tensorflow} (an open-source machine learning framework developed by Google).

8.2.3 Time Series Analysis

1. {forecast}: For forecasting functions.
2. {prophet}: Specifically designed for time series forecasting with an emphasis on flexibility and ease of use. Developed by Facebook, prophet can handle various time series patterns, including seasonality, holiday effects, and trend changes, making it suitable for modelling infectious disease trends over time.
3. {fpp3}:[4] This package is part of the Forecasting: Principles and Practice (3rd edition) book, offering data and tools for forecasting time series data, such as the import of the {fable} package with the `ARIMA()` model which is relevant for modelling disease spread over time.

8.2.4 Bayesian Analysis

1. {brms}: For Bayesian generalised multivariate non-linear multilevel models using Stan.
2. {rstan}: For Bayesian inference using Stan.

8.2.5 Specialized Tools

1. {spdep} is a powerful tools for spatial statistics, it provides a set of functions for analysing spatial dependencies and autocorrelation in spatial data, particularly relevant in infectious disease modelling. It also incorporates spatial effects into models and allows for a better understanding of how infectious diseases spread across space.
2. {INLA}:[5] Integrated Nested Laplace Approximations (INLA) is a package for Bayesian inference using the INLA method. It is particularly useful for spatial and spatio-temporal modelling, which can be relevant for studying the spread of infectious diseases.

These packages offer a diverse set of tools and techniques for modelling infectious disease spread and assessing its impact on health metrics like DALYs. These packages provide valuable insights into the dynamics of infectious diseases and can be used to inform public health interventions and policies. However, whether these packages are the most suitable depends on various factors, including:

- the specific requirements of the analysis
- the expertise of the researcher
- the nature of the data being used

Each package has its strengths and weaknesses, and the choice of package often depends on factors such as:

- the complexity of the modelling task

[4] *Forecasting: Principles and Practice (3rd Ed)*, n.d., https://otexts.com/fpp3/.
[5] "R-INLA Project - What Is INLA?" n.d., https://www.r-inla.org/what-is-inla.

- the type of data available
- the preferred modelling approach (e.g., frequentist vs. Bayesian).

For example, `tidymodels` provides a tidy and consistent workflow for modelling tasks, while `mlr3` offers extensive support for machine learning algorithms and hyperparameter tuning.

It's also worth considering other packages that may be relevant for specific aspects of the analysis, such as spatial modelling (e.g., `spdep`) or time series forecasting (e.g., `prophet`).

The features and capabilities of each package should carefully be evaluated in relation to their specific research objectives before choosing the one that best meets research needs and objectives. And it is worth considering that experimenting with different packages and techniques may be beneficial to identify the most effective approach for a given analysis.

8.3 Model Framework Application Examples

In this section we provide some examples of the application of different model frameworks. Data are used, as introduced in Chapter 7, to demonstrate the application of model frameworks such as `mlr3`, `h2o`, and `keras` for machine learning tasks.

We have already shown an application of the `{tidymodels}` meta-package in Chapter 6 and Chapter 7, particularly useful for testing out different types of models with the help of key functions such as the `workflow()`, `workflow_set()`, and `workflow_map()`.

8.3.1 Example: DALYs Due to Dengue with mlr3

The dataset for this example is from the `{hmsidwR}` package, which contains data on Deaths, DALYs, YLDs, YLLs, Prevalence, and Incidence due to selected infectious diseases from 1980 to 2021.

```
library(tidyverse)
hmsidwR::infectious_diseases %>% names
#>  [1] "year"          "location_name" "location_id"   "cause_name"
#>  [5] "Deaths"        "DALYs"         "YLDs"          "YLLs"
#>  [9] "Prevalence"    "Incidence"
```

Let's have a look at the locations where Dengue has been reported:

```
hmsidwR::infectious_diseases %>%
  filter(cause_name == "Dengue") %>%
  distinct(location_name)
#> # A tibble: 5 x 1
#>   location_name
#>   <chr>
#> 1 Malawi
#> 2 Central African Republic
#> 3 Lesotho
#> 4 Eswatini
#> 5 Zambia
```

And look at how the health metrics shape up over the years for Dengue:

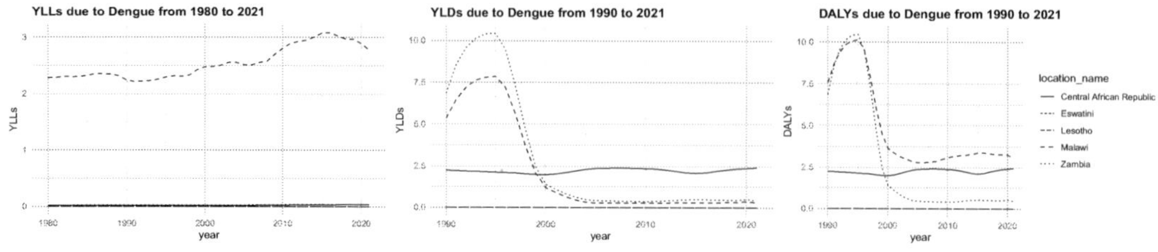

(a) YLLs (b) YLDs (c) DALYs

Figure 8.1 Health Metrics due to Dengue

The trend of the metrics in some locations is quite flat ranging around zero, while in others it is more evident. YLLs are the leading cause of DALYs, but YLDs are also contributing to the burden of disease.

We will focus on DALYs due to **Dengue** in three locations, Malawi, Zambia, and Central African Republic from 1990 to 2016 (26 years). The data from 2017 to 2021 is not included in the analysis and held out to be used as new data for testing the model's performance, as shown in Chapter 9.

Data are preprocessed to remove missing values, the values of DALYs only appeared in 1990, and then grouped by location id; the location name is removed.

```
dalys_dengue <- hmsidwR::infectious_diseases %>%
  arrange(year) %>%
  filter(cause_name == "Dengue",
         year<=2016,
         !location_name %in% c("Eswatini", "Lesotho")) %>%
  drop_na() %>%
  group_by(location_id) %>%
  select(-location_name, -cause_name)

dalys_dengue %>%
  head()
#> # A tibble: 6 x 8
#> # Groups:   location_id [3]
#>    year location_id   Deaths DALYs  YLDs   YLLs Prevalence Incidence
#>   <dbl>       <dbl>    <dbl> <dbl> <dbl>  <dbl>      <dbl>     <dbl>
#> 1  1990         182 0.0330    7.59  5.35 2.24         33.7      560.
#> 2  1990         191 0.00135   6.88  6.86 0.0229       42.4      713.
#> 3  1990         169 0.000760  2.25  2.24 0.0186       13.1      222.
#> 4  1991         191 0.00135   8.57  8.54 0.0230       52.5      884.
#> 5  1991         182 0.0327    8.68  6.47 2.21         40.9      681.
#> 6  1991         169 0.000760  2.23  2.22 0.0185       13.0      218.
```

The {mlr3} is a meta-package particularly useful for its syntax, as it guides the user through the machine learning steps by providing a consistent naming convention. It is also useful for benchmarking different models. In addition to the {mlr3} package, the {mlr3learners}, {mlr3viz}, and {mlr3verse}, and {data.table} packages are also loaded. Each of these packages provides additional functionality for machine learning tasks. More information on these packages can be found in the respective documentation, and further details can be found in the mlr3 book. In this example we use two types of models:

- `regr.cv_glmnet`: A cross-validated `glmnet` model with an alpha of 0.5 and a lambda of 0.1.
- `regr.xgboost`: An `xgboost` model with 1000 rounds, a maximum depth of 6, and an eta of 0.01. For this model the `{xgboost}` package is required.

```
library(mlr3)
library(mlr3learners)
library(mlr3viz)
library(mlr3verse)
library(data.table)
# library(xgboost)
```

Define the task, where the `id`, `backend`, and `target` are specified. The `backend` is the data that will be used for training the models. The `task` is the interface between the data and the learners; in this use-case the preprocessing steps are done beforehand, by removing missing and categorical values.

```
task <- TaskRegr$new(id = "DALYs",
                     backend = dalys_dengue,
                     target = "DALYs")

task$data() %>%
  select(year, DALYs, YLDs, YLLs) %>%
  head()
#>     year    DALYs     YLDs       YLLs
#>    <num>    <num>    <num>      <num>
#> 1:  1990 7.591334 5.354059 2.23727545
#> 2:  1990 6.882299 6.859449 0.02285062
#> 3:  1990 2.253677 2.235120 0.01855750
#> 4:  1991 8.565327 8.542325 0.02300233
#> 5:  1991 8.682844 6.469088 2.21375567
#> 6:  1991 2.234340 2.215861 0.01847933
```

The learners are the model's specifications. A full list of learners can be obtained with the function `as.data.table(mlr_learners)`.

```
learner_cv_glmnet <- lrn("regr.cv_glmnet",
                         alpha = 0.5,
                         s = 0.1)
learner_xgboost <- lrn("regr.xgboost",
                       nrounds = 1000,
                       max_depth = 6,
                       eta = 0.01)
```

Then define a **resampling strategy** to estimate the generalization performance, then create a **benchmark design** to compare different learners:

```
resampling <- rsmp("cv", folds = 5)

design <- benchmark_grid(tasks = task,
                         learners = list(learner_cv_glmnet,
                                         learner_xgboost),
                         resamplings = resampling)
design
#>      task          learner resampling
#>    <char>           <char>     <char>
#> 1:  DALYs regr.cv_glmnet         cv
#> 2:  DALYs   regr.xgboost         cv
```

Run the benchmark:

```
set.seed(19052024)
bmr <- benchmark(design,
                 store_models = TRUE,
                 store_backends = TRUE)
```

To access the content of an object such as `bmr`, use the `$` operator, or for more options use the `View()` function.

The `score()` function is used to extract the performance metrics of the models, in this case the mean squared error (MSE) is used.

```
bmr$score()[, .(learner_id,
                task_id,
                iteration,
                regr.mse)]
#>         learner_id task_id iteration    regr.mse
#>             <char>  <char>     <int>       <num>
#>  1: regr.cv_glmnet   DALYs         1 0.009638128
#>  2: regr.cv_glmnet   DALYs         2 0.008946393
#>  3: regr.cv_glmnet   DALYs         3 0.013166374
#>  4: regr.cv_glmnet   DALYs         4 0.012098411
#>  5: regr.cv_glmnet   DALYs         5 0.008993369
#>  6:   regr.xgboost   DALYs         1 0.140507087
#>  7:   regr.xgboost   DALYs         2 0.087534489
#>  8:   regr.xgboost   DALYs         3 0.522633289
#>  9:   regr.xgboost   DALYs         4 0.207629600
#> 10:   regr.xgboost   DALYs         5 0.031557756
```

Here we see the results of the benchmark, the `regr.mse` is the mean squared error of the models. The `regr.rmse` and `regr.mae` are also available.

```
set.seed(349)
autoplot(bmr, measure = msr("regr.rmse"))
autoplot(bmr, measure = msr("regr.mae"))
```

Aggregate the results:

```
measures <- msrs(c("regr.rmse", "regr.mae"))
aggr <- bmr$aggregate(measures)
```

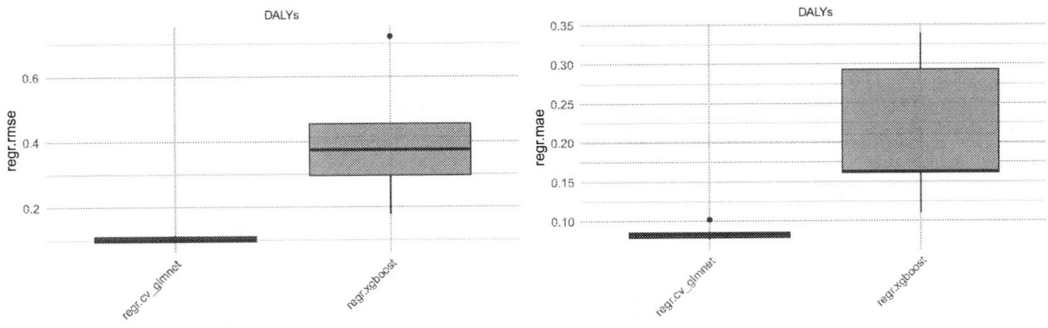

(a) BMR Regression RMSE **(b)** BMR Regression MAE

Figure 8.2 BMR Regression RMSE and MAE

```
rr1 <- aggr$resample_result[[1]]
rr2 <- aggr$resample_result[[2]]
```

Create a data frame with the results, for plotting with ggplot2, consider data are shuffled in the resampling process, and need to be reordered:

```
regr.cv_glmnet <- as.data.table(rr1$prediction()) %>%
  mutate(learner = "regr.cv_glmnet") %>%
  # order data to match the original order
  cbind(rr1$task$data()[rr1$prediction()$row_ids])

regr.xgboost <- as.data.table(rr2$prediction()) %>%
  mutate(learner = "regr.xgboost") %>%
  # order data to match the original order
  cbind(rr2$task$data()[rr2$prediction()$row_ids])


dat <- rbind(regr.cv_glmnet, regr.xgboost)
```

Plot the results:

```
dat %>%
  ggplot(aes(x = truth, y = response,
             group = learner)) +
  geom_abline() +
  geom_point(aes(color = learner)) +
  scale_color_manual(values = c("regr.cv_glmnet" = "navy",
                                "regr.xgboost" = "orange")) +
  facet_wrap(~learner) +
  labs(x = "Truth", y = "Response") +
  theme(legend.position = "none")
```

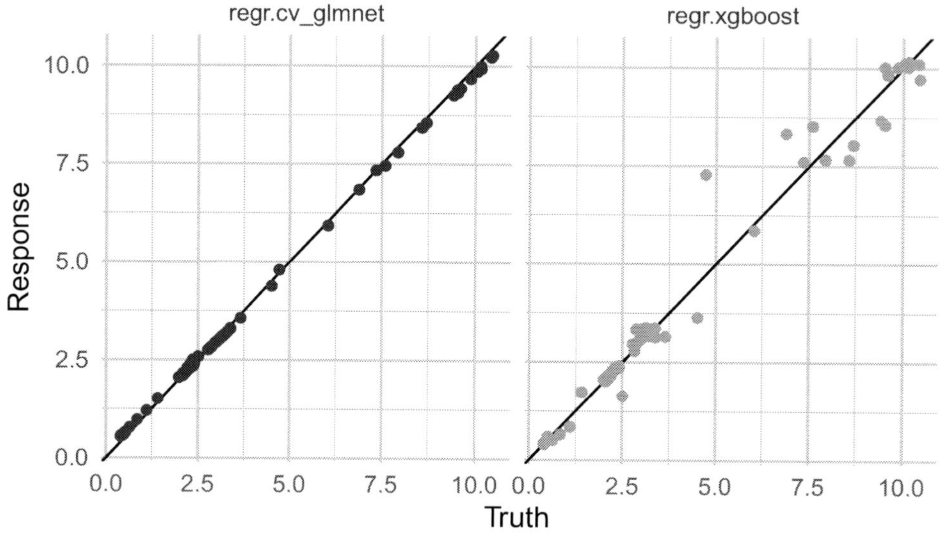

Figure 8.3 Truth vs Response for cv.glmnet and xgboost

```
dat %>%
  group_by(location_id, learner) %>%
  ggplot(aes(x = year)) +
  geom_point(aes(y = truth),
             size = 0.2) +
  geom_line(aes(y = response,
                linetype = learner),
            linewidth = 0.3) +
  # create facets for each location and
  # rename the location_id with the location_name
  # with the labeller function
  facet_wrap(vars(location_id),
    labeller = as_labeller(c(`182` = "Malawi",
                             `191` = "Zambia",
                             `169` = "Central African Republic")),
    scales = "free") +
  labs(title = "Dalys due to Dengue 1990-2016: Truth vs Responses",
       caption = "Scale Free - Dots represent the Truth Values",
       x = "Year", y = "DALYs", linetype = "Model") +
  theme(plot.title = element_text(hjust = 0.5))
```

In the next Chapter 9 we will see an application of these two models on remaining years from 2017 to 2021, to test the model performance as it was on new data.

8.3.2 Example: DALYs Due to Rabies with H2O

The following example shows how to use the {h20} r package for running H2O via its REST API.

```
options(timeout = 6000)
install.packages("h2o")
```

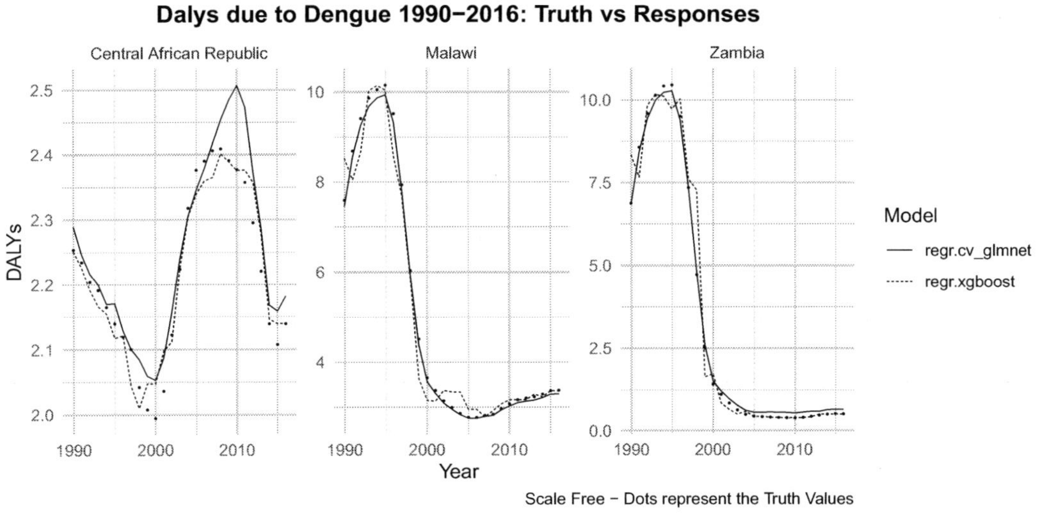

Figure 8.4 Models results on observed DALYs due to Dengue 1990-2016; Test Resampled Data with cv.glmnet and xgboost.

```
library(h2o)
```

```
# Initialize the H2O cluster
h2o.init()
```

We use the **rabies** dataset from the {hmsidwR} package, which has been used in Section 7.4. The dataset contains information on the number of deaths and dalys due to rabies in different countries and regions. The dataset is preprocessed to remove unnecessary columns and pivoted to create a wide format with the relevant health metrics.

```
library(tidyverse)

rabies <- hmsidwR::rabies %>%
  select(-upper, -lower) %>%
  pivot_wider(names_from = measure, values_from = val) %>%
  filter(cause == "Rabies",!is.na(DALYs)) %>%
  rename(dx_rabies = Deaths, dalys_rabies = DALYs) %>%
  select(-cause) %>%
  mutate(across(where(is.character), as.factor))

rabies %>% head
#> # A tibble: 6 x 4
#>   location  year dx_rabies dalys_rabies
#>   <fct>    <dbl>     <dbl>        <dbl>
#> 1 Asia      1990     0.599         33.1
#> 2 Asia      1992     0.575         31.9
#> 3 Asia      1994     0.554         30.7
#> 4 Asia      1991     0.585         32.3
#> 5 Asia      1995     0.551         30.5
#> 6 Asia      1997     0.502         27.9
```

The h2o_rabies object is created by importing the rabies data frame to H2O with the as.h2o() function.

```
# Upload data to H2O
h2o_rabies <- as.h2o(rabies)
```

Set a response variable and predictors.

```
response <- "dalys_rabies"
```

```
predictors <- setdiff(names(rabies), response)
```

```
# Split data into training and testing sets
splits <- h2o.splitFrame(h2o_rabies,
                         ratios = 0.8,
                         seed = 1234)
train <- splits[[1]]
test <- splits[[2]]
```

Train three models:

- a linear regression model (family = "gaussian" or standard ordinary least squares (OLS) linear regression)
- a GBM model (Gradient Boosting Machine)
- a random forest model

```
model_lm <- h2o.glm(x = predictors,
                    y = response,
                    training_frame = train,
                    family = "gaussian")
model_gbm <- h2o.gbm(x = predictors,
                     y = response,
                     training_frame = train,
                     validation_frame = test,
                     ntrees = 1000,
                     max_depth = 6,
                     learn_rate = 0.01,
                     seed = 1234)
model_rf <- h2o.randomForest(x = predictors,
                             y = response,
                             training_frame = train,
                             ntrees = 100,
                             max_depth = 20,
                             seed = 1234)
```

Evaluate the models with the h2o.performance() function to evaluate the performance of the models by calculating the metrics.

```
perf_lm <- h2o.performance(model_lm, newdata = test)
perf_gbm <- h2o.performance(model_gbm, newdata = test)
perf_rf <- h2o.performance(model_rf, newdata = test)
```

Then extract the RMSE and MAE metrics:

```
h2o.rmse(<model>)
```

```
h2o.mae(<model>)
```

```
#>   model     rmse       mae
#> 1    lm 2.732294 2.2957256
#> 2   gbm 1.373425 0.9379672
#> 3    rf 1.399058 1.1779029
```

The best model is the one with the lowest RMSE and MAE values. In this case, the `gbm` model is the best performing model among the three.

To predict on the test data, we use the `gbm` model in the `h2o.predict()` function:

```
# Predict on test data
predictions <- h2o.predict(model_gbm,
                           newdata = test)
```

Convert the predictions and actual values to data frames for plotting:

```
pred_df <- as.data.frame(predictions)
actual_df <- as.data.frame(test)
```

```
# Combine actual and predicted values
results_df <- data.frame(Actual = actual_df[, response],
                         Predicted = pred_df[, 1])
```

The check for normality of the residuals is done with the `qqnorm()` and `qqline()` functions. The residuals are calculated as the difference between the actual and predicted values.

```
# Calculate residuals
results_df$Residuals <- results_df$Actual - results_df$Predicted
# Plot Residuals vs Predicted
ggplot(results_df,
       aes(x = Predicted, y = Residuals)) +
  geom_point(color = "navy", alpha = 0.5) +
  geom_hline(yintercept = 0,
             color = "orange", linetype = "dashed") +
  labs(title = "Residuals vs Predicted Values",
       x = "Predicted", y = "Residuals")
# Normality Test of the Residuals
qqnorm(results_df$Residuals)
qqline(results_df$Residuals, col = 2)
```

```
# Adding time to the results data frame
results_df$Time <- actual_df$year
```

```
# Plot Actual vs Predicted
p1 <- ggplot(results_df,
             aes(x = Actual, y = Predicted)) +
  geom_point(color = "blue", alpha = 0.5) +
  geom_abline(slope = 1, intercept = 0,
              color = "red", linetype = "dashed") +
  labs(title = "Actual vs Predicted Values",
       x = "Actual", y = "Predicted")
# Plot Actual vs Predicted over time
p2 <- ggplot(results_df, aes(x = Time)) +
```

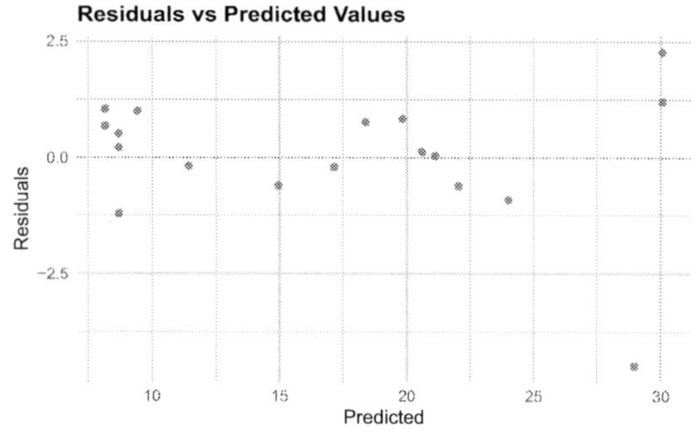

(a) Residuals vs Predicted Values

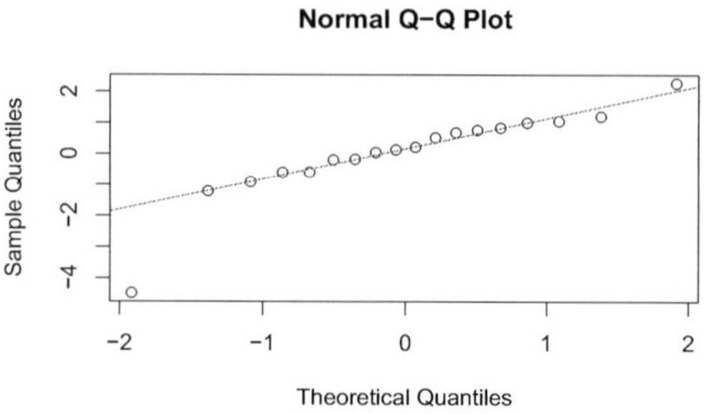

(b) Normality Test of the Residulas

Figure 8.5 H2O - GBM Model Results on DALYs due to Rabies; Residuals Distribution and Normality Test

```
  geom_line(aes(y = Actual,
                color = "Actual"),
            linetype = 1) +
  geom_line(aes(y = Predicted,
                color = "Predicted"),
            linewidth = 1,
            linetype = "dashed") +
  labs(title = "Actual vs Predicted Values Over Time",
       x = "Time", y = "Value") +
  scale_color_manual(name = "Legend",
                     values = c("Actual" = "navy",
                                "Predicted" = "orange"))
```

In conclusion, the H2O GBM model performed well on the rabies dataset, with a low RMSE and MAE. The residuals were normally distributed, indicating that the model's predictions were accurate. The actual vs predicted values plot shows a good fit, and the time series plot indicates that the model captured the trend in the data.

```
h2o.shutdown(prompt = FALSE)
```

8.3.3 Example: General Infection with Keras

The following example shows how to use the `{keras}`, a package that facilitates the creation and training of **neural networks** and **deep learning** models. It provides a user-friendly interface to build models, whether they are simple neural networks or complex deep learning architectures, particularly useful for handling network connections. More detailed explanation of how a neural network works can be found in

In this case the **SEIR** model (susceptible, exposed, infected and recovered) is used, as seen in Chapter 6 chapter, to simulate the spread of a general infection in a population of 1000 individuals over 160 days. For some types of infections, the latency period is significant as it is the time during which infected individuals are not yet infectious themselves. During this period the individual is in compartment E (for exposed).

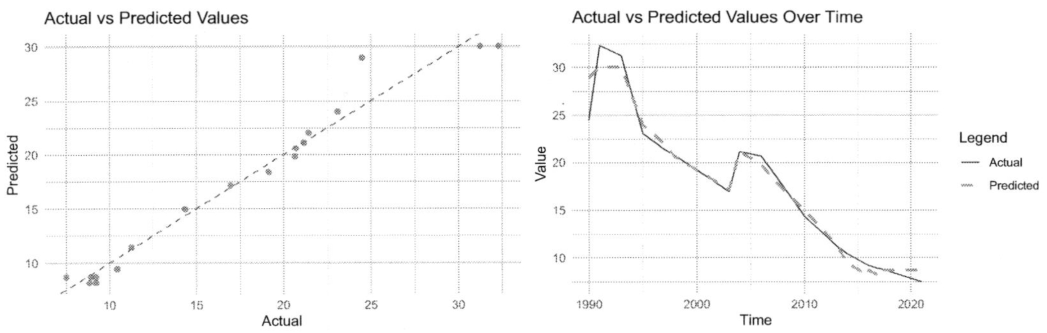

(a) Actual vs Predicted Values **(b)** Actual vs Predicted Over Time

Figure 8.6 H2O - GBM Model Results on DALYs due to Rabies

Once the simulation of the infected population is done, the **deep learning** model acts by training social media data to predict the probability of infection based on social media activity. The model results are then used to adjust the SEIR parameters based on the predicted infection status and re-run again on new data.

```
install.packages("keras3")
keras3::install_keras(backend = "tensorflow")
```

```
library(keras3)
library(deSolve)
library(ggplot2)
```

To setup the SEIR compartments we start by defining the differential equations built by considering the rates of change of each compartment (S, E, I, R), the parameters (β, σ, γ), the initial state value of the population $(N = 1000)$, and the length of time in days $(t = 160)$. Finally the `ode()` function is used to solve the differential equations and provide the output dataset.

```
SEIR <- function(time, state, parameters) {
  with(as.list(c(state, parameters)), {
    # Differential equations
    dS <- -beta * S * I / N
    dE <- beta * S * I / N - sigma * E
    dI <- sigma * E - gamma * I
    dR <- gamma * I
    # Return the rates of change
    list(c(dS, dE, dI, dR))
  })
}
# Parameters
parameters <- c(beta = 0.3, # Infection rate
                sigma = 0.2, # Incubation rate
                gamma = 0.1 # Recovery rate
                )
# Initial state values
N <- 1000
initial_state <- c(S = 999, E = 1, I = 0, R = 0)
```

```
# Time points
times <- seq(0, 160, by = 1)
# Solve the model
output <- ode(y = initial_state,
              times = times,
              func = SEIR,
              parms = parameters
              )
# Convert output to a data frame
output <- as.data.frame(output)
```

The social media data is simulated and consists of 1000 individuals (n) over 10 (p) days, with an infection vector, and 10 features (x_i), including social distancing adherence, mask usage (always, sometimes, never), hand hygiene frequency (times per day washing or sanitizing), work or study environment (remote versus in-person), participation in gatherings (number of gatherings attended recently), and contact tracing status (exposure to a confirmed case), among others. All values are standardized obtained from a normal distribution.

```
set.seed(123)
n <- 1000 # number of samples
p <- 10 # number of features
# Generate random features and labels
social_features <- matrix(rnorm(n * p),
                          nrow = n, ncol = p)
infection_labels <- sample(0:1, n, replace = TRUE)
# Combine into a data frame
social_data <- data.frame(social_features)
social_data$infection <- infection_labels

social_data[1:4,c(1:3,11)]
#>            X1          X2         X3 infection
#> 1 -0.56047565 -0.99579872 -0.5116037         0
#> 2 -0.23017749 -1.03995504  0.2369379         0
#> 3  1.55870831 -0.01798024 -0.5415892         0
#> 4  0.07050839 -0.13217513  1.2192276         1
```

Define the model by using the `keras_model_sequential()` function, and add layers with the `layer_dense()` and `layer_activation()` functions. On each layer the model will apply a transformation to the input data, and the activation function will introduce non-linearity to the model.

Here we use a simple model with just two layers and a **ReLU** and a **Sigmoid** as activation functions. These functions have specific shapes that allow the model to learn complex patterns in the data. Any time one layer is done the output is passed to the next layer.

Although the `layer_dropout()` is not actually used in this application, it could be added to the model as a layer that drops out output results under specified requirements. The function is used to prevent overfitting by randomly setting a fraction of input units to zero during training.

The model concludes with one more `layer_dense()` with `activation` used to finally activate the output with a tailored function. In this case a **sigmoid**, but also a **softmax** function could be used.

The decision of which activation function to use depends on the task type (classification or regression), or due to performance considerations, such as the ReLU is computationally simple and efficient. The **sigmoid** function is used in binary classification problems, where the output is a probability between 0 and 1. The **softmax** function is used in multi-class classification problems, where the output is a probability distribution over multiple classes. Sometimes, you try a few and see which works best through cross-validation or tuning.

Given an input vector $x = [x_1, x_2, ..., x_p]$ of size p, the model is composed of:

1. **First Dense Layer Transformation**:

$$z^{(1)} = \sum_{i=1}^{p} W_i^{(1)} x_i + b^{(1)} \tag{8.1}$$

where $W \epsilon R^{1 \times p}$ are the weights, b is the bias, and z is the output.

2. **First Activation (ReLU)**:

$$a^{(1)} = ReLu(z^{(1)}) = max(0, z^{(1)}) \tag{8.2}$$

3. **Second Dense Layer Transformation**:

$$z^{(2)} = \sum_{i=1}^{p} W_i^{(2)} x_i + b^{(2)} \tag{8.3}$$

4. **Output Activation (Sigmoid)**:

$$a^{(2)} = Sigmoid(z^{(2)}) = \frac{1}{1 + e^{-z^{(2)}}} \tag{8.4}$$

```
model <- keras_model_sequential(input_shape = c(p))
# simple model
model %>%
  layer_dense(units = 1) %>%
  layer_activation("relu") %>%
  layer_dense(units = 1, activation = "sigmoid")
```

The model is then compiled using the `compile()` function which with the use of a **loss function** optimises the results matching them against a minimum required value, and specified metrics to reduce the error.

$$y = \hat{y} + \epsilon \tag{8.5}$$

where y is the true value, $\hat{y}$ is the predicted value, and ϵ is the error.

The loss function is used to measure how well the model is performing, in this case a **binary crossentropy** loss function is used, to match the difference between original data and the model output, and apply model adjustments in case the difference is too high. The formula for binary crossentropy is:

$$L(y, \hat{y}) = -\frac{1}{n} \sum_{i=1}^{n} y_i \log(\hat{y}_i) + (1 - y_i) \log(1 - \hat{y}_i) \tag{8.6}$$

where L is the loss, y is the true value, $\hat{y}$ is the predicted value, and n is the number of samples.

The `optimizer_adam()` function, used to update the model's weights during training, in **Keras** specifies the use of the **Adaptive Moment Estimation (Adam)** optimization algorithm for training a neural network. It updates the parameters of the neural network.

Then finally, the model is evaluated on performance with the **accuracy** metric.

```
# Compile the model
model %>% compile(loss = "binary_crossentropy",
                  optimizer = optimizer_adam(),
                  metrics = c("accuracy"))
```

Once the model is defined and compiled, the model is then trained using the `fit()` function with the training data, number of **epochs**, **batch size**, and **validation** split specified. The number of epochs is the number of times the model will go through the training data, the batch size is the number of samples used in each training step, and the validation split is the fraction of the training data that will be used for validation.

A particular object that is created in this type of models is the `history` object, which is used to store the training history of the model. This object contains information about the loss and accuracy of the model on the training and validation data during training.

```
history <- model %>% fit(x = as.matrix(social_data[, 1:p]),
                         y = social_data$infection,
                         epochs = 30,
                         batch_size = 128,
                         validation_split = 0.2
                         )
```

The subsequent times the `history` object is created, the model is trained with half the number of epochs and batch size. And this specifications can further be adjusted as needed.

```
history2 <- model %>% fit(x = as.matrix(social_data[, 1:p]),
                          y = social_data$infection,
                          epochs = 30 / 2,
                          batch_size = 128 / 2,
                          validation_split = 0.2
                          )
```

Here are two attempts of the trained model with different parameters, the first with 30 epochs and a batch size of 128, and the second with 15 epochs and a batch size of 64. The training history of both models is then plotted to compare their performance.

The model is then used to predict the probability of infection based on the social media data. The predictions are then converted to binary values using a threshold of 0.5, where values greater than 0.5 are classified as 1 (infected) and values less than or equal to 0.5 are classified as 0 (not infected).

```
new_social_data <- matrix(rnorm(p * 160),
                          nrow = 160, ncol = p)
```

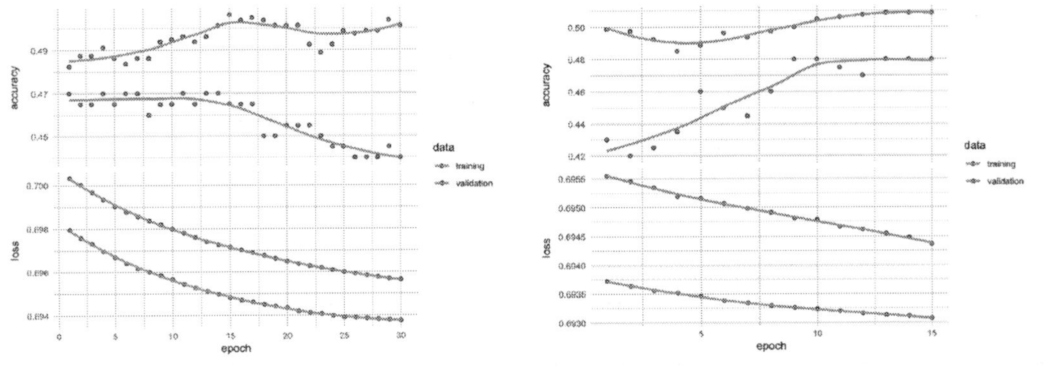

(a) Model 1 History

(b) Model 2 History

Figure 8.7 Model 1 and Model 2 Training History

```
predicted_infections <- model %>%
  predict(new_social_data)
predicted_infections <- ifelse(predicted_infections > 0.5, 1, 0)
```

The adjustment is then done on the SEIR parameters based on predicted results. The beta parameter is adjusted by multiplying it by the mean of the predicted infections.

```
adjusted_parameters <- parameters
adjusted_parameters["beta"] <-
  adjusted_parameters["beta"] * (1 + mean(predicted_infections))
```

The SEIR model is then re-run with the adjusted parameters to simulate the spread of the infection in the population.

```
adjusted_output <- ode(y = initial_state,
                       times = times,
                       func = SEIR,
                       parms = adjusted_parameters
                       )
# Convert output to a data frame
adjusted_output <- as.data.frame(adjusted_output)
```

The output shows the impact of the social media adjustments on the spread of the infection.

```
ggplot() +
  geom_line(data = output,
            aes(x = time, y = I,
                color = "Original Infections")) +
  geom_line(data = adjusted_output,
            aes(x = time, y = I,
                color = "Adjusted Infections")) +
  labs(title = "SEIR Model - Social Media Adjustments",
       y = "Infectious Population",
       color = "Scenario") +
```

```
  scale_color_manual(values = c(
    "Original Infections" = "navy",
    "Adjusted Infections" = "orange"))
```

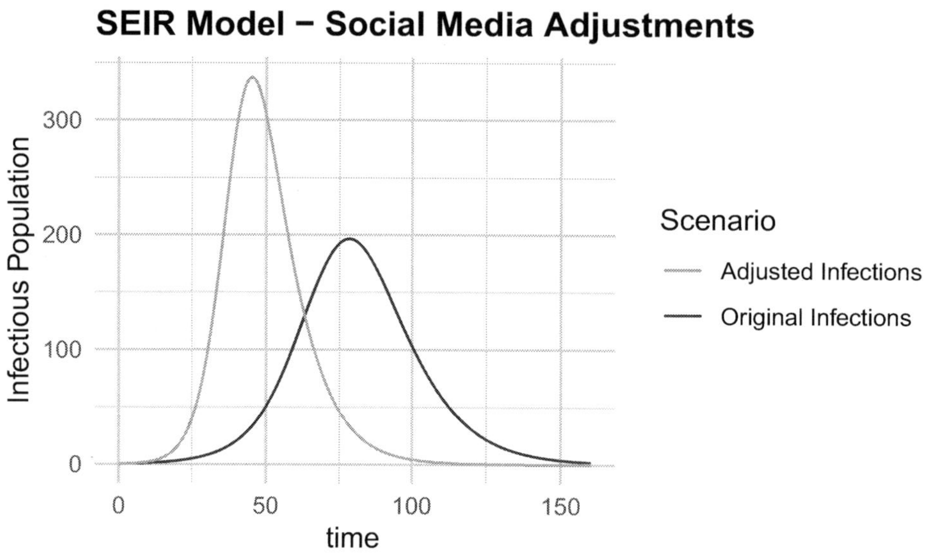

Figure 8.8 SEIR Model with and without Social Media Adjustments

This is just a simple example of how the `{keras}` package can be used to train a deep learning model on social media data to predict the probability of infection. The model can be tested on using different layers, more specifications are found in the keras documentation.

8.4 How to Find a New R-Package

Finding a new R-package can be a daunting task, given the vast number of packages available on CRAN and other repositories. A strategy to identify relevant packages for your specific needs would be to use some prebuilt packages which provide search functionalities.

For example, the `package_search()` function from the `{pkgsearch}` package takes a text string as input and uses basic text mining techniques to search all of CRAN.

```
library(tidyverse) # for data manipulation
library(dlstats) # for package download stats
library(pkgsearch) # for searching packages
```

We search for packages related to *"excess of mortality"* and "infectious diseases":

```
excessPkg <- pkg_search(query = "excess of mortality", size = 200)
```

```
head(excessPkg$maintainer_name)
#> [1] "Rafael A. Irizarry" "Mathieu Fauvernier" "Juste Goungounga"
#> [4] "Yohann Foucher"     "Joonas Miettinen"   "Rob Hyndman"
```

```
excessPkgShort <- excessPkg %>%
  filter(maintainer_name != "ORPHANED", score > 100) %>%
  select(score, package, downloads_last_month) %>%
  arrange(desc(downloads_last_month))

head(excessPkgShort)
#> # A data frame: 5 x 3
#>   score package     downloads_last_month
#> * <dbl> <chr>                      <int>
#> 1  183. popEpi                      1867
#> 2  682. survPen                     1172
#> 3  274. RISCA                        483
#> 4 1009. excessmort                   317
#> 5  673. xhaz                         180
```

```
excess_shortList <- excessPkgShort$package
```

```
excess_downloads <- cran_stats(excess_shortList)
```

```
ggplot(excess_downloads, aes(end, downloads,
                             group = package,
                             color = package)) +
  geom_line() +
  geom_point(aes(shape = package)) +
  scale_y_continuous(trans = "log2")
```

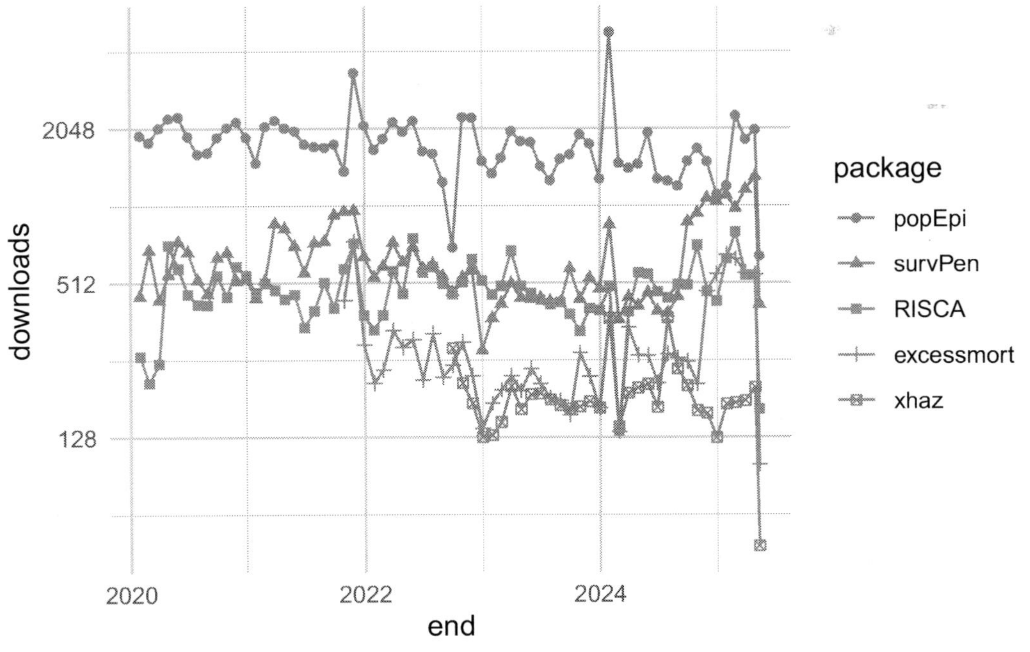

Figure 8.9 Excess of Mortality Packages Downloads

Another example is the {cranly} package, which provides a simple interface to search for packages on CRAN. The package provides comprehensive methods for cleaning up and organising the information in the CRAN package database, making it easier to find relevant packages for your specific needs.

```
library(cranly)
p_db <- tools::CRAN_package_db()
package_db <- clean_CRAN_db(p_db)
```

```
package_db %>%
  filter(grepl("infectious diseases",
               description,
               ignore.case = TRUE)) %>%
  select(package)
#>         package
#> 1  EpiDynamics
#> 2    epitweetr
#> 3        pempi
#> 4         rts2
#> 5    seqDesign
#> 6 SMITIDstruct
#> 7       spaero
#> 8         ssrn
```

9

Predictive Modelling and Beyond

Learning Objectives

- Use model predictions to make informed decisions on new or unseen data
- Apply time series analysis to forecast the Socio-Demographic Index (SDI)
- Estimate Years Lived with Disability (YLDs) using mixed-effects models

In the dynamic landscape of public health, the ability to forecast and predict future trends is essential for effective decision-making and the implementation of timely interventions. This chapter provides an overview of **predictive modelling**, focusing on the challenges of applying predictions to new data, the use of **time series analysis**, and **mixed models** to anticipate the trajectory of infectious diseases and health metrics. By exploring the underlying patterns and analysing historical data, we estimate the disease burden and evaluate the impact of interventions on population health. We demonstrate how time series analysis and mixed models can be tailored to address specific research questions, such as predicting disease outbreaks, estimating disease burden, and assessing the impact of interventions on population health.

9.1 Predictions About the Future

The previous chapters provided an attempt at estimating future outcomes based on the application of various type of statistical and machine learning techniques. Here we look at how to use these predictions on new data.

When making predictions on new data, it is important to consider the **generalisability** of the model. A model that performs well on the training data may not necessarily generalise well to new, unseen data. To evaluate the performance of the model we used the **cross-validation** technique, but there are more such as **hold-out validation**, **k-fold cross-validation**, **leave-one-out cross-validation**, and **bootstrapping**. These methods help assess the model's ability to make accurate predictions on data not used during training, providing a more reliable estimate of the model's performance in real-world scenarios.

Once the model has been trained and evaluated, it is used to make predictions on new data. This process involves applying the model to the new data to generate forecasts or estimates of the outcome of interest. For example, in the case of infectious diseases, predictive models can be used to forecast the trajectory of an outbreak, estimate the number of cases, or evaluate the impact of interventions on disease transmission. By leveraging historical data and the insights gained from the model, we can effectively evaluate the model performance and make informed decisions based on the predictions.

DOI: 10.1201/9781032625935-9

9.2 Example: Dengue Test Predictions for 2017-2021

Predictive modelling is a powerful tool for forecasting future trends. Here we test the Dengue's model made with `{mlr3}` meta-package in Chapter 8. The model was trained on data from 1990 to 2016 and now tested for years 2017 to 2021.

First we load the original data and name it `old_data`.

```
library(tidyverse)
library(data.table)
```

```
old_data <- hmsidwR::infectious_diseases %>%
  arrange(year)%>%
  filter(cause_name == "Dengue",
         year<=2017,
         !location_name %in% c("Eswatini", "Lesotho")) %>%
  drop_na() %>%
  group_by(location_id) %>%
  select(-location_name, -cause_name)
```

Then, we load Dengue data from 2017 to 2021 and name it `new_data`.

```
new_data <- hmsidwR::infectious_diseases %>%
  arrange(year)%>%
  filter(cause_name == "Dengue",
         year>=2017,
         !location_name %in% c("Eswatini", "Lesotho")) %>%
  drop_na() %>%
  group_by(location_id) %>%
  select(-location_name, -cause_name)
```

In the next step, we use the trained models from Chapter 8 to make predictions on the new data. The predictions are stored in `new_pred_regr.cv_glmnet` and `new_pred_regr.xgboost`. The resampling results: `rr1$learners` and `rr2$learners`, contain the trained models, in particular the first of 5 folds cross validation sample is used for the predictions.

```
new_pred_regr.cv_glmnet <-
  rr1$learners[[1]]$predict_newdata(new_data,
                                    task = rr1$task)
```

This object contains the predictions for the new data, and we can access the response data by:

```
new_pred_regr.cv_glmnet$`data`$response
```

With the support of `data.table::as.data.table()` we can see the data, and create a new column `ape` to evaluate the `Absolute Percentage Error (APE)`. Here are shown the first 6 rows of the data:

```
data.table::as.data.table(new_pred_regr.cv_glmnet) %>%
  mutate(ape = round(abs(truth - response)/truth,3)*100) %>%
  head()
```

```
#>     row_ids      truth  response    ape
#>       <int>      <num>     <num>  <num>
#> 1:        1 3.3219788 3.2615171    1.8
#> 2:        2 2.2361377 2.2855594    2.2
#> 3:        3 0.5021275 0.6403621   27.5
#> 4:        4 3.2737870 3.2193092    1.7
#> 5:        5 0.4893329 0.6327542   29.3
#> 6:        6 2.3045710 2.3715899    2.9
```

And calculate some metrics to evaluate the model performance on new data. We calculate the **Mean Absolute Percent Error (MAPE)**, the **Mean Squared Error (MSE)**, and the **Root Mean Squared Error (RMSE)**. The MAPE is a measure of prediction accuracy, while the MSE and RMSE are measures of the average squared difference between predicted and actual values.

```
data.table::as.data.table(new_pred_regr.cv_glmnet) %>%
  mutate(ape = round(abs(truth - response)/truth,3)*100) %>%
  summarise(mape = mean(ape),
            mse =  mean((truth - response)^2),
            rmse = sqrt(mean((truth - response)^2))) %>%
  round(3)
#>     mape  mse  rmse
#> 1 11.413 0.01 0.098
```

The model performs fairly well, with relatively low error:

- An average relative error of ~11% is typically considered acceptable in many forecasting or prediction tasks.
- The small RMSE (0.098) and MSE (0.01) suggest that large errors are rare or small.

Much more can be done to improve the models, such as **hyperparameter tuning**, **feature engineering**, and **model ensembles**, but this is a good point to start. We could also look at the confidence intervals of the predictions, to see how certain we are about the predictions, and so on.

This is the result of the `cv_glmnet` application on new data:

```
regr.cv_glmnet_new <- as.data.table(new_pred_regr.cv_glmnet) %>%
  mutate(learner = "regr.cv_glmnet") %>%
  cbind(new_data)

regr.cv_glmnet_new %>%
  ggplot(aes(x = year)) +
  geom_line(data = old_data, aes(y = DALYs))+
  geom_line(aes(y = DALYs), color = "brown") +
  geom_line(aes(y = response), linetype = "dashed") +
  facet_wrap(vars(location_id),
             labeller = as_labeller(c(`182` = "Malawi",
                                      `191` = "Zambia",
                                      `169` = "Central African Republic")),
             scales = "free_y") +
  labs(title = "Dengue Predictions for 2017-2021: cv_glmnet",
       x = "Time (Year)")
```

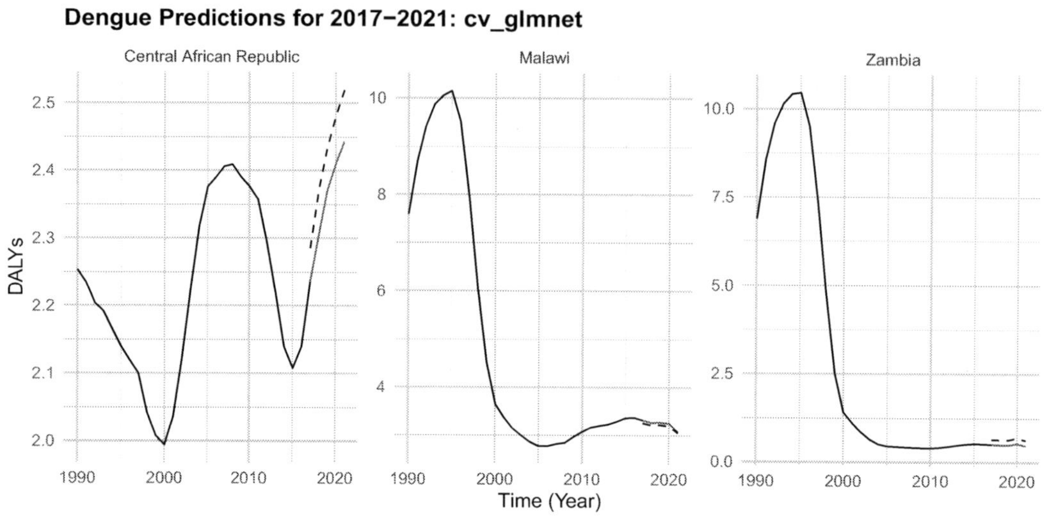

Figure 9.1 Dengue Predictions for 2017-2021: cv_glmnet. The solid line shows the historical data, the brown line shows the new data, and the dashed line the predictions.

The same steps are taken for the `xgboost`, and the results are shown below to compare the two models.

```
new_pred_regr.xgboost <-
  rr2$learners[[1]]$predict_newdata(new_data,
                                    task = rr2$task)
```

```
regr.xgboost_new <- as.data.table(new_pred_regr.xgboost) %>%
  mutate(learner = "regr.xgboost") %>%
  cbind(new_data)
```

```
rbind(regr.cv_glmnet_new,
      regr.xgboost_new) %>%
  mutate(ape = round(abs(truth - response)/truth, 3)*100) %>%
  group_by(learner) %>%
  summarise(mape = mean(ape),
            mse =  mean((truth - response)^2),
            rmse = sqrt(mean((truth - response)^2)))
#> # A tibble: 2 x 4
#>   learner         mape     mse   rmse
#>   <chr>          <dbl>   <dbl>  <dbl>
#> 1 regr.cv_glmnet  11.4 0.00963 0.0981
#> 2 regr.xgboost    20.1 0.0567  0.238
```

The `glmnet` performs better than `xgboost`. The xgboost model may be overfitting or it is just poorly tuned, given its higher error despite being a more complex model.

```
regr.xgboost_new %>%
  ggplot(aes(x = year)) +
  geom_line(data = old_data, aes(y = DALYs))+
```

```
geom_line(aes(y = DALYs), color = "brown") +
geom_line(aes(y = response), linetype = "dashed") +
facet_wrap(vars(location_id),
           labeller = as_labeller(c(`182` = "Malawi",
                                    `191` = "Zambia",
                                    `169` = "Central African Republic")),
           scales = "free_y") +
labs(title = "Dengue Predictions for 2017-2021: xgboost")
```

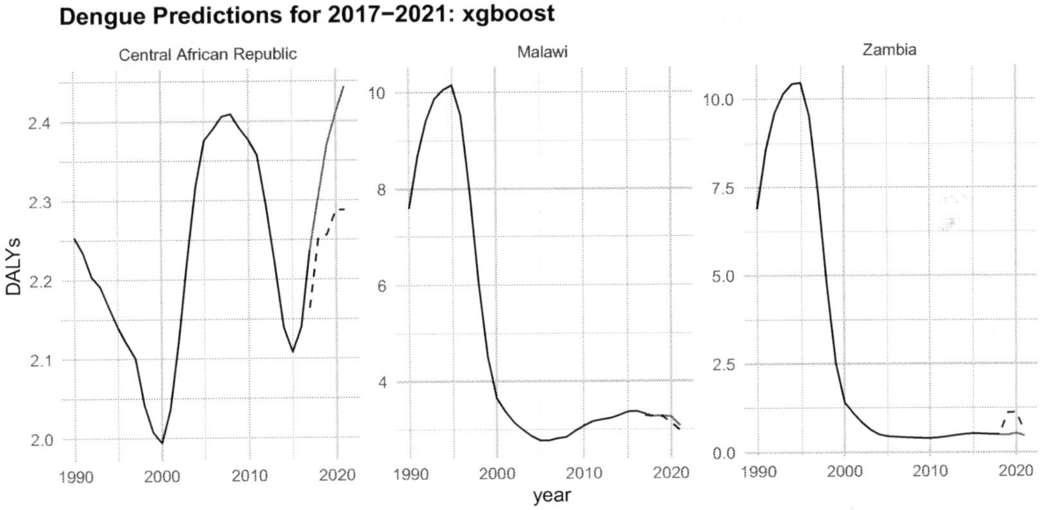

Figure 9.2 Dengue Predictions for 2017-2021: xgboost. The solid line shows the historical data, the brown line shows the new data, and the dashed line the predictions.

In conclusion, predictive modelling is a valuable tool for forecasting future trends and making informed decisions based on historical data. By leveraging the insights gained from the models, we can anticipate the trajectory of infectious diseases, estimate disease burden, and evaluate the impact of interventions on population health. The models can be further refined and optimised to improve their predictive performance and provide more accurate forecasts.

By combining predictive modelling with time series analysis and mixed models, we can gain a comprehensive understanding of the complex dynamics of public health and make data-driven decisions to improve population health outcomes.

9.3 Time Series Analysis

One important side of the analysis is to consider the evolution of the phenomenon in time. We can do this by using `time` as a factor in the model. **Time series** analysis serves as a tool for understanding and forecasting temporal patterns. Techniques such as **AutoRegressive**

Integrated Moving Average (ARIMA) models offer a systematic approach to modelling time-dependent data, capturing seasonal variations, trends, and irregularities to generate accurate forecasts.

Mixed models, on the other side, provide a versatile framework for incorporating various sources of variability and correlation within the data. Also known as **hierarchical models**, **multilevel models**, or **random effects models**, are a type of statistical model that include both fixed effects and random effects. By combining fixed effects with random effects, mixed models accommodate complex data structures, such as hierarchical or longitudinal data, while accounting for individual-level and group-level factors that may influence the outcome of interest.

To analyse temporal data, where observations are collected at regular intervals over time, time series analysis allows for studying the patterns, trends, and dependencies present in the data to make forecasts or infer relationships. Time series data often exhibit inherent characteristics such as trend, seasonality, cyclic patterns, and irregular fluctuations, which can be explored using various methods such as **decomposition**, **smoothing**, and **modelling**. This analysis is widely used in fields like economics, finance, epidemiology, and environmental science to understand and predict future trends, identify anomalies, and make informed decisions based on historical patterns.

Decomposition methods play a crucial role by pulling out the underlying structure of temporal data. The components of a time series are `trend`, `seasonality`, and `random fluctuations`. Understanding the trend allows for the identification of long-term changes or shifts in the data, while detecting seasonal patterns helps uncover recurring fluctuations that may follow seasonal or cyclical patterns.

By separating these components, through decomposition methods, it is possible to discover the temporal dynamics within the data, facilitating more accurate forecasting and predictive modelling. Moreover, decomposing time series data can aid in anomaly detection, trend analysis, and seasonal adjustment, making it a fundamental tool for interpreting complex temporal phenomena.

Modelling time series data often requires a combination of techniques to capture its complex nature. **Mixed models**, **Splines**, and **ARIMA** are powerful tools commonly used for this purpose. Splines provide a flexible way to capture nonlinear relationships and smooth out the data, which is particularly useful for capturing trends or seasonal patterns. ARIMA models, on the other hand, are best at capturing the autocorrelation structure present in the data, including both short-term and long-term dependencies.

Time series analysis can also be performed on estimated values produced by a machine learning model. This involves using vectors of estimates, actual values (ground truth), and time (such as years). By incorporating these elements, the time series analysis can help identify trends, seasonal patterns, and other temporal structures within the data. This approach enhances the robustness and accuracy of the predictions by combining the strengths of machine learning models with traditional time series techniques.

9.4 Example: SDI Time Series Analysis

In this example, we provide a brief overview of the **Socio-Demographic Index (SDI)**, its components, and how it can be predicted using time series analysis. From projecting the spread of emerging pathogens to assessing the long-term effects of public health policies, predictive modelling offers valuable insights into the future of global health. As discussed in Chapter 5, incorporating indicators such as the **SDI** can offer a more comprehensive understanding of how social and economic determinants influence health outcomes.

The SDI is a **composite index** developed by the Global Burden of Disease (GBD) Study to capture a country's level of socio-demographic development, that combines various social and demographic factors to provide a comprehensive measure of a population's health and well-being.

It is based on three components:

1. Total fertility rate (TFR) among women under age 25 (TFU25)
2. Average educational attainment in the population over age 15 (EDU15+)
3. Income per capita (lag-distributed)

It ranges from 0 to 1 but it is usually multiplied by 100 for a scale of 0 to 100.

Standard Calculation of SDI

The SDI is calculated as the geometric mean of these three components:

$$SDI = \sqrt[3]{TFU25 \times EDU15 + \times LDI} \tag{9.1}$$

Each component TFU25, EDU15+, and LDI is normalised before taking the geometric mean to ensure they are on a comparable scale.

In particular, **Total Fertility Rate (TFR)** defined as the average number of children a woman would have over her lifetime given current age-specific fertility rates—is a key demographic indicator with broad implications for national well-being.

Standard Calculation of TFR

$$\text{TFR} = \sum(\text{ASFR}_i \times 5) \tag{9.2}$$

where ASFR_i represents the age-specific fertility rates for age group i , and the sum is typically calculated over all childbearing age groups (often 5-year intervals from ages 15-49).

The TFR formula is specific to calculating fertility rates, while the SDI formula incorporates a specific **subset of the TFR (TFU25)** along with education and income metrics to create a broader socio-demographic index.

In general, the level of this index helps identify key drivers in the development of health outcomes. SDI can be used as a predictor in predictive models to estimate the burden of diseases, mortality rates, and other health metrics.

For example, the relationship between SDI and the incidence of a disease can be modelled using a logistic regression model:

$$\log\left(\frac{p}{1-p}\right) = \beta_0 + \beta_1 \times \text{SDI} + \beta_2 \times X_2 + \cdots + \beta_k \times X_k \tag{9.3}$$

Where, p is the probability of the incidence of the disease, $\log\left(\frac{p}{1-p}\right)$ is the log-odds (logit) of the disease incidence, β_0 is the intercept term, $\beta_1, \beta_2, \ldots, \beta_k$ are the coefficients for the predictor variables, and $X_2, \ldots, X_k$ are other potential predictor variables that might influence the disease incidence.

To convert the `log-odds` back to the **probability of disease incidence** given the value of SDI:

$$p = \frac{1}{1 + e^{-(\beta_0 + \beta_1 \times \text{SDI})}} \tag{9.4}$$

9.4.1 SDI Data and Packages

In this example we use the SDI values from 1990 to 2019, for 3 locations plus the Global region and evaluate the difference in SDI average across the time.

We start by loading the data and required libraries. We use the `{hmsidwR}` package, which contains the SDI data from 1990 to 2019, the data is available in the `sdi90_19` object, and the `{fpp3}`[1] package for time series analysis mentioned in Section 8.2.3. We also show how to use the `|>` native pipe operator to filter and manipulate the data, instead of the `%>%` pipe operator from the `{dplyr}` package.

```
library(tidyverse)
library(hmsidwR)
library(fpp3)
```

```
hmsidwR::sdi90_19 |> head()
#> # A tibble: 6 x 3
#>   location  year value
#>   <chr>    <dbl> <dbl>
#> 1 Global    1990 0.511
#> 2 Global    1991 0.516
#> 3 Global    1992 0.521
#> 4 Global    1993 0.525
#> 5 Global    1994 0.529
#> 6 Global    1995 0.534
```

```
sdi90_19 |>
  filter(location %in% c("Global", "Italy",
                         "France", "Germany")) |>
  ggplot(aes(x = year, y = value,
             linetype = location)) +
  geomtextpath::geom_textline(aes(label = location),
                              hjust = 0, vjust = 0) +
  labs(title = "Social Demographic Index (SDI) from 1990 to 2019")+
  theme(legend.position = "none")
```

[1] *Forecasting*.

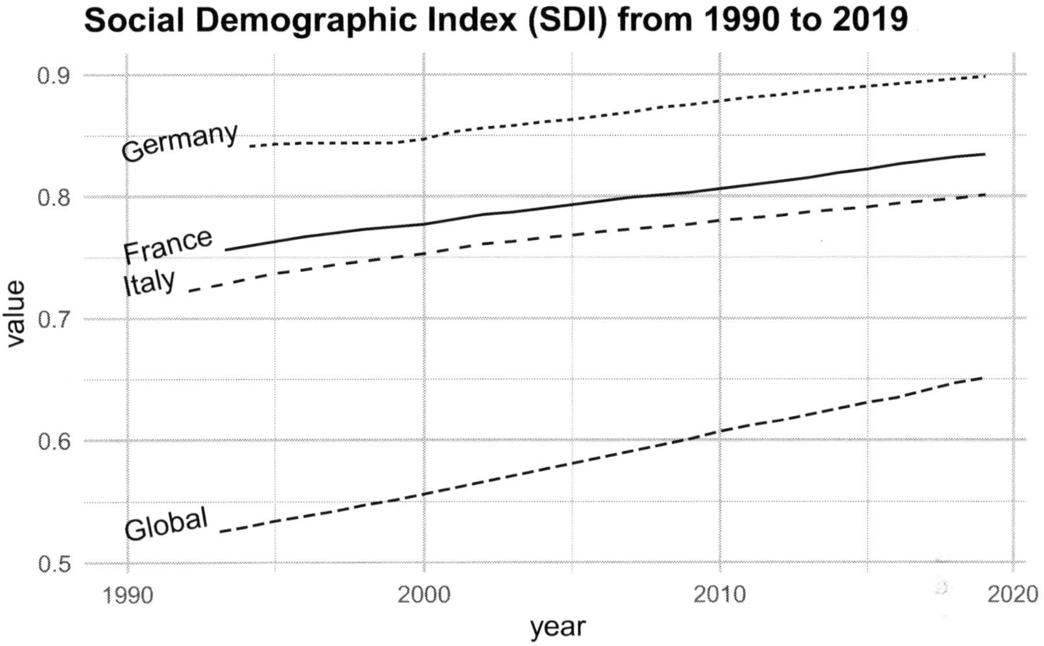

Figure 9.3 Social Demographic Index (SDI) from 1990 to 2019

Grouping the data by location and calculating the average SDI, we can note that the highest average value is found in Germany, followed by France, Italy, and the Global average.

```
sdi90_19 |>
  group_by(location) |>
  reframe(avg = round(mean(value), 3)) |>
  arrange(desc(avg)) |>
  filter(location %in% c("Global", "Italy", "France", "Germany"))
#> # A tibble: 4 x 2
#>   location   avg
#>   <chr>    <dbl>
#> 1 Germany  0.863
#> 2 France   0.79
#> 3 Italy    0.763
#> 4 Global   0.58
```

Focusing on France as the location of interest, we analyse the time series by decomposing the series into its components and evaluating the autocorrelation function to assess underlying temporal patterns, and apply an `ARIMA(1,0,0)` model.

```
sdi_fr <- sdi90_19 |>
  filter(location == "France")

sdi_fr |>
  head() |>
  str()
#> tibble [6 x 3] (S3: tbl_df/tbl/data.frame)
#>  $ location: chr [1:6] "France" "France" "France" "France" ...
```

```
#>  $ year    : num [1:6] 1990 1991 1992 1993 1994 ...
#>  $ value   : num [1:6] 0.738 0.743 0.75 0.755 0.759 0.763
```

The {fpp3} package is a meta-package and contains other packages such as: `tsibble`, `tsibbledata`, `feasts`, `fable`, and `fabletools`.

The {tsibble} package is used to set the data ready to be used inside the model. The `tsibble::as_tsibble()` function coerce our data to be a `tsibble` object:

```
library(tsibble)
sdi_fr_ts <- tsibble::as_tsibble(sdi_fr, index = year)
sdi_fr_ts |> head()
#> # A tsibble: 6 x 3 [1Y]
#>   location  year value
#>   <chr>    <dbl> <dbl>
#> 1 France    1990 0.738
#> 2 France    1991 0.743
#> 3 France    1992 0.75
#> 4 France    1993 0.755
#> 5 France    1994 0.759
#> 6 France    1995 0.763
```

```
sdi_fr_ts |> autoplot()
```

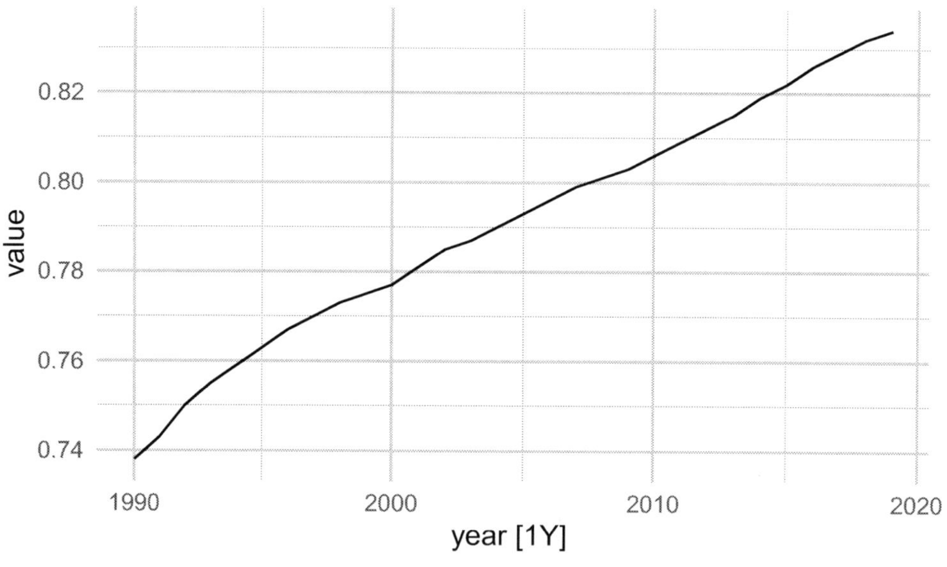

Figure 9.4 Social Demographic Index (SDI) in France

Then, the `fabletools::model()` function is used to train and estimate models. In this case we use the `STL()` (Multiple seasonal decomposition by Loess) function, which decomposes a time series into seasonal, trend and remainder components.

```
dcmp <- sdi_fr_ts |>
  model(stl = STL(value))
```

```
components(dcmp) |> head()
#> # A dable: 6 x 6 [1Y]
#> # Key:      .model [1]
#> # :         value = trend + remainder
#>   .model  year value trend remainder season_adjust
#>   <chr>  <dbl> <dbl> <dbl>     <dbl>         <dbl>
#> 1 stl     1990 0.738 0.738 -0.000400         0.738
#> 2 stl     1991 0.743 0.744 -0.000560         0.743
#> 3 stl     1992 0.75  0.749  0.00128          0.75
#> 4 stl     1993 0.755 0.754  0.00136          0.755
#> 5 stl     1994 0.759 0.758  0.000800         0.759
#> 6 stl     1995 0.763 0.762  0.000680         0.763
```

There are three main types of time series patterns: trend, seasonality, and cycles. When a time series is decomposed into components, the trend and cycle are typically combined into a single trend-cycle component, often referred to simply as the trend for the sake of simplicity. As a result, a time series can be understood as comprising three components: a trend-cycle component, a seasonal component, and a remainder component, which captures any other variations in the series.[2]

The components of a time series can be additive or multiplicative, depending on the nature of the data:

$$y_t = S_t + T_t + R_t \tag{9.5}$$

$$y_t = S_t * T_t * R_t \tag{9.6}$$

$$log(y_t) = log(S_t) + log(T_t) + log(R_t) \tag{9.7}$$

where:

- y_t is the observed value of the time series at time t,
- S_t represents the seasonal component, capturing regular fluctuations that repeat over fixed periods (e.g., annually or quarterly),
- T_t is the trend component, reflecting the long-term progression or direction in the data (such as gradual increases or declines),
- R_t denotes the remainder or residual component, accounting for short-term noise or random variation not explained by seasonality or trend.

The equation Equation 9.5 assumes that the components combine additively and are independent of one another, which is suitable when the seasonal variation remains relatively constant over time. The equation Equation 9.6 is used when seasonal or residual effects vary proportionally with the trend (e.g., higher variability during periods of higher values). Finally, The equation Equation 9.7 represents a log-transformed multiplicative model, which stabilizes variance and allows for additive decomposition in the logarithmic scale—often preferred when dealing with exponential growth or heteroscedasticity.

The `autoplot()` function is from the `{fabletools}` package and allows for the visualization of the components. In particular, the **remainder** component shown in the bottom panel is what is left over when the seasonal and trend-cycle components have been subtracted from the data.

[2] *Forecasting*.

```
components(dcmp) |> fabletools ::autoplot()

components(dcmp) |>
  as_tsibble() |>
  autoplot(value) +
  geom_line(aes(y = trend),
            linetype="dashed")+
labs(title = "Trend line of SDI in France")
```

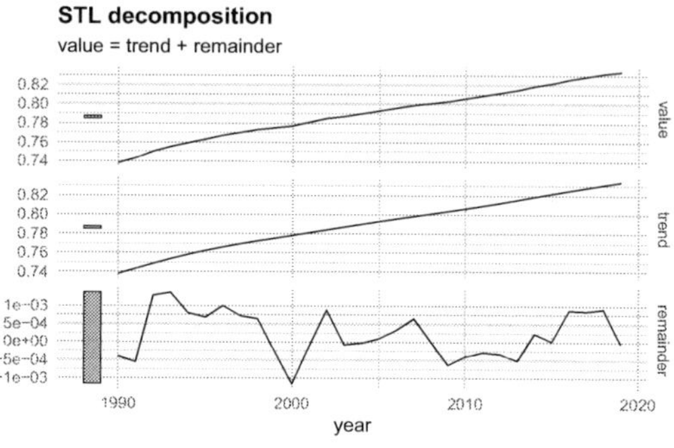

(a) Components of SDI in France

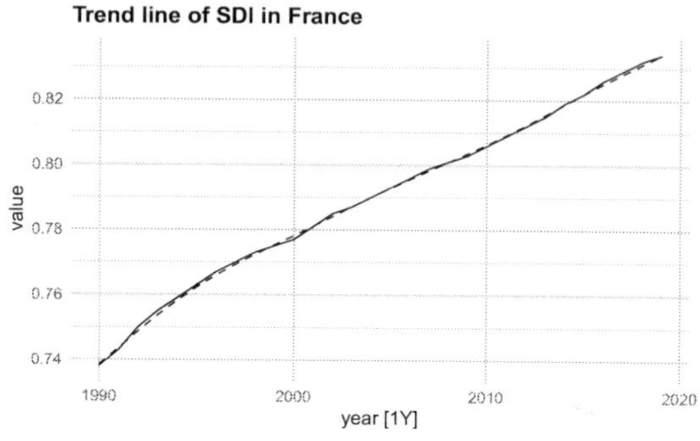

(b) Trend line of SDI in France

Figure 9.5 Components of SDI in France

9.4.2 Autocorrelation and Stationarity

Autocorrelation is very important in time series analysis as it explains whether past values influence future values. If a variable today is similar to what it was yesterday or last month, we say it has autocorrelation at lag 1 or lag k.

$$r_k = \frac{\sum_{t=k+1}^{T}(y_t - \bar{y})(y_{t-k} - \bar{y})}{\sum_{t=1}^{T}(y_t - \bar{y})^2} \tag{9.8}$$

where:

- $r_k$is the autocorrelation coefficient at lag k,
- y_t is the value of the time series at time t,
- $\bar{y}$ is the mean of the series,
- T is the total number of time points.

Time series that exhibit **no autocorrelation**, or no predictable relationship between observations at different time points, are referred to as **white noise series**, where each value is essentially a random draw from the same distribution, with constant mean and variance, with no pattern recognition.

On the contrary, the presence of **autocorrelation**, or statistically significant correlations between current and past values, indicates the absence of white noise. This means the time series has temporal structure, which can be modelled for prediction. For example, positive autocorrelation suggests that high (or low) values tend to be followed by similarly high (or low) values, while negative autocorrelation implies an alternating pattern.

$$r_k = \begin{cases} > 0 & \text{positive autocorrelation (e.g., trends)} \\ < 0 & \text{negative autocorrelation (e.g., alternating pattern)} \\ \approx 0 & \text{no autocorrelation (white noise)} \end{cases} \tag{9.9}$$

To check for autocorrelation in our data, we can use the `ACF()` function from the `{feasts}` package:

```
sdi_fr_ts |>
  ACF(value) |>
  autoplot()
```

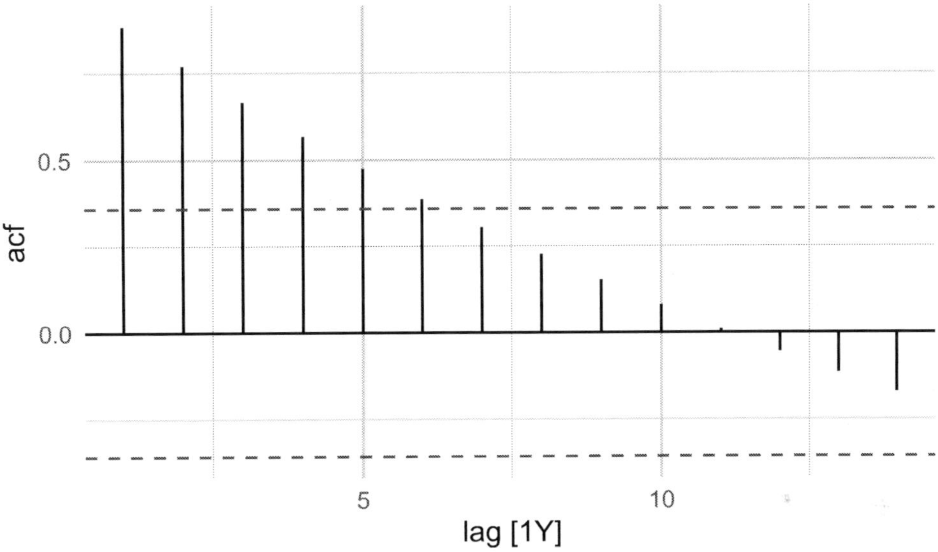

Figure 9.6 Autocorrelation Function of SDI in France. The blue dashed lines represent the 95% confidence interval for the null hypothesis: `There is no autocorrelation at lag k.`

The output clearly shows that our data displays autocorrelation, this validates the use of time series models such as ARIMA, which rely on autocorrelated structure.

To assess whether the series is **stationary**, we use a specific test, the **KPSS test**[3] or **Augmented Dickey-Fuller test**. If this test, generally defined as **unit root test**, indicates non-stationarity, we can apply a **first-order difference** to remove the trend and convert it into a stationary series.

To apply the KPSS test we use the `features()` function from `{fabletools}` package and specify the feature to be: `unitroot_kpss`. The `{urca}` might be needed for this task; if needed `install.packages("urca")`.

```
sdi_fr_ts |>
  features(value,
```

[3]"KPSS Test," October 12, 2023, https://en.wikipedia.org/w/index.php?title=KPSS_test&oldid=1179751435.

```
          features = unitroot_kpss)
#> # A tibble: 1 x 2
#>   kpss_stat kpss_pvalue
#>       <dbl>       <dbl>
#> 1      1.09        0.01
```

A $p - value = 0.01$, which is less than 0.05, indicates strong evidence against the null hypothesis of stationarity.

In summary, the presence of autocorrelation combined with the **non-stationarity** result from the KPSS test suggests that the series has a trend or random walk component, and is not stationary.

> A fundamental concept in time series analysis is **stationarity**. A time series is said to be stationary when its statistical properties do not change over time. This means the mean, variance, and autocorrelation structure remain constant throughout the series. On the other hand, a **non-stationary** time series exhibits properties that change over time—for example, a long-term trend, changing variability, or evolving seasonal patterns.

In this case we apply the first-order differencing (differences = 1) to the data before applying models that assume stationarity, such as ARIMA.

$$y'_t = y_t - y_{t-1} \tag{9.10}$$

Differencing transforms the series by subtracting each observation from its previous value, thereby removing trends and stabilizing the mean over time. This transformation often makes the mean and variance more stable, and is essential because non-stationary time series can lead to unreliable or misleading model results.

```
# Apply first-order differencing to remove trend
sdi_fr_diff <- sdi_fr_ts |>
  mutate(diff_value = difference(value, differences = 1))
sdi_fr_diff |> head()
#> # A tsibble: 6 x 4 [1Y]
#>   location  year value diff_value
#>   <chr>    <dbl> <dbl>      <dbl>
#> 1 France    1990 0.738   NA
#> 2 France    1991 0.743    0.00500
#> 3 France    1992 0.75     0.00700
#> 4 France    1993 0.755    0.00500
#> 5 France    1994 0.759    0.00400
#> 6 France    1995 0.763    0.00400
```

```
sdi_fr_diff |>
  ggplot(aes(x = year, y = diff_value)) +
  geom_line() +
  labs(title = "First-order Differenced SDI (France)",
       x = "Year", y = "Differenced SDI")
```

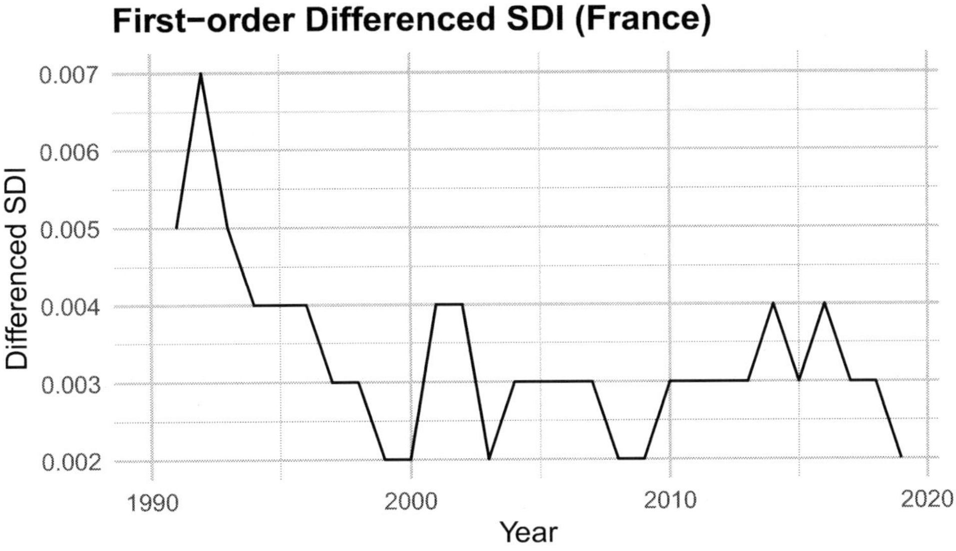

Figure 9.7 First-order Differenced SDI (France)

9.4.3 Partial Autocorrelations

The **Partial Autocorrelation Function (PACF)** removes the effects of intermediate lags. It is a measures of the direct relationship between a time series and its own lagged values. The PACF allows for a more specific identification of how many lags to include in the AR part of the `ARIMA` model. The number of autoregressive (AR) terms (p) is determined by the number of significant lags in the PACF plot.

```
sdi_fr_ts |>
  PACF(value) |>
  autoplot()

sdi_fr_ts |>
  gg_tsdisplay(y = value, plot_type = "partial")
```

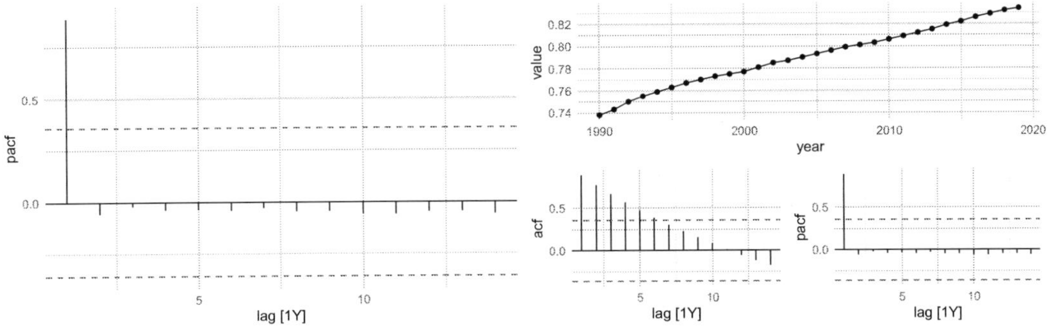

(a) PACF **(b)** gg_tsdisplay

Figure 9.8 Partial Autocorrelations of SDI in France

In this plot we can see that the PACF shows a significant spike at lag 1, indicating that the first lag is important for predicting the current value. The subsequent lags are not significant, suggesting that only the first lag should be included in the ARIMA model.

9.4.4 ARIMA model

The **ARIMA** model forecasts time series values based on past observations.

> In time series analysis, the terms forecast and predict are sometimes used interchangeably, but there's a subtle distinction:
>
> - Forecast typically refers to estimating future values based on a model trained on historical data.
> - Predict can refer more generally to estimating outcomes, including within-sample estimates (e.g., fitting values during model training).

Auto-ARIMA model is used to establish the best fit by combining autoregressive, moving average, and differencing components. However, careful analysis of stationarity, autocorrelations, and the residuals is required to fine-tune the model and improve forecasting accuracy.

The `ARIMA(value)` function automatically selects the best p, d, and q values.

In general, the ARIMA model is defined as:

$$\text{ARIMA}(p, d, q) = \text{AR}(p) + \text{I}(d) + \text{MA}(q) \tag{9.11}$$

where:

- $\text{AR}(p)$ is the autoregressive part of the model, which uses past values of the time series to predict future values,
- $\text{I}(d)$ is the integrated part of the model, which represents the differencing of the time series to make it stationary,
- $\text{MA}(q)$ is the moving average part of the model, which uses past forecast errors to predict future values.

The `ARIMA()` function from the `{fable}` package automatically selects the appropriate degree of differencing needed to achieve stationarity and fits the ARIMA model accordingly. The `report()` function provides a summary of the fitted model, including parameter estimates and diagnostic statistics.

```
fit <- sdi_fr_ts |>
  model(ARIMA(value))

fit |> report()
#> Series: value
#> Model: ARIMA(1,1,0) w/ drift
#>
#> Coefficients:
#>          ar1  constant
#>       0.5971    0.0013
#> s.e.  0.1562    0.0002
#>
```

```
#> sigma^2 estimated as 8.634e-07:  log likelihood=162.46
#> AIC=-318.92   AICc=-317.96   BIC=-314.82
```

The model suggests that the differenced series follows a stable upward trend, with moderate autocorrelation and low residual variance, implying a strong and reliable forecast model for the observed data.

In particular, selected `ARIMA(1,1,0)` indicates:

- One autoregressive (AR) term ($ar1 = 0.5971$): There is moderate persistence; the differenced value at time t is positively correlated with the previous time point
- First-order differencing ($d = 1$) was applied to achieve stationarity
- No moving average (MA) term ($q = 0$)
- The model includes a drift term (constant $= 0.0013$), which accounts for a consistent upward trend in the differenced series.
- Standard errors (s.e.) for both coefficients are small, suggesting estimates are fairly precise.
- $\sigma^2 = 8.634e - 07$: Very low variance of the residuals, indicating a good fit.
- Log-likelihood $= 162.46$: Used for model comparison.
- AIC $= -318.92$, AICc $= -317.96$, BIC $= -314.82$: All are low values, which generally indicate a better-fitting model when compared to alternatives.

9.4.5 ARIMA Forecast

The `forecast()` function from the `{fable}` package is used to generate forecasts based on the fitted ARIMA model. The `h` parameter specifies the forecast horizon, which is the number of future time points to predict. In this case we used $h = 10$ for the next 10 years.

```
fit |>
  forecast(h = 10) |>
  ggplot(aes(x = year, y = .mean)) +
  geom_line(data = sdi_fr_ts,
            aes(y = value)) +
  geom_line(color = "purple", linetype = "dashed")+
  labs(title = "Forecast of SDI in France")
```

9.4.6 Model Ensembles

In time series analysis, an individual model trained on historical data to generate forecasts is known as a **single learner**, such as a single ARIMA model. However, a single learner may not be sufficient to capture the full complexity of the data, especially when dealing with intricate patterns, nonlinear relationships, or multiple influencing factors, leading to poor generalisation on unseen data.

Single approaches often fail to account for crucial factors like external shocks, structural changes, or nonlinear relationships, making them insufficient for capturing all aspects of the data, including trend and seasonality.

This is where **ensemble learning** comes into play.

By aggregating the predictions from **multiple single learners**, we can form a **model ensemble**, to improve predictive performance and generate more robust forecasts.

Ensemble learning is a machine learning technique that leverages the diversity of individual models to make more accurate predictions and reduce overfitting. Ensemble methods can

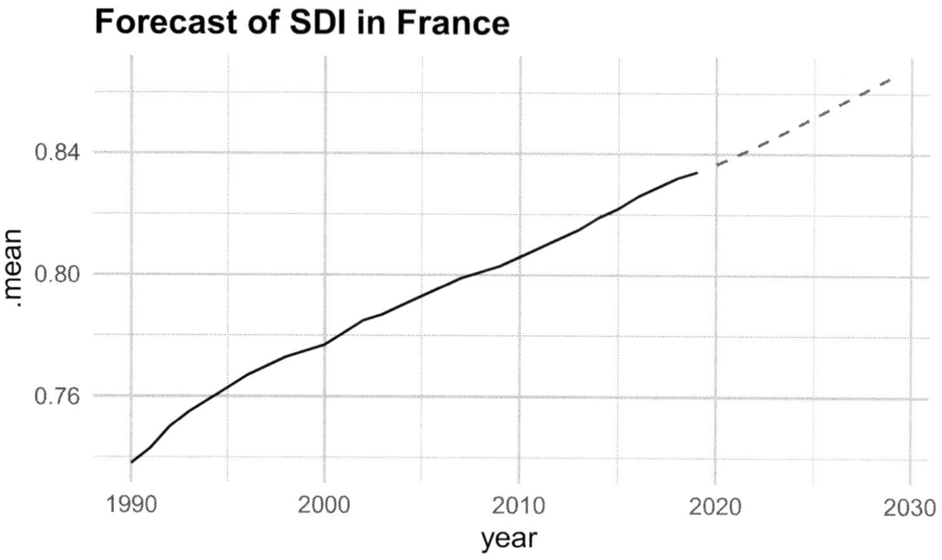

Figure 9.9 Forecast of SDI in France

reduce the variance and bias of the predictions, examples are techniques such as bagging, boosting, and stacking that leverage the diversity of individual models to create a stronger collective model that outperforms its components.

These methods are widely used in machine learning and predictive modelling to enhance the predictive power of the model and achieve better generalisation performance on unseen data.

In this example, we will use the `ARIMA()` function to fit multiple ARIMA models with different orders and compare their performance using the `glance()` function from the `{broom}` package.

```
caf_fit <- sdi_fr_ts |>
  model(
    arima210 = ARIMA(value ~ pdq(2, 1, 0)),
    arima013 = ARIMA(value ~ pdq(0, 1, 3)),
    stepwise = ARIMA(value),
    search = ARIMA(value, stepwise = FALSE)
    )
```

```
caf_fit |>
  pivot_longer(cols = everything(),
               names_to = "Model name",
               values_to = "Orders")
#> # A mable: 4 x 2
#> # Key:     Model name [4]
#>   `Model name`                  Orders
#>   <chr>                        <model>
#> 1 arima210     <ARIMA(2,1,0) w/ drift>
#> 2 arima013     <ARIMA(0,1,3) w/ drift>
#> 3 stepwise     <ARIMA(1,1,0) w/ drift>
#> 4 search       <ARIMA(1,1,0) w/ drift>
```

```
glance(caf_fit) |>
  arrange(AICc) |>
  select(.model:BIC)
#> # A tibble: 4 x 6
#>   .model         sigma2 log_lik   AIC  AICc   BIC
#>   <chr>           <dbl>   <dbl> <dbl> <dbl> <dbl>
#> 1 stepwise 0.000000863    162. -319. -318. -315.
#> 2 search   0.000000863    162. -319. -318. -315.
#> 3 arima210 0.000000896    162. -317. -315. -311.
#> 4 arima013 0.000000950    162. -314. -312. -308.
```

The results of the model ensemble analysis reveal that both the **stepwise** and **search** ARIMA models outperform the others in terms of model fit, as indicated by their lower AIC and AICc values. These two models exhibit identical log-likelihood values and minimal residual variance, suggesting that they provide the most accurate forecasts while maintaining model simplicity. In contrast, the **arima210** and **arima013** models show slightly higher AIC and AICc values, indicating that they are less efficient at capturing the underlying patterns in the data.

Based on these findings, we select the **search** model with ARIMA(1,1,0), and visualize the residuals of the fitted model.

```
caf_fit |>
  select(search) |>
  gg_tsresiduals()


caf_fit |>
  forecast(h = 5) |>
  filter(.model == "search") |>
  ggplot(aes(x = year, y = .mean)) +
  geom_line(data = sdi_fr_ts,
            aes(y = value)) +
  geom_line(color = "purple", linetype = "dashed")
```

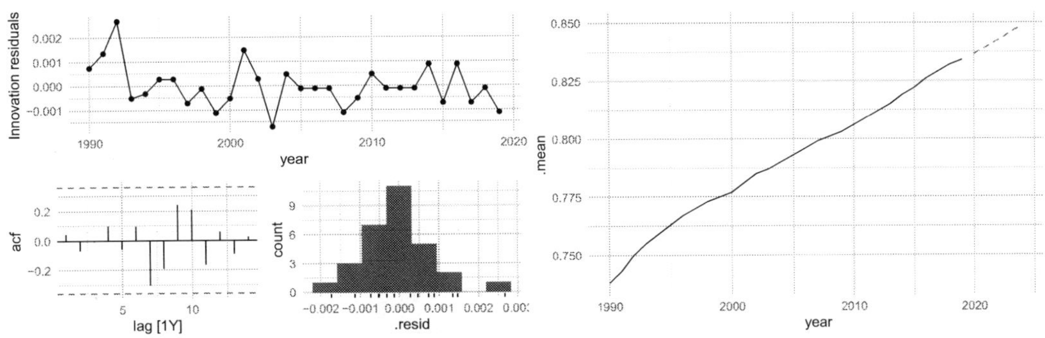

(a) Residuals of ARIMA Models **(b)** Forecast of SDI in France

Figure 9.10 Residuals of ARIMA Models

In conclusion, the analysis of the **Socio-Demographic Index (SDI)** in France from 1990 to 2019 demonstrates the effectiveness of time series analysis and mixed models in understanding and forecasting complex health-related data. By employing techniques such as decomposition, autocorrelation analysis, and ARIMA modelling, we can gain valuable insights into the underlying patterns and trends in the data. The use of ensemble learning further enhances the predictive performance of the models, allowing for more accurate forecasts and better-informed decision-making in public health. However, additional model validation and diagnostic checks, such as residual analysis and cross-validation, should be conducted to ensure that these models generalize well to unseen data and are not overfitting.

9.5 Mixed Models

Mixed models are a powerful statistical tool for analysing data with a hierarchical or nested structure, where observations are grouped within higher-level units. By incorporating both **fixed** and **random effects**, mixed models can account for the variability within and between groups, providing a flexible framework for modelling complex data structures. Mixed models are widely used in various fields, and particularly useful in fields like healthcare and infectious diseases where data might be collected across different subjects or time points.

In the following section, we will discuss the application of mixed models in estimating the **Years Lived with Disability (YLDs)** and the different ratios used in forecasting non-fatal disease burden.

9.5.1 Mixed-Effects Models in Estimating YLDs

Mixed-effects models are particularly useful in estimating YLDs because they can handle data that is hierarchically structured data.

Fixed Effects: These are the primary effects of interest and include variables such as age, gender, year, and specific interventions or treatments.

Random Effects: These capture the variability that is not explained by the fixed effects, such as differences between patients, clinics, or regions.

By using mixed-effects models, we can better account for the within-subject and between-subject variability, providing more accurate estimates of YLDs.

9.6 Example: YLDs due to Tuberculosis - Mixed-Effects Models

In this example, we will demonstrate how estimated **Years Lived with Disability (YLDs)** due to **Tuberculosis** can be used to predict future values using mixed-effects models.

We use the `{lme4}` package to fit **mixed-effects models**, enabling us to account for both fixed effects (e.g., year, prevalence) and random effects (e.g., variability across countries). This approach is particularly valuable for analysing grouped or repeated measures data, such as longitudinal health data, where observations are not independent over time or across different levels of analysis.

Data are from the `g7_hmetrics` dataset in the `{hmsidwR}` package, which contains rates (per 100,000 population) for **YLDs**, **deaths**, **incidence**, and **prevalence** of **Respiratory infections and tuberculosis** in 2010 and 2019 for selected countries.

```
library(lme4)
library(tidyverse)

tuberculosis <- hmsidwR::g7_hmetrics %>%
  filter(measure %in% c("Prevalence",
                        "YLDs"),
         str_detect(cause, "Tuberculosis"),
         !year == 2021,
         !location == "Global",
         metric == "Rate",
         sex == "both") %>% # per 100,000 population
  select(year, location, measure, val) %>%
  pivot_wider(names_from = measure,
              values_from = val)

tuberculosis %>% head()
#> # A tibble: 6 x 4
#>    year location  YLDs Prevalence
#>   <dbl> <chr>    <dbl>      <dbl>
#> 1  2010 Japan     3.07     17720.
#> 2  2019 Japan     2.03     14215.
#> 3  2010 Germany   1.79      7758.
#> 4  2019 Germany   1.55      6706.
#> 5  2010 UK        2.67      8670.
#> 6  2019 UK        1.84      7534.
```

We can see how the level of YLDs due to tuberculosis has decreased in all selected countries over the 10-year period.

```
library(ggpattern)
ggplot(tuberculosis,
       aes(x = fct_reorder(location, YLDs),
           y = YLDs, group = year)) +
  ggpattern::geom_col_pattern(aes(pattern = factor(year)),
                              position = "dodge",
                              fill= 'white',
                              colour= 'black') +
  labs(title="YLDs for Tuberculosis by Location and Year",
       x = "Location", pattern = "Year")
```

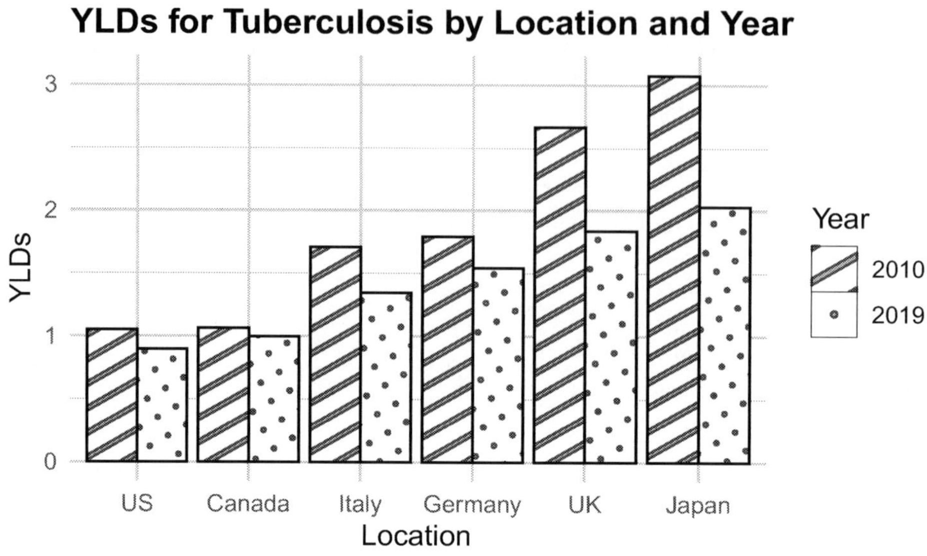

Figure 9.11 YLDs for Tuberculosis by Location and Year

The disability weight for tuberculosis in 2019 is set at 0.333 for the Global region. The duration, derived from the GBD 2021 and based on a systematic review, was adjusted for treated and untreated cases: it was estimated to be 3 years for untreated cases and 6 months for treated cases.[4]

The formula $YLDs\ Prevalence + year + (1|location)$ specifies a linear mixed-effects model for predicting Years Lived with Disability (YLDs) due to tuberculosis. The model includes fixed effects for prevalence and year, as well as a random intercept for location ($(1|location)$). This allows for the estimation of YLDs while accounting for variability across different locations.

```
# Define the formula
formula <- YLDs ~ Prevalence + year + (1 | location)

# Fit the mixed-effects model
model <- lmer(formula, data = tuberculosis)
model
#> Linear mixed model fit by REML ['lmerMod']
#> Formula: YLDs ~ Prevalence + year + (1 | location)
#>    Data: tuberculosis
#> REML criterion at convergence: 34.6921
#> Random effects:
#>  Groups   Name        Std.Dev.
#>  location (Intercept) 0.6202
#>  Residual             0.1773
#> Number of obs: 12, groups:  location, 6
#> Fixed Effects:
```

[4] Edine W. Tiemersma et al., "Natural History of Tuberculosis: Duration and Fatality of Untreated Pulmonary Tuberculosis in HIV Negative Patients: A Systematic Review," *PLOS ONE* 6, no. 4 (April 4, 2011): e17601, doi:10.1371/journal.pone.0017601.

```
#> (Intercept)   Prevalence        year
#>  67.7989019    0.0001619   -0.0336388
#> fit warnings:
#> Some predictor variables are on very different scales: consider rescaling
```

```
# Extract fixed effects
fixed_effects <- fixef(model)

fixed_effects
#>   (Intercept)    Prevalence          year
#> 67.7989018583  0.0001619458 -0.0336387726
```

Considering only the fixed effects the model function becomes:

$$Y\hat{LD}s = 67.79889 + 0.00016 * Prevalence - 0.03364 * year \tag{9.12}$$

In particular, a prevalence coefficient of 0.00016 means that for each unit increase in prevalence, YLDs increase by 0.00016, while a year coefficient of -0.03364 means that for each unit increase in year, YLDs decrease by 0.03364.

Looking at the random effects, we can see how the model accounts for the variability across different locations.

```
# Extract random effects
random_effects <- ranef(model)

random_effects
#> $location
#>         (Intercept)
#> Canada  -0.40736806
#> Germany  0.44667833
#> Italy   -0.09317570
#> Japan   -0.06401586
#> UK       0.87190488
#> US      -0.75402360
#>
#> with conditional variances for "location"
```

The model function with random_effects for each location becomes:

$$\begin{aligned} Y\hat{LD}s &= 67.79889 \\ &+0.00016 \cdot \text{Prevalence} \\ &-0.03365 \cdot \text{year} \\ &+ \text{random effect for each location} \end{aligned} \tag{9.13}$$

Then, predictions are made for the YLDs due to tuberculosis using the mixed-effects model on observed data and new data. The predictions are compared with the actual YLDs to evaluate the model's performance.

```
# Predict YLDs for observed data
predictions <- predict(model,
                       tuberculosis,
```

```
                    allow.new.levels = TRUE)

tuberculosis$predicted_YLD <- predictions
```

Predicted versus Estimated YLDs due to Tuberculosis are shown in the following plot:

```
ggplot(tuberculosis %>%
         filter(!location=="Global"),
       aes(x = YLDs, y = predicted_YLD,
       group = location)) +
  geom_point(aes(shape = factor(location))) +
  geom_abline() +
  facet_wrap(~ year) +
  labs(title = "YLDs due to Tuberculosis",
       subtile = "Predicted vs Estimated",
       x = "YLDs",
       y = "Predicted YLD",
       shape = "Location")
```

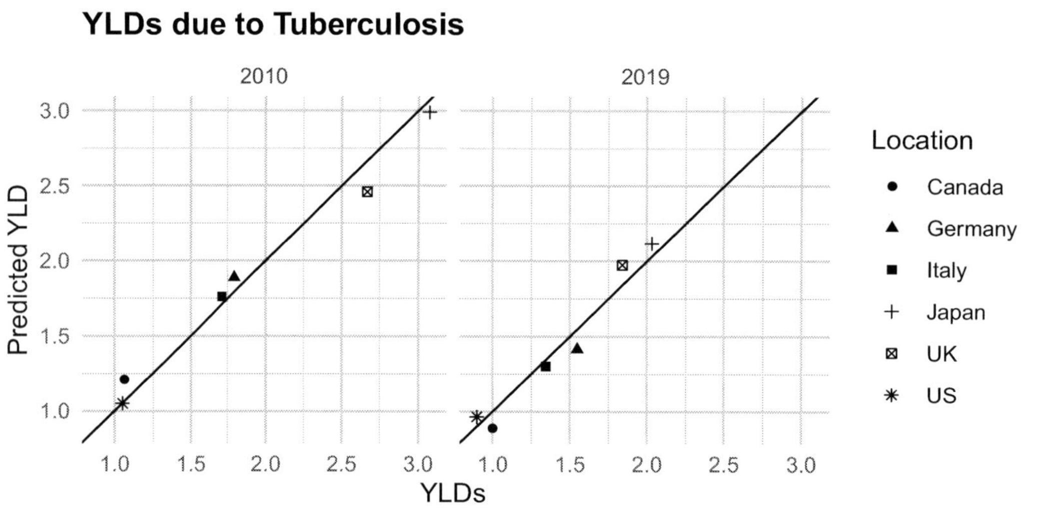

Figure 9.12 Predicted vs Estimated YLDs due to Tuberculosis

The plot shows a good fit between the predicted and estimated YLDs, indicating that the model is able to capture the underlying trends in the data. The error is calculated as the absolute difference between the predicted and estimated YLDs, divided by the estimated YLDs, multiplied by 100 to express it as a percentage.

```
tuberculosis %>%
  mutate(ape = abs(predicted_YLD - YLDs) / YLDs * 100) %>%
  summarise(mape = mean(ape, na.rm = TRUE))
#> # A tibble: 1 x 1
#>    mape
#>   <dbl>
#> 1  6.21
```

The **mean absolute percent error (MAPE)** is 6.2%, indicating that the model is able to predict YLDs with a reasonable level of accuracy.

The **residual sum of squared error (RSE)** is also calculated as the square root of the sum of squared residuals divided by the number of observations minus the number of parameters in the model. The RSE is a measure of how well the model fits the data, and a lower value indicates a better fit.

```
tuberculosis %>%
  mutate(residuals = predicted_YLD - YLDs) %>%
  summarise(
    rse = sqrt(sum(residuals^2) / (nrow(tuberculosis) - length(fixef(model)))))
#> # A tibble: 1 x 1
#>     rse
#>   <dbl>
#> 1 0.126
```

A RSE of 0.1262147 indicates that the model is able to predict YLDs with a reasonable level of accuracy.

Let's use the data for 2021 which we have left aside, and fit the model.

```
tuberculosis_2021 <- hmsidwR::g7_hmetrics %>%
  filter(measure %in% c("Prevalence",
                        "YLDs"),
         str_detect(cause, "Tuberculosis"),
         year == 2021,
         !location == "Global",
         metric == "Rate",
         sex == "both") %>% # per 100,000 population
  select(year, location, measure, val) %>%
  pivot_wider(names_from = measure,
              values_from = val)

tuberculosis_2021
#> # A tibble: 6 x 4
#>    year location  YLDs Prevalence
#>   <dbl> <chr>    <dbl>      <dbl>
#> 1  2021 Japan    1.98      13567.
#> 2  2021 Germany  1.54       6507.
#> 3  2021 UK       1.53       7308.
#> 4  2021 US       0.925     11313.
#> 5  2021 Italy    1.38       9061.
#> 6  2021 Canada   1.02       8767.
```

```
# Predict YLDs for new data
predictions_2021 <- predict(model,
                            tuberculosis_2021,
                            allow.new.levels = TRUE)
```

Check how the model performed on the 2021 data. The predictions are compared with the actual YLDs to evaluate the model's performance.

```
tuberculosis_2021$predicted_YLD <- predictions_2021

tuberculosis_2021 <- tuberculosis_2021 %>%
  select(-Prevalence) %>%
  mutate(residuals = predicted_YLD - YLDs)

tuberculosis_2021
#> # A tibble: 6 x 5
#>    year location  YLDs predicted_YLD residuals
#>   <dbl> <chr>    <dbl>         <dbl>     <dbl>
#> 1  2021 Japan    1.98          1.95    -0.0283
#> 2  2021 Germany  1.54          1.32    -0.229
#> 3  2021 UK       1.53          1.87     0.344
#> 4  2021 US       0.925         0.893   -0.0316
#> 5  2021 Italy    1.38          1.19    -0.190
#> 6  2021 Canada   1.02          0.827   -0.193
```

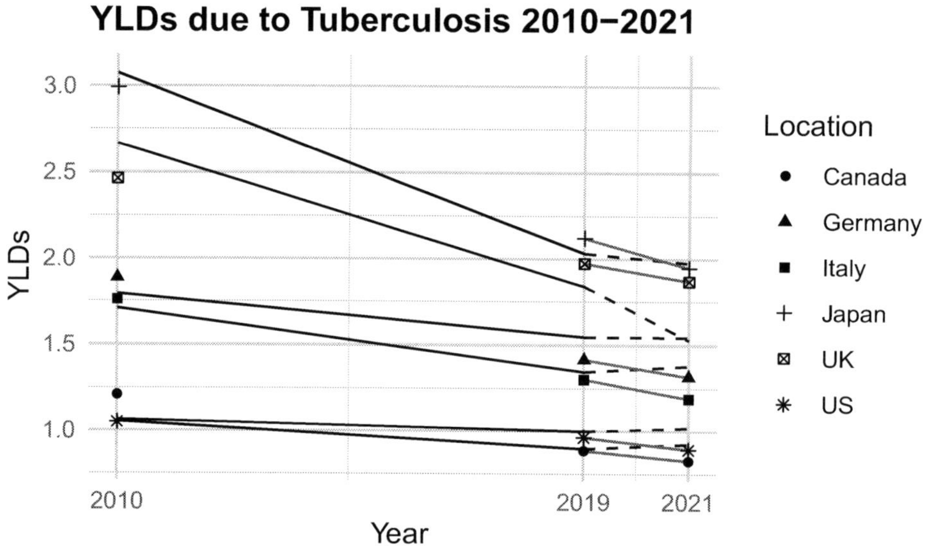

Figure 9.13 YLDs due to Tuberculosis - Mixed-Model Results. Solid lines show the original values, the dashed lines show the original values for 2021, and the dots shaped are by location the predicted values.

The plot shows the estimated YLDs due to tuberculosis for 2010, 2019, and 2021. The dashed lines represent the estimated YLDs for 2010 and 2019, while the solid lines represent the predicted YLDs for 2021. The points represent the actual YLDs for 2021. The model is able to predict YLDs with a reasonable level of accuracy, as indicated by the close fit between the predicted and actual values.

9.7 Summary

Predictive modelling is a valuable tool for forecasting future trends and making informed decisions based on historical data. By leveraging the insights gained from the models, we can anticipate the trajectory of infectious diseases, estimate disease burden, and evaluate the impact of interventions on population health. The models can be further refined and optimised to improve their predictive performance and provide more accurate forecasts. By combining predictive modelling with time series analysis and mixed models, we can gain a comprehensive understanding of the complex dynamics of public health and make data-driven decisions to improve population health outcomes.

Part III

Data Visualization

10

Introduction to Data Visualisation

Data visualisation is a powerful tool for transforming complex datasets into clear and insightful graphical representations. It plays a central role in **Exploratory Data Analysis (EDA)**, helping to reveal important patterns, trends, and hidden insights that are often obscured in raw data. The information contained within data highlights important patterns and trends, and uncover hidden insights that might not be apparent from raw data alone. In the context of health metrics and infectious diseases, data visualisation plays a critical role in tracking disease outbreaks, understanding health trends, and communicating findings to policymakers and the public.

We have already seen how to create various types of plots using the `{ggplot2}` package. In this chapter, we will discuss the history and evolution of data visualisation, delve deeper into the topic, introducing the concept of the **Grammar of Graphics**, exploring techniques for customising plots, adding annotations, labels, and themes, and creating interactive visualisations.

10.1 History of Data Visualisation

The history of data visualisation spans centuries. The roots of data visualisation can be traced back to ancient times with rudimentary visual representations, but its modern form began to take shape with the growth of statistics and graphical methods in the 17th and 18th centuries. One notable milestone was the publication of **William Playfair**'s **"Commercial and Political Atlas"**[1] in 1786, which introduced innovative graphical techniques like the line graph, bar chart, and pie chart.

Throughout the 19th and 20th centuries, pioneers such as **Florence Nightingale** (1820-1910), **John Snow** (1813-1858), and **Jacques Bertin** further advanced the field, using visualisations to communicate complex data and uncover insights with his **Semiology of Graphics** - 1967.

Data visualisation was largely done manually or with the help of basic plotting tools. One example are the hand-drown visualisations made by **W.E.B. Du Bois** (1868-1963) in the early 20th century to illustrate the social and economic conditions of African Americans in the United States. These visualisations are now considered iconic examples of data visualisation and have been widely studied and digitally reproduced.

The Digital Revolution

The digital revolution of the late 20th century, with the advent of powerful computing technologies, enabled the creation of interactive and dynamic visualisations. Early programming

[1] "William Playfair," March 9, 2025, https://en.wikipedia.org/w/index.php?title=William_Playfair&oldid=1279573846.

DOI: 10.1201/9781032625935-10

languages like Fortran and BASIC were used to create simple plots, then the development of specialised software like SAS and SPSS provided more robust tools for data analysis and visualisation.

The emergence of the internet and web technologies in the 1990s led to the introduction of more sophisticated statistical software and programming environments. Tools like R, Python, and JavaScript, along with libraries like `ggplot2`, `matplotlib`, and `D3.js`, revolutionised the field of data visualisation, making it more accessible and powerful.

In summary, data visualisation plays a crucial role in fields like data science, business analytics, scientific research, journalism, and public policy. It serves as a potent tool for communicating data while visualising patterns, trends, and relationships that might not be apparent from raw data alone. For instance, in public health, tracking disease outbreaks in real time, such as with COVID19, tools like dashboards and interactive maps are used extensively to monitor the spread of the virus and communicate the effectiveness of interventions.

10.2 The Grammar of Graphics

One of the fundamental concepts in modern data visualisation is the **Grammar of Graphics**, which provides a structured approach to creating visualisations layer by layer. This concept is clearly interpreted in tools like the `{ggplot2}` R package, part of the `{tidyverse}` ecosystem, developed by **Hadley Wickham** in 2005.

The Grammar of Graphics allows for the creation of complex visualisations by combining simple building blocks such as **data**, **aesthetics**, and **geoms** (geometric objects) in a structured manner. It provides a flexible framework for customising visualisations and supports the creation of a wide range of plots, from basic scatter plots to intricate multi-layered visualisations.

It starts with the `ggplot()` function, which initialises the plot. The function takes a data frame as its first argument and then additional arguments to specify the aesthetics of the plot, such as the x and y variables, colour, shape, and size.

```
ggplot()
```

The aesthetics are defined using the `aes()` function, which maps variables in the data frame to visual properties of the plot, such as x and y coordinates, colour, shape, and size. The `aes()` function is the mapping part of the plot, and it can be called with the `mapping` argument in the layers of the plot.

```
ggplot(data = df,
       mapping = aes(x = x, y = y, color = z))
```

Data can also be called outside of the `ggplot()` function.

```
data %>%
  ggplot(aes(x = x, y = y, color = z))
```

And then additional layers are added using functions like `geom_point()` for a scatterplot, or `geom_line()` for a line plot, and so on. Then, with the `labs()` function, we can add titles, labels, and captions to the plot.

```
ggplot(data = df, aes(x = x, y = y, color = z))+
  geom_point()+
  labs(title = "Scatter Plot")
```

The `{ggplot2}` package provides a wide range of geoms, scales, and themes to customise the appearance of the plot. By combining these elements, you can create visually appealing and informative visualisations that effectively communicate your data.

It allows the user to create complex visualisations by combining simple building blocks, with each layer of the plot allowing for an aesthetic mapping of data to visual properties, such as colour, fill, shape, and size, making it easy to create a wide range of visualisations, or even new data. In this example there is also the use of an alternative to the `labs()` function with the `ggtitle()` function, which differs in the way the title is placed in the plot.

```
ggplot(data = df, aes(x = x, y = y, color = z))+
  geom_point()+
  geom_point(data = df2, aes(x = x2, y = y2, color = z2))+
  ggtitle("Scatter Plot")
```

In addition to functions provided by `{ggplot2}`, there are ggplot **extensions**, other functions and packages that can be used to create visualisations, such as `{plotly}`, `{ggplotly}`, `{leaflet}`, `{tmap}`, and `{shiny}`. These tools provide additional functionality for creating interactive plots, maps, and dashboards, allowing for more engaging and dynamic data visualisations.

10.3 General Guidelines for Data Visualisation

There are many types of plots that can be used to visualise different types of data, such as cross tabulations for categorical variables, scatter plots for continuous variables, side-by-side box plots, and other summaries.

Here are some specifications about the usage of common types of plots:

10.4 Example: Visualising Lung Cancer Deaths by Age in Germany

This is an example of visualising lung cancer deaths by age in Germany. It is a line plot showing the number of deaths by age group. We have already seen how to create a line plot using `{ggplot2}` in previous chapters, the focus here is on customising the plot to make it more visually appealing and informative.

This is a basic output, and we will enhance it by customising patterns, colours, legend, and adjusting the layout. We will also explore how to save the plot as an image file for sharing or publication.

```
library(ggplot2)
library(ggpattern)
```

Plot	Type of Plot	Description
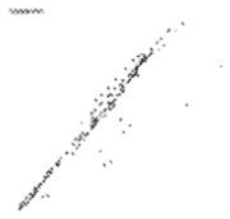	Scatter Plots	Used to show the relationship between two variables.
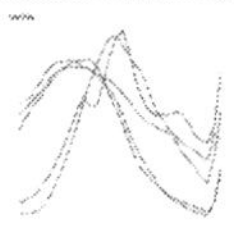	Line Plots	Used to show trends over time or across categories.
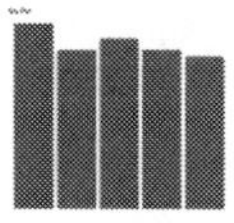	Bar Plots	Used to compare values across categories.
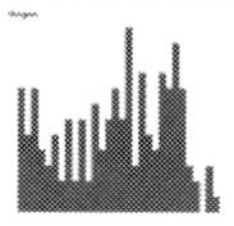	Histograms	Used to show the distribution of a single variable.
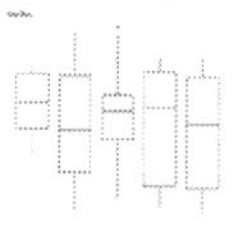	Box Plots	Used to show the distribution of a variable across categories.
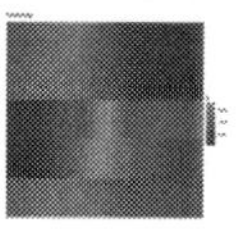	Heatmaps	Used to show the relationship between two categorical variables.
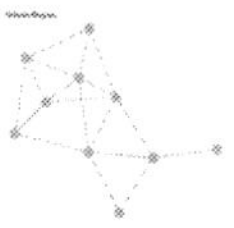	Network Diagrams	Used to show the relationships between nodes in a network.
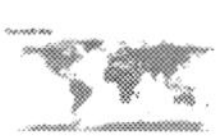	Choropleth Maps	Used to show the distribution of a variable across geographic regions.
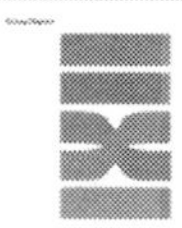	Sankey Diagrams	Used to show the flow of data between different categories.
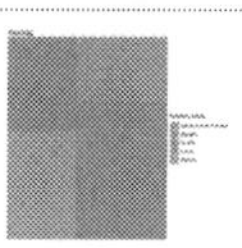	Treemaps	Used to show hierarchical data as a series of nested rectangles.

Figure 10.1 Basic Data Visualisation Rules

```
scatterplot <- hmsidwR::germany_lungc |>
  ggplot(aes(x = age, y = dx)) +
  geom_point(aes(shape =sex)) +
  labs(title = "Lung Cancer Deaths by Age in Germany",
       x = "Age",
       y = "Deaths")

lineplot <- hmsidwR::germany_lungc |>
  ggplot(aes(x = age, y = dx, group = sex)) +
  geom_line(aes(linetype=sex)) +
  geom_point() +
  labs(title = "Lung Cancer Deaths by Age in Germany",
       x = "Age",
       y = "Deaths")

barplot <- hmsidwR::germany_lungc |>
  ggplot(aes(x = age, y = dx, group = sex))  +
  ggpattern::geom_col_pattern(aes(pattern=sex),
                              position="stack",
                              fill= 'white',
                              colour= 'black') +
  labs(title = "Lung Cancer Deaths by Age in Germany",
       x = "Age",
       y = "Deaths")
```

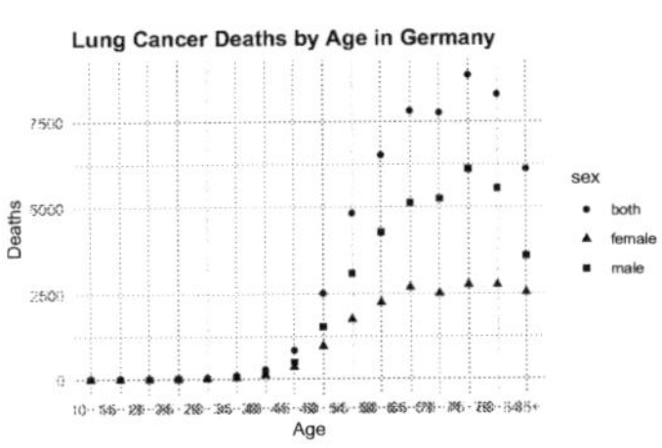

(a) Scatterplot: Lung Cancer Deaths by Age in Germany

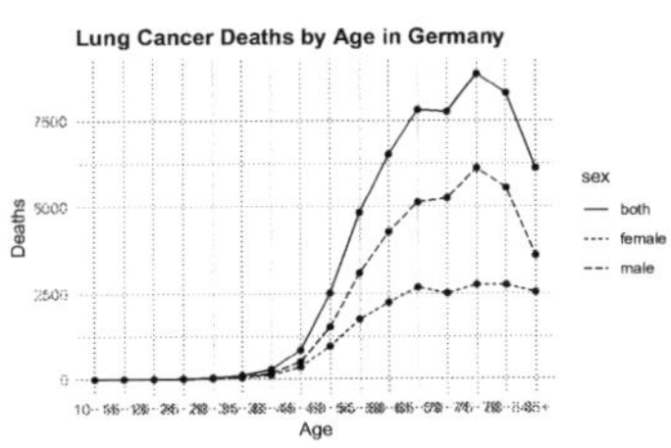

(b) Lineplot: Lung Cancer Deaths by Age in Germany

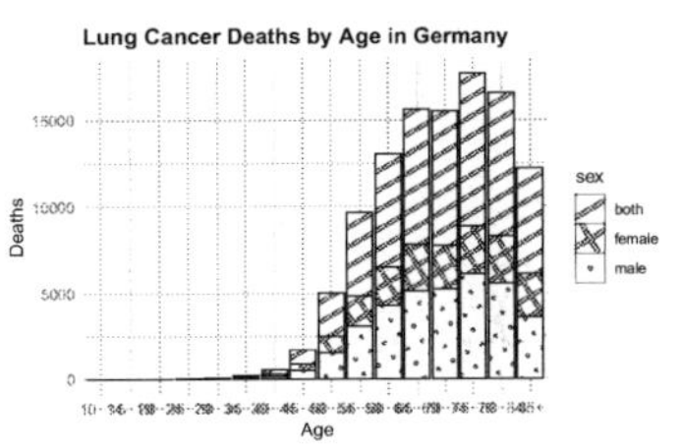

(c) Barplot: Lung Cancer Deaths by Age in Germany

Figure 10.2 Scatterplot and Barplot of Lung Cancer Deaths by Age in Germany

All of these three plots have a grammar of graphic structure, which means that they are built using layers of data, aesthetics, and geometric objects. The `ggplot()` function initializes the plot, and then we add layers using `geom_point()`, `geom_line()`, and `geom_col()`, (or `geom_col_pattern()` in this particular example), to create the visualisations. We can further customise these plots by adding titles, labels, and adjusting the appearance of the plot elements.

Finally, another way to visualise Lung Cancer Deaths by Age in Germany is to use the `geom_col()` function and create a bar plot for each sex category. This is a basic bar plot, and we will enhance it by adjusting the layout. The `facet_<>` functions are used to create a grid of plots, where each plot represents a different subset of the data. In this case, we are using `facet_grid()` to create a grid of plots based on the `sex` variable.

```
hmsidwR::germany_lungc |>
  ggplot(aes(x = age, y = dx, group = sex)) +
  geom_col(position="identity",
           fill= 'white',
           colour= 'black') +
  # adjust the layout with three barplot one for each category
  facet_grid(sex ~ .) +
  labs(title = "Lung Cancer Deaths by Age in Germany",
       x = "Age",
       y = "Deaths") +
  theme(axis.text.x = element_text(angle = 45, hjust = 1))
```

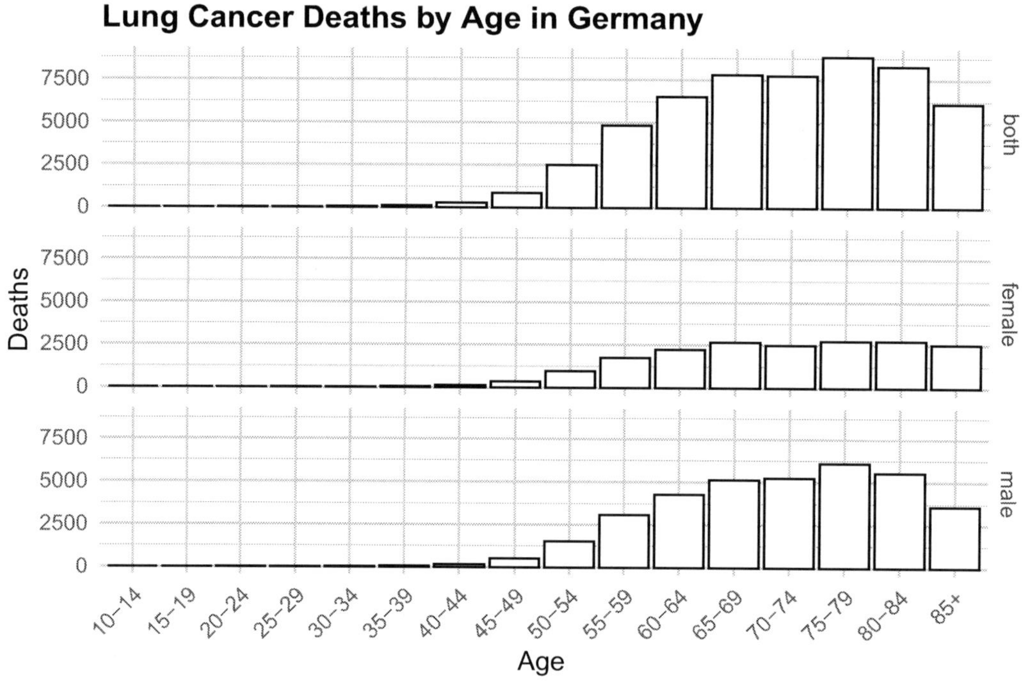

Figure 10.3 Barplots Layout - Lung Cancer Deaths by Age in Germany

10.4.1 Colors and Patterns

Choosing the right colours for your visualisations is crucial. Colors can highlight important aspects of your data and improve readability. Many tools provide built-in color palettes, but you can also customise your own. Here we just add the `scale_color_manual()` function to customise the original plot, with a new color palette.

By typing `?scale_color_manual()` in the R console, you can access the documentation and explore other options for customising colours using the `scale_<..>_<..>()` functions.

```
# Example: customising colours in a bar chart
lineplot +
  scale_color_manual(values = c("brown", "navy", "orange"))
```

In addition to colours, patterns can be used to differentiate between the groups in the plot. The {ggpattern} package provides a variety of patterns that can be used to fill the bars in a bar plot. Here we have used the `geom_col_pattern()` function to add patterns to the bars in the plot. An example is in show in the plot with the barplot. Another way is to use the `linetype` or `shape` aesthetics to differentiate between groups in a line plot or scatter plot.

10.4.2 Theme, Legends, and Guides

Legends and guides are essential for interpreting visualisations. They help the audience understand what different colours, shapes, or sizes represent in the plot. Here we have just changed the title of the legend, but much more can be done, such as changing the position, and labels. To change the position of the legend we can use the `theme()` function as shown below.

In the R console, typing `?theme()` will provide more information on customising the appearance of your plots. In this case it is useful to adjust the angle of the text in the x-axis, and even this can be done specifying the `angle` parameter in the `theme()` function.

The `guides()` function can be used to customise the legend, such as reversing the order of the legend items.

```
# Customising a legend to a plot
lineplot1 <- lineplot +
  labs(linetype = "Sex",
    subtitle = "Year 2019",
    caption = "DataSource: hmsidwR::germany_lungc") +
  guides(linetype = guide_legend(reverse = TRUE)) +
  theme(legend.position = "top",
        axis.text.x = element_text(angle = 45, hjust = 1),
        plot.title = element_text(hjust = 0.5, face = "bold"))

lineplot2 <- lineplot1 +
  scale_y_log10() +
  coord_cartesian(clip = "off") +
  annotate("text", x = Inf, y=Inf,
           hjust = 1, vjust = 0,
           label = "Log Scale")
```

10.4.3 Plot Layouts

The layout of your plots can significantly impact their effectiveness. Arranging multiple plots in a grid can help compare different aspects of your data side-by-side. We can use the `grid.arrange()` function from the {gridExtra} package to arrange multiple plots in a grid layout. Or, we can use the `layout()` function to specify the layout of the plots. There are other packages that can be used such as {patchwork} and {cowplot}, which provide additional functionalities for arranging plots.

```
# Example: Arranging multiple plots
library(gridExtra)

grid.arrange(lineplot, lineplot1, lineplot2, ncol = 3)
```

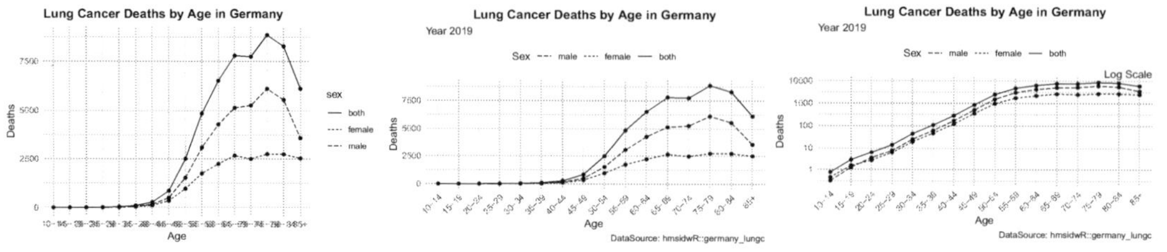

(a) Basic Lineplot

(b) Customised Lineplot

(c) Customised Lineplot on a Log Scale

Figure 10.4 Customised Lineplots and Logarithmic Scale Transformation

10.4.3.1 Exercise

Replicate the plots above, customizing the legend and axis text to improve readability. Apply a logarithmic scale to the y-axis for better data visualization, and consider adding a caption to indicate the data source.

10.4.4 Saving as an Image

Once you've created your visualisation, you might want to save it as an image file for sharing or publication.

```
ggsave("lineplot.png", plot = lineplot2, width = 6, height = 4)
```

10.5 Practising Data Visualisation

To practise making data visualisations, there are numerous free resources available that provide valuable information and opportunities to enhance your skills. By engaging with these platforms, you can practise your abilities, share your final results, and receive feedback from the community. While the feedback may sometimes be critical, it is an essential part of the learning process and will help you improve if you stay persistent.

Participating in competitions and challenges such as **#TidyTuesday**, **#30DayChartChallenge**, and **#30DayMapChallenge** offers a great way to refine your skills. These competitions encourage you to create and share visualisations on various themes, pushing you to experiment with different techniques and styles. By consistently participating in these challenges and actively seeking feedback, you will steadily enhance your proficiency. Over time, you will find yourself becoming more adept and confident in your data visualisation skills.

11

Interpreting Model Results Through Visualisation

Learning Objectives

- Visualize predicted vs. observed values and assess residuals
- Interpret model metrics with VIP, accuracy, and partial dependency plots
- Create and customize ROC curves and compute AUC for classification models

In the introduction to data visualisation (Chapter 10), we explored foundational techniques for effectively communicating model results and data insights through plots. We reviewed essential plots used to visualise predictions and outcomes, such as scatter plots, line graphs, and bar charts. The chapter also covered how to customise these plots using colours, palettes, legends, and guides to improve clarity and visual appeal. Additionally, we discussed how to craft compelling data stories by organising multiple plots in a layout and saving them as image files for reports or presentations.

In this chapter, which is an essential part of the data visualisation section, we focus on how to effectively interpret and use the results from machine learning models in the context of health metrics and infectious diseases.

We will explore how to visualise the results of:

- **Regression models** with a linear regression, and a generalized additive model (GAM)
- **Classification models** with decision trees, and random forest models.

11.1 Practical Insights and Examples

The practice of visualising model results is essential for communicating insights from a model to stakeholders.

Considerations for visualising model results include:

- **Understanding the data**: Before visualising the results, it is important to understand the data and the model used. This includes understanding the variables, their relationships, and the assumptions of the model.
- **Choosing the right visualisation**: Different types of data and models require different types of visualisations. It is important to choose the right visualisation to effectively communicate the results.

DOI: 10.1201/9781032625935-11

11.1.1 Example: Deaths due to Meningitis

Data are from the **Institute for Health Metrics and Evaluation (IHME)** and include **death rates due to meningitis**, as well as two exposure levels of risk factors—particulate matter (PM2.5) and smoking—in the Sub-Saharan Africa (Central African Republic, Zambia, Eswatini, Lesotho, and Malawi) from 1990 to 2021. The data are in the `{hmsidwR}` package and can be loaded as `hmsidwR::meningitis`.

```
install.packages("hmsidwR")
# or
# install the development version of book package
devtools::install_github("Fgazzelloni/hmsidwR")
```

Let's have a look at the first few rows of the data:

```
# Load libraries and data
library(tidyverse)
library(hmsidwR)
meningitis %>% head
#> # A tibble: 6 x 6
#>    year location                 deaths dalys smoking  pm25
#>   <dbl> <chr>                     <dbl> <dbl>   <dbl> <dbl>
#> 1  1990 Eswatini                   12.6  669.    5.91  55.0
#> 2  1990 Malawi                     52.7 3160.    7.57  78.7
#> 3  1990 Zambia                     54.9 3101.    6.71  66.9
#> 4  1990 Lesotho                    10.1  541.   10.6   61.2
#> 5  1990 Central African Republic   33.7 2142.    6.61  80.0
#> 6  1991 Zambia                     55.4 3101.    6.71  66.6
```

Meningitis[1] is a serious global health concern characterised by inflammation of the membranes surrounding the brain and spinal cord. It can arise from both infectious and non-infectious causes and is often associated with a high risk of mortality and long-term complications.

In this example, we explore how two environmental risk factors — **particulate matter (PM2.5)** and **smoking** — may influence meningitis mortality. These variables represent **aggregate exposure levels** that could potentially contribute to meningitis-related deaths.

Meningitis death rates vary considerably across countries and over time. To begin, we visualise how these rates have changed from 1990 to 2021 in five Sub-Saharan African countries. A scatter plot will show annual death rates by country, while a smooth line will reveal the overall trend, helping to contextualize patterns before moving to modelling.

```
meningitis %>%
  ggplot(aes(x = year, y = deaths)) +
  geom_line(aes(group = location,
                linetype = location)) +
  geom_smooth() +
  labs(title = "Deaths due to Menigitis",
       subtitle = "from 1990 to 2021 in Sub-Saharan Africa",
       y = "Death Rates", x = "Time (Year)") +
  theme(legend.position = "bottom",
        legend.title = element_blank())
```

[1]"Meningitis," n.d., https://www.who.int/news-room/fact-sheets/detail/meningitis.

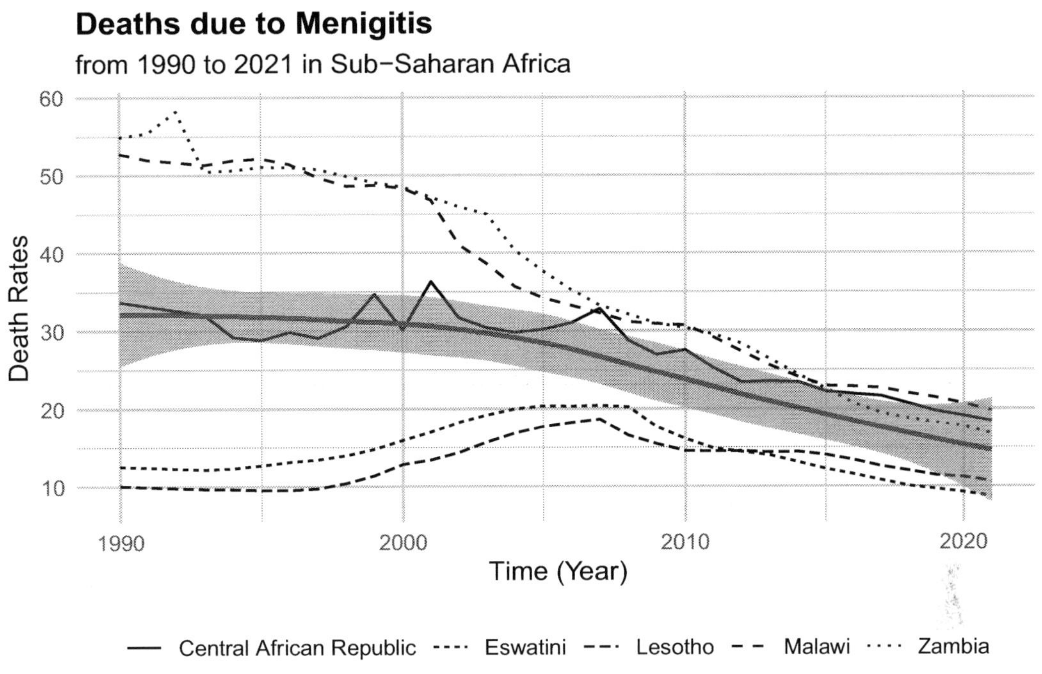

Figure 11.1 Deaths due to Menigitis from 1990 to 2021 in Sub-Saharan Africa. The solid ticker line represents the smooth line revealing the overall trend, while the other lines represent the death rates for each country.

To gain an idea of the estimated average of death rates in the population, we can fit a simple linear regression model with `lm()` function, with the formula `deaths ~ 1`, which means that we are fitting a model with only an intercept (i.e., no predictors). Then we draw a simple **Q-Q plot**[2] (a scatterplot created by plotting two sets of quantiles against one another) to check the normality of the residuals.

```
mod0 <- lm(deaths ~ 1, data = meningitis)
summary(mod0)
#>
#> Call:
#> lm(formula = deaths ~ 1, data = meningitis)
#>
#> Residuals:
#>     Min      1Q  Median      3Q     Max
#> -17.092 -11.372  -3.745   6.822  32.369
#>
#> Coefficients:
#>             Estimate Std. Error t value Pr(>|t|)
#> (Intercept)   25.826      1.062   24.32   <2e-16 ***
#> ---
#> Signif. codes:  0 '***' 0.001 '**' 0.01 '*' 0.05 '.' 0.1 ' ' 1
```

[2]"Q–Q Plot," March 20, 2025, https://en.wikipedia.org/w/index.php?title=Q%E2%80%93Q_plot&oldid=1281381233.

```
#>
#> Residual standard error: 13.43 on 159 degrees of freedom
```

The summary of this model shows the intercept value to be the estimate average of the death rates. We can look at the distribution of the death rates with an histogram:

```
hist1 <- meningitis %>%
  ggplot(aes(x = deaths)) +
  geom_histogram(bins = 10,
                 fill = "grey70", color = "grey40") +
  geom_vline(aes(xintercept = mean(deaths)),
             color = "black",
             size = 2,
             linetype = "dashed") +
  labs(title = "Histogram of Death Rates due to Meningitis",
       x = "Death Rates", y = "Count") +
  theme(legend.position = "bottom",
        legend.title = element_blank())

# Add log scale to x axis
hist2 <- hist1 +
  scale_x_log10()
```

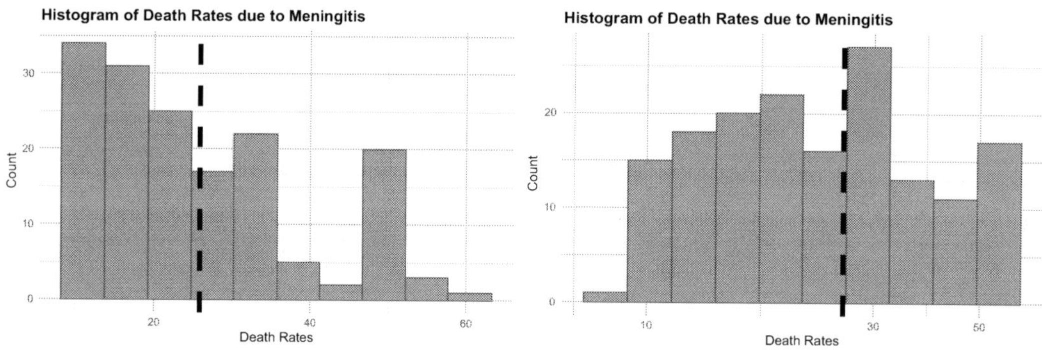

(a) Histogram of Death Rates due to Meningitis

(b) Histogram of Death Rates due to Meningitis (log scale)

Figure 11.2 The histogram of Death Rates due to Meningitis clearly show the right-skewness of the data. The dashed line represents the mean value of the death rates.

To investigate the non linear relationship between the number of deaths and the two risk factors, we can use a **Generalized Additive Model (GAM)** with `s()` function from the `{mgcv}` package. The `s()` function is used to fit smooth terms in the model, which allows us to capture non-linear relationships between the predictors and the response variable.

```
library(mgcv)
mod1 <- gam(deaths ~ s(smoking), data = meningitis)
mod2 <- gam(deaths ~ s(smoking) + s(pm25),
            data = meningitis)
```

To summarise, the models results in a table format, with the estimated coefficients for each model, we can see that the values for the intercept and the coefficients for smoking and

PM2.5 are all positive and statistically significant ($p < 0.05$), indicating that **higher levels of these risk factors are associated with higher death rates due to meningitis**.

Table 11.1 Estimated coefficients for the models

Model	Beta0	Beta1	Beta2
mod0 - linear model	25.83	NA	NA
mod1 - gam 1 predictor	25.83	25.99	NA
mod2 gam 2 predictors	25.83	14.68	1.18

```
plot(mod1)
plot(mod2)
```

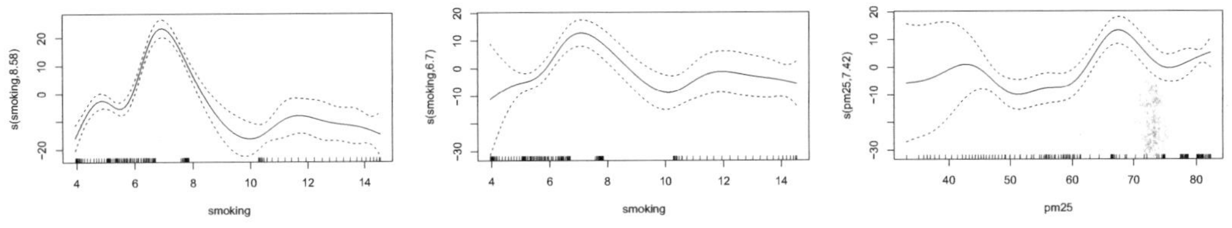

(a) Smocking - mod1 **(b)** Smocking - mod2 **(c)** PM2.5 - mod2

Figure 11.3 Summary Exposure Values: Smocking and PM2.5

A further comparison is done with the `AIC()` function:

```
AIC(mod1, mod2)
#>            df      AIC
#> mod1 10.57829 1102.339
#> mod2 16.11216 1060.531
```

The second GAM model (mod2) is clearly better than the first one (mod1):

- The AIC drops by ~42 points, which is a substantial improvement (a drop of >10 is considered strong evidence).
- The additional smooth term s(pm25) significantly improves model fit, even after accounting for increased complexity (degrees of freedom increase from 10.6 to 16.1).

Let's now include the `year` variable in the model, to account for the temporal trend in the data. We can also include an interaction term between `year` and `location` to account for the different trends in different countries. The `by` argument in the `s()` function allows us to fit separate smooth terms for each level of the `location` variable.

We set the location to be a factor variable:

```
meningitis$location <- as.factor(meningitis$location)
```

Then we can fit the third model:

```
mod3 <- gam(deaths ~ s(smoking) + s(pm25) + s(year, by = location),
            data = meningitis)
```

The `s(year, by = location)` term allows for different smooth terms:

```
par(mfrow = c(2, 3))
for (i in 1:5) {
  plot(mod3, select = i + 2, shade = TRUE,
       main = levels(meningitis$location)[i])
}
```

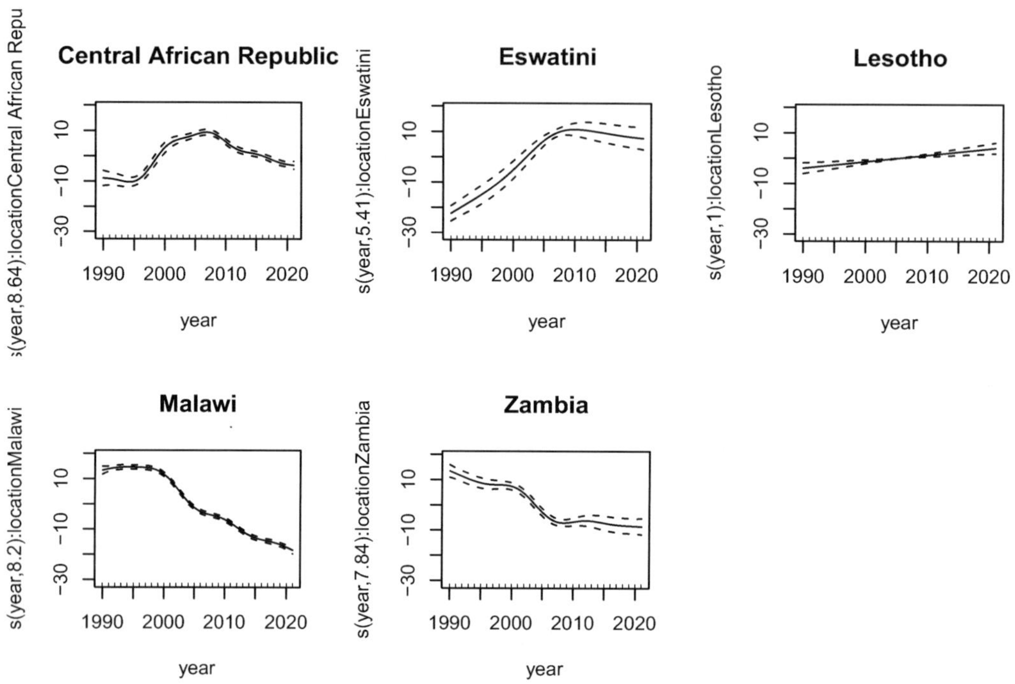

Figure 11.4 Meningitis Death Rates by Country. The solid line represents the smooth line revealing the overall trend, while the other lines represent the death rates for each country.

Table 11.2 Model Metrics

Model	R2	DevExp
mod0 - linear model	0.7030403	0.7190617
mod1 - gam 1 predictor	0.7784592	0.7981222
mod2 gam 2 predictors	0.9957811	0.9968419

In conclusion, we began with a generalised additive model with just smoking as influencing factor, then we fit a second model where both smoking and PM2.5 were modelled as smooth functions. This second model explained nearly 80% of the variance in meningitis death rates. However, by incorporating country-specific nonlinear time trends, we dramatically improved the model fit to over 99% of variance explained. This highlights the importance of accounting for temporal and spatial structure in health data, particularly when modelling long time spans across multiple countries.

There is still a consideration to be made related to the exposure effect of smocking and PM2.5 on meningitis death rates.

Table 11.3 Model p-values

term	p.value_mod1	p.value_mod2	p.value_mod3
s(smoking)	0	7.69e-05	0.0000000
s(pm25)	0	0.00e+00	0.6979803

In the second model (mod2), both the smoking and PM2.5 terms have p-values below 0.05, indicating that they are statistically significant predictors of meningitis mortality. However, when incorporating temporal and spatial effects in mod3, the significance of these exposure variables changes — most notably, PM2.5 is no longer statistically significant. This shift suggests that the apparent association in the simpler model may be confounded by time trends or country-level differences, highlighting the importance of accounting for structured variation in space and time.

Let's use both models to predict the number of deaths due to meningitis in the dataset. We can use the `predict()` function to obtain the predicted values for the model. The predicted values are added to the original dataset as a new column called `predicted`.

```
meningitis$predicted_mod2 <- predict(mod2)
meningitis$predicted_mod3 <- predict(mod3)
```

```
ggplot(meningitis,
       aes(x = year, y = deaths, color = location)) +
  geom_line() +
  geom_line(aes(y = predicted_mod2),
            linetype = "dashed") +
  facet_grid(location ~ ., scale = "free") +
  labs(title = "Meningitis Death Rates by Country",
       subtitle = "Observed vs Predicted",
       y = "Death Rate", x = "Year") +
  theme(legend.position = "none")

ggplot(meningitis,
       aes(x = year, y = deaths, color = location)) +
  geom_line() +
  geom_line(aes(y = predicted_mod3),
            linetype = "dashed") +
  facet_grid(location ~ ., scale = "free") +
  labs(title = "Meningitis Death Rates by Country",
       subtitle = "Observed vs Predicted",
       y = "Death Rate", x = "Year") +
  theme(legend.position = "none")
```

We can notice that the model fits the data well, with the predicted values closely following the observed values, with mod3 clearly overfitting the data.

Let's check the residuals of mod2:

```
meningitis %>%
  # calculate the residuals to see how well the model fits the data
  mutate(residuals = deaths - predicted_mod2) %>%
  select(deaths, predicted_mod2, residuals) %>%
```

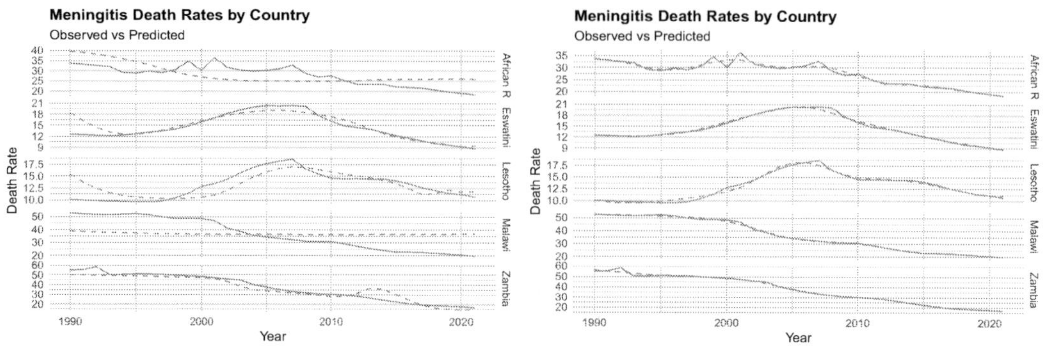

(a) Observed vs Predicted - Mod2 **(b)** Observed vs Predicted - Mod3

Figure 11.5 Meningitis Death Rates by Country. The dashed line represents the predicted values from the model, while the solid lines represent the observed values.

```
  head()
#> # A tibble: 6 x 3
#>   deaths predicted_mod2 residuals
#>    <dbl>       <dbl[1d]> <dbl[1d]>
#> 1   12.6            18.3     -5.76
#> 2   52.7            38.8     13.9
#> 3   54.9            50.3      4.62
#> 4   10.1            15.4     -5.31
#> 5   33.7            39.5     -5.83
#> 6   55.4            50.0      5.40
```

The residuals column represents the difference between the observed and predicted values. A positive residual indicates that the model underestimates the number of deaths, while a negative residual indicates an overestimate.

To evaluate model performance, we can visualize the residuals against the predicted values. In this plot, the dashed line marks the zero-residual baseline. Points above the line correspond to underestimation, and those below represent overestimation. The fact that most points cluster closely around the zero line suggests that the model provides a reasonably good fit to the data.

```
meningitis %>%
  mutate(residuals = deaths - predicted_mod2) %>%
  ggplot(aes(x = predicted_mod2, y = residuals)) +
  geom_point() +
  geom_hline(yintercept = 0, linetype = "dashed") +
  facet_grid(location ~ ., scale = "free") +
  labs(title = "Residuals vs Predicted",
       x = "Predicted Values", y = "Residuals") +
  theme(legend.position = "none")

meningitis %>%
  mutate(residuals = deaths - predicted_mod2) %>%
  ggplot(aes(sample = residuals)) +
```

```
  geom_qq() +
  geom_qq_line() +
  facet_grid(location ~ ., scale = "free") +
  labs(title = "QQ-plot of the residuals",
       x = "Theoretical Quantiles", y = "Sample Quantiles") +
  theme(legend.position = "none")
```

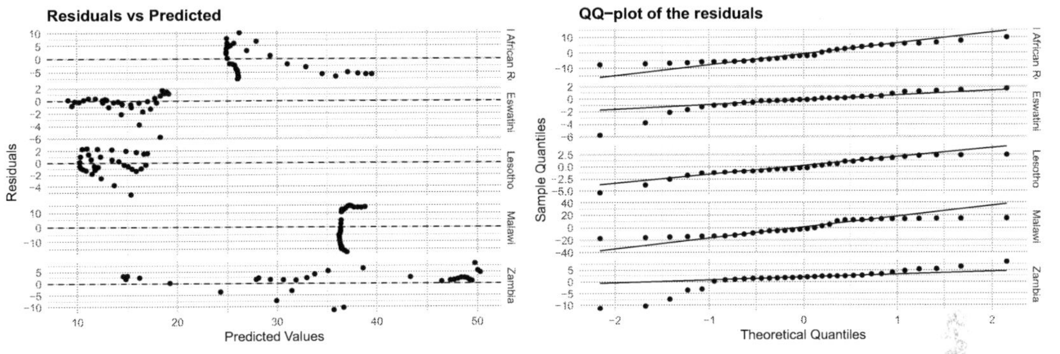

(a) Residuals vs Predicted

(b) QQ-plot of the residuals

Figure 11.6 Residuals vs Predicted

Heteroskedasticity is a common problem in regression analysis, and it occurs when the variance of the residuals is not constant across all levels of the predictor variables. This can lead to biased estimates of the coefficients and incorrect conclusions about the significance of the predictors. In this case, we can see that the residuals are not evenly distributed around zero, indicating that there may be some **heteroskedasticity** in the data.

11.1.1.1 Exercise: One Country Focus

Improve the model specifically for Lesotho by refining the smooth terms and including year as a covariate to capture temporal patterns:

1. Subset the data to include only observations from Lesotho
2. Adjust the smooth functions as needed for a better fit
3. Refit the model incorporating the year variable
4. Perform cross-validation by splitting the data into training and test sets, and simulate model performance across multiple samples

Evaluate the model fit and compare it to previous results. Consider visualizing the residuals and predicted values for further insight.

```
Lesotho_data <- meningitis %>%
  filter(location == "Lesotho")

Lesotho_data$predicted_mod2 <- predict(mod2, newdata = Lesotho_data)
```

```
Lesotho_data %>%
  ggplot() +
  geom_point(aes(year, deaths)) +
```

```
  geom_line(aes(year, predicted_mod2),
            linetype = "dashed") +
  labs(title = "Lesotho_data: Observed vs. Predicted",
       x = "Time(Year)", y = "Death Rates")

Lesotho_data %>%
  ggplot(aes(x = year, y = deaths)) +
  geom_point() +
  geom_line(aes(year, predicted_mod2),
            linetype = "dashed") +
  geom_segment(aes(xend = year,
                   yend = predicted_mod2),
               linewidth = 0.1) +
  labs(title = "Lesotho: Observed vs. Predicted",
       subtitle = "Segments represent the residuals",
       x = "Time(Year)", y = "Death Rates")
```

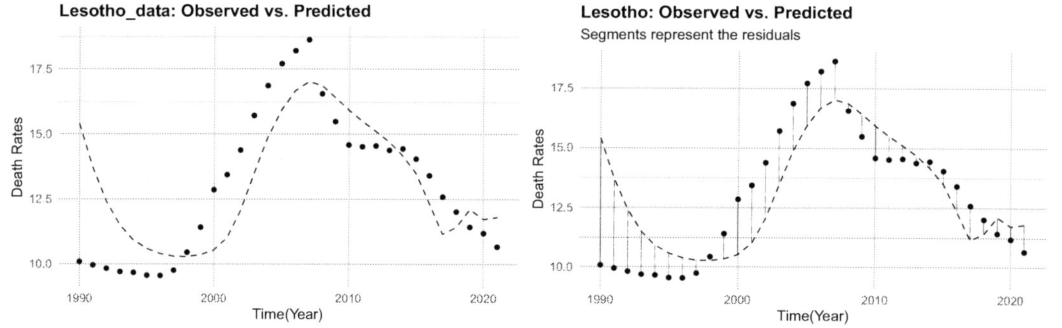

(a) Observed vs Predicted - Mod2 **(b)** Observed vs Predicted - Mod3

Figure 11.7 Lesotho Death Rates by Country. The dashed line represents the predicted values from the model, while the solid lines represent the observed values.

11.1.2 Example: Ischemic Stroke Decision Tree

In this example we have a look at how to visualise the results of a decision tree model for predicting Ischemic Stroke.

Load necessary libraries and the data for the Ischemic Stroke.[3]

```
# Ischemic Stroke decision tree
library(tidymodels)
library(rpart)
library(rpart.plot)
```

[3]"FES/Data_Sets/Ischemic_Stroke at Master · Topepo/FES," n.d., https://github.com/topepo/FES/tree/master/Data_Sets/Ischemic_Stroke.

Data are already split into training and test sets, we will combine them for the analysis. The `stroke_train` and `stroke_test` datasets contain 89, 37 observations respectively and 29 variables. Within the variables we have information on volume, proportion, area, thickness of the arterial wall, among others. The target variable is `Stroke`, which indicates whether the patient has had a stroke or not.[4]

We select the variables of interest for the analysis with `any_of()`, a function to select the variables based on their names.

`?any_of()` for more infromation about the function.

```
selected_train <- stroke_train %>%
  dplyr::select(any_of(VC_preds), Stroke)
```

To check which columns in `stroke_train` dataset were not selected:

```
setdiff(names(stroke_train), names(selected_train))
#> [1] "NASCET"                   "age"
#> [3] "sex"                      "SmokingHistory"
#> [5] "AtrialFibrillation"       "CoronaryArteryDisease"
#> [7] "DiabetesHistory"          "HypercholesterolemiaHistory"
#> [9] "HypertensionHistory"
```

Set up the recipe for the data with the `recipe()` function from the `tidymodels` package. We will use the `step_corr()` function to remove highly correlated predictors, `step_center()` and `step_scale()` to standardise the predictors, `step_YeoJohnson()` to transform the predictors, and `step_zv()` to remove zero variance predictors.

```
is_recipe <- recipe(Stroke ~ ., data = selected_train) %>%
  #step_interact(int_form)  %>%
  step_corr(all_predictors(), threshold = 0.75) %>%
  step_center(all_predictors()) %>%
  step_scale(all_predictors()) %>%
  step_YeoJohnson(all_predictors()) %>%
  step_zv(all_predictors())

is_recipe %>%
  prep() %>%
  bake(new_data=NULL) %>%
  select(1:5) %>%
  head(5)
#> # A tibble: 5 x 5
#>   CALCVolProp MATXVol MATXVolProp MaxCALCAreaProp MaxDilationByArea
#>         <dbl>   <dbl>       <dbl>           <dbl>             <dbl>
#> 1      -0.143  0.106       -0.161          0.0541            0.0249
#> 2      -1.35  -0.0530       0.858         -0.931            -0.748
#> 3      -0.784  1.03         0.218          0.284            -0.320
#> 4       1.06   0.587       -0.144          1.05              0.423
#> 5      -0.708 -0.107       -0.307         -0.203            -0.738
```

[4] Max Kuhn Johnson and Kjell, *2 Illustrative Example: Predicting Risk of Ischemic Stroke | Feature Engineering and Selection: A Practical Approach for Predictive Models*, n.d., https://bookdown.org/max/FES/stroke-tour.html.

Set up the decision tree model with the `decision_tree()` function from the `tidymodels` package. We will use the `rpart` engine for the decision tree model and set the mode to classification.

```
class_tree_spec <- decision_tree() %>%
  set_engine("rpart") %>%
  set_mode("classification")
```

Finally, we will fit the model with the `fit()` function from the `tidymodels` package and visualise the results with the `rpart.plot` package.

```
is_wfl <- workflow() %>%
  add_model(class_tree_spec) %>%
  add_recipe(is_recipe)

is_dt_fit_wfl <- is_wfl %>%
  fit(data = selected_train,
      control = control_workflow())

is_dt_fit_wfl%>%
  extract_fit_engine() %>%
  rpart.plot::rpart.plot(roundint = FALSE)
```

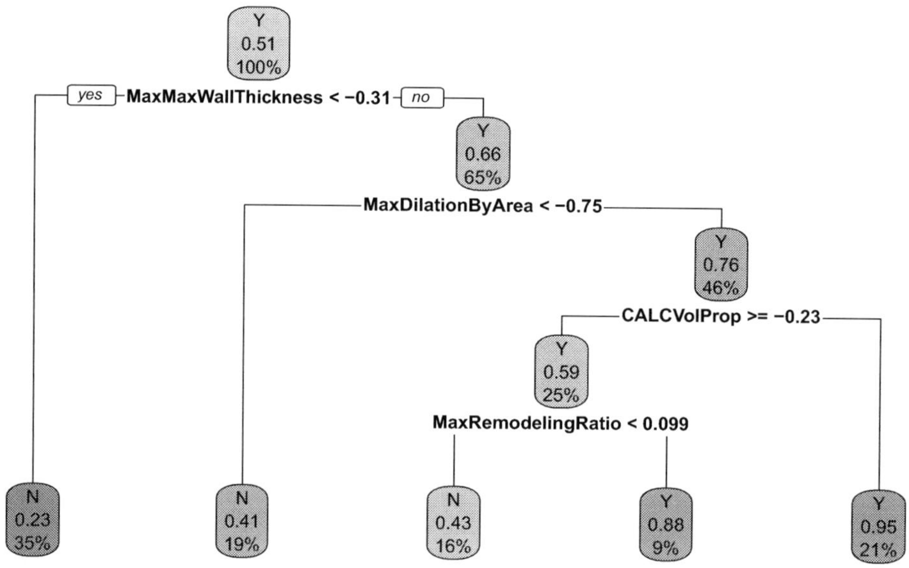

Figure 11.8 Decision Tree for Ischemic Stroke

In this plot, the decision tree is visualised with the `rpart.plot` and the information released evidences the importance of some specific predictors, such as max wall thickness, max dilatation by area, volume proportion, and max remodelling ratio. The decision tree is a useful tool for visualising the results of the model and understanding the relationships between the predictors and the target variable.

The interpretation of the decision tree is straightforward: each node represents a decision based on the value of a predictor, and the leaves represent the final classification. The tree can be pruned to reduce its complexity and improve its interpretability. The decision tree can be used to make predictions on new data by following the path from the root to a leaf node based on the values of the predictors.

11.1.3 Example: Ischemic Stroke Classification

In this second example we will demonstrate **classification** (stroke vs. no stroke) using patient and plaque imaging features, and visualise model insights for stakeholder communication.

The objective is to visualise how well the model predict whether a patient experienced a stroke (Stroke) based on imaging features (e.g., MaxStenosisByArea, CALCVolProp) and risk factors (e.g., age, DiabetesHistory).

Visualise:

- Variable importance
- Prediction performance (e.g., ROC curve)
- Partial dependence of key features

Load necessary libraries, and fit a **random forest** model to the data with the `rand_forest()` function from the `{tidymodels}` package. We will use the `ranger` engine for the random forest model and set the mode to classification.

```
library(tidyverse)
library(tidymodels)
library(vip)
library(DALEXtra)
library(pROC)
```

The model specify the number of trees to grow, the minimum number of observations in a node before a split is attempted, and the maximum depth of the tree. The `set_engine()` function specifies the engine to use for the model, in this case `ranger`, and the `set_mode()` function specifies the mode of the model, in this case classification.

```
rf_spec <- rand_forest(trees = 500, min_n = 5) %>%
  set_engine("ranger", importance = "impurity") %>%
  set_mode("classification")

rf_wf <- workflow() %>%
  add_formula(Stroke ~ .) %>%
  add_model(rf_spec)

rf_fit <- rf_wf %>% fit(data = stroke_train)
```

11.1.3.1 Variable Importance

The object `rf_fit` contains the fitted model. We can extract the the model specification and use the `vip()` function to visualise what are the predictors that most influence the model. The `vip()` function creates a variable importance plot, which shows the importance of each predictor in the model. The importance is calculated based on the **Mean Decrease in Impurity (MDI)** for each predictor.

```
rf_fit %>%
  extract_fit_parsnip() %>%
  vip::vip(num_features = 10)
```

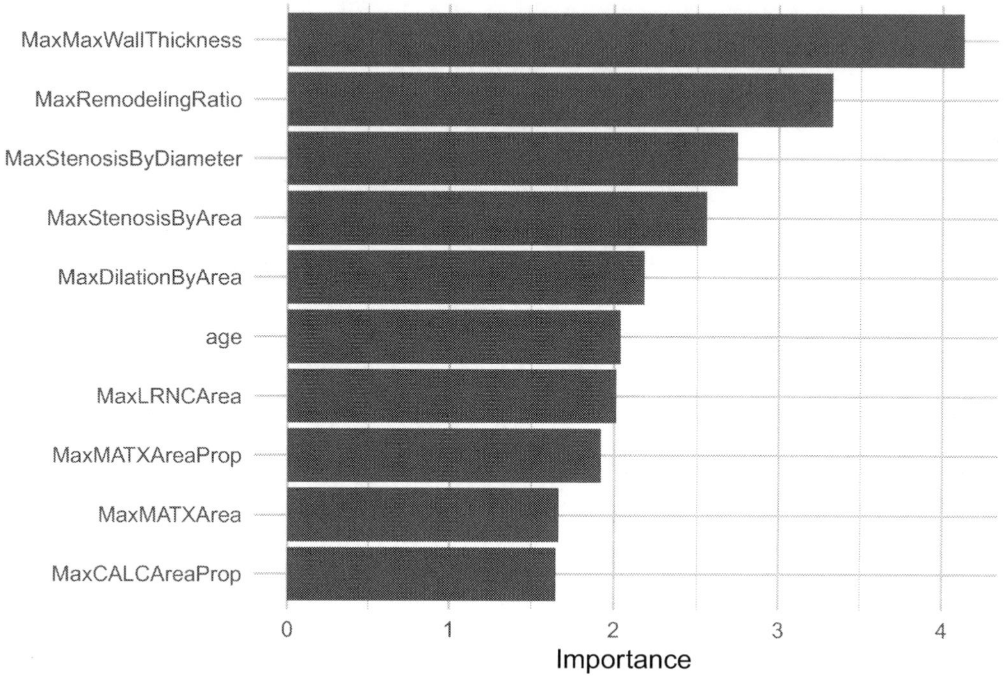

Figure 11.9 Variable Importance for Ischemic Stroke

We can conclude that for this data set, the most important predictors are `MaxStenosisByArea`, `CALCVolProp`, `MaxWallThickness`, and `MaxRemodellingRatio`.

Next step is to evaluate the model performance. We will use the `predict()` function to make predictions on the test data set (`stroke_test`) and calculate the **accuracy** of the model.

```
set.seed(05122025)
rf_preds <- predict(rf_fit, stroke_test,
                    type = "prob") %>%
  bind_cols(predict(rf_fit, stroke_test)) %>%
  bind_cols(stroke_test %>% select(Stroke))

rf_preds %>% head()
#> # A tibble: 6 x 4
#>   .pred_N .pred_Y .pred_class Stroke
#>     <dbl>   <dbl> <fct>       <fct>
#> 1   0.507   0.493 N           N
#> 2   0.395   0.605 Y           Y
#> 3   0.884   0.116 N           Y
#> 4   0.846   0.154 N           N
#> 5   0.839   0.161 N           N
```

```
#> 6    0.683    0.317 N            N
```

11.1.3.2 Accuracy

The accuracy of the model is calculated as the proportion of correct predictions. The `accuracy()` function from the `yardstick` package calculates the accuracy of the model based on the predicted and observed values.

```
rf_preds %>%
  accuracy(truth = Stroke, .pred_class)
#> # A tibble: 1 x 3
#>   .metric  .estimator .estimate
#>   <chr>    <chr>          <dbl>
#> 1 accuracy binary         0.703
```

In this case, the accuracy of the model is 0.70, which means that the model correctly predicts whether a patient experienced a stroke or not 70% of the time. The accuracy is calculated as the number of correct predictions divided by the total number of predictions.

11.1.3.3 ROC Curve

The **Receiver Operating Characteristic (ROC)** curve is a graphical representation of the performance of a binary classifier system as its discrimination threshold is varied. The ROC curve plots the true positive rate (TPR) against the false positive rate (FPR) at various threshold settings.

We can use the `roc_curve()` function from the `yardstick` package to calculate the ROC curve and the area under the curve (AUC). The `roc_curve` object contains the specificity and sensitivity values for each threshold, which can be used to calculate the **AUC**.

```
roc_curve <- yardstick::roc_curve(data = rf_preds,
                                  truth = Stroke, .pred_N)
roc_curve %>% head()
#> # A tibble: 6 x 3
#>   .threshold specificity sensitivity
#>        <dbl>       <dbl>       <dbl>
#> 1  -Inf           0                1
#> 2     0.0863      0                1
#> 3     0.226       0.0526           1
#> 4     0.284       0.105            1
#> 5     0.309       0.158            1
#> 6     0.319       0.211            1
```

The relationship between the **True Positive Rate (TPR)** and **False Positive Rate (FPR)** is visualised in the ROC curve. The area under the curve (AUC) is a measure of the model's performance, with values closer to 1 indicating better performance. The **specificity** and **sensitivity** of the model indicate the proportion of true positives and true negatives, respectively, and we can use the `autoplot()` function to visualise the ROC curve.

```
autoplot(roc_curve)
```

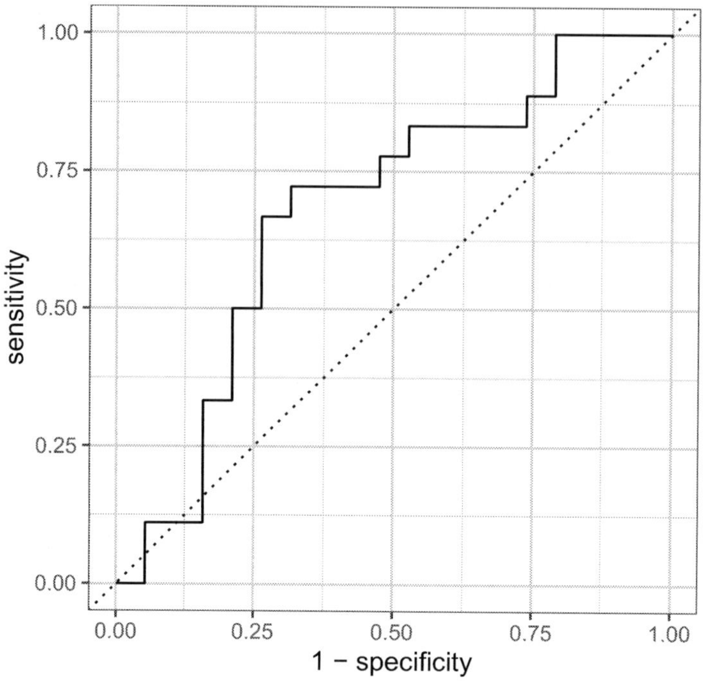

Figure 11.10 ROC Curve for Ischemic Stroke

Another way to extract the ROC curve is to use the `pROC` package and the `roc()` function. The `roc()` function takes the observed values and the predicted probabilities as arguments and returns an object containing the ROC curve.

```
roc_obj <- pROC::roc(rf_preds$Stroke,
                     rf_preds$.pred_N)
roc_obj %>%
  pROC::auc() %>%
  round(2)
#> [1] 0.68
```

The `roc_obj` object provides information about the area under the ROC curve. In this case we have an AUC is 0.68. The AUC is a measure of the model's performance, values closer to 1 indicate better performance.

11.1.3.4 Partial Dependence

> "How does the prediction change when a specific feature changes, holding all others constant?"

Finally, we attempt an explanation of the model using `DALEX` and `DALEXtra` packages, and some specific functions, such as: `explain_tidymodels()` and `model_profile()`.

```
explainer_rf <-
  DALEXtra::explain_tidymodels(rf_fit,
                               data = select(stroke_train, -Stroke),
                               y = stroke_train$Stroke)
```

The `explainer_rf` object contains the model, the data, and the target variable and it will be used to create the partial dependence plot with the `model_profile()` function.

A **Partial Dependence Plot (PDP)** is a tool used in machine learning to help interpret black-box models like random forests. It shows the marginal effect of one (or two) features on the predicted outcome, while averaging out the influence of all other features.

In this case we specify the `MaxStenosisByArea` variable, to see how changes in `MaxStenosisByArea` influence the model's predicted outcome, on average. A higher value of MaxStenosisByArea indicates more severe arterial narrowing, which is a risk factor for stroke or heart attack.

```
DALEX::model_profile(explainer_rf,
                     variables = "MaxStenosisByArea") %>%
  plot() +
  labs(
    title = "Partial Dependence Plot for Ischemic Stroke",
    subtitle = "",
    x = "Value",
    y = "AVG Prediction") +
  theme_minimal()
```

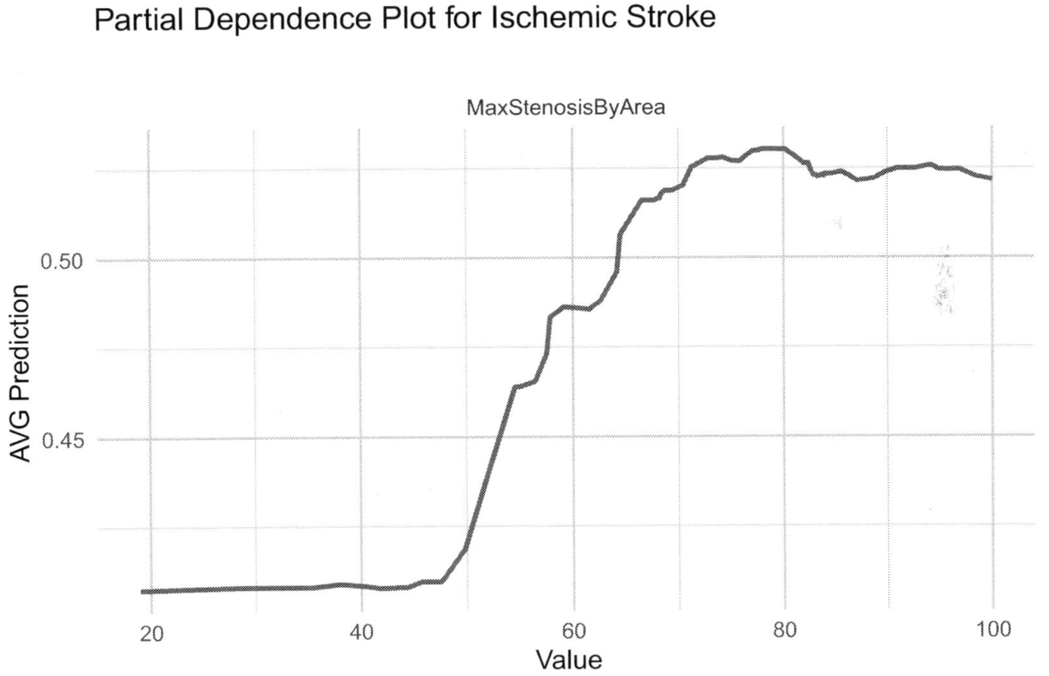

Figure 11.11 Partial Dependence Plot for Ischemic Stroke: MaxStenosisByArea (arterial narrowing)

The plot shows the partial dependence of the `MaxStenosisByArea` variable on the predicted probability of having a stroke. The results indicate that `MaxStenosisByArea` has a positive influence on stroke risk, though this effect plateaus beyond a certain threshold.

11.2 Summary

In this chapter, we have learned how to visualise the results of a model. There are several important considerations when visualising the results of a model, and differences might arise due to the type of model used. We have seen how to use several packages and functions, such as `ggplot2`, `vip`, `pROC`, and `DALEX` to visualise the results of a model. We have also seen how to interpret the results of a model and how to communicate them effectively. The examples provided in this chapter demonstrate how to use visualisation techniques to enhance decision-making and communicate findings to various stakeholders.

12

Spatial Data Modelling and Visualisation

Learning Objectives

- Learn how to model and visualise spatial data
- Understand the concepts of spatial data, spatial data models, and spatial models
- Create maps, simulate infections, and predict the spatial distribution of phenomena

In the previous chapters, we explored the fundamentals of **data visualisation** with various techniques for creating static and interactive plots. In this chapter, we will learn how to model and visualise **spatial data**, which involves analysing and representing data with spatial components. We will explore the concepts of spatial data, spatial data models, and **spatial models**, and learn how to create maps, simulate infections, and predict the spatial distribution of phenomena such as disease spread. By combining spatial data with machine learning techniques, we can model the spatial dynamics of disease transmission and assess the risks associated with the spread of infections. We will use various packages such as `sf`, `ggplot2`, and `gstat` to create spatial models and visualisations, and gain insights into the spatial distribution of infections in a specific region.

12.1 Spatial Data, Spatial Data Models, and Spatial Models

Understanding the spatial distribution of phenomena such as disease spread, land cover changes, or climate patterns requires the use of spatial data and spatial models. These tools are essential for analysing and predicting spatial processes and for informing data-driven decisions in public health, environmental management, and urban planning.

A notable example is the **Ebola Virus Disease outbreak in West Africa (2014–2016)**. The virus spread across countries like Guinea, Liberia, and Sierra Leone, driven by factors such as population density, healthcare infrastructure, and human mobility. By analysing spatial data on cases, fatalities, and healthcare facilities and applying spatial models to simulate the virus's spread, researchers gained valuable insights into the dynamics of the outbreak. This analysis helped identify high-risk areas for targeted interventions.[1]

But what exactly distinguishes spatial data, spatial data models, and spatial models?

- **Spatial Data**: This refers to data that includes geographic coordinates, addresses, or boundaries, representing the physical location of objects or events. Spatial data can be stored in two main formats: vector and raster. Vector data models use geometric shapes

[1]Null null, "Ebola Virus Disease in West Africa — the First 9 Months of the Epidemic and Forward Projections," *New England Journal of Medicine* 371, no. 16 (October 16, 2014): 1481–95, doi:10.1056/NEJMoa1411100.

DOI: 10.1201/9781032625935-12

(points, lines, polygons) to represent features such as roads, cities, and boundaries. Raster data models, on the other hand, use a grid of cells or pixels, each with a value representing a variable like temperature, land cover, or elevation.
- **Spatial Data Models**: These are frameworks for organizing and representing spatial data. They provide the structure for connecting real-world phenomena with their digital representation through algorithms and spatial primitives (like spatial relationships and topology). Spatial data models form the foundation for managing and processing spatial information, enabling meaningful analysis and visualization.
- **Spatial Models**: Unlike spatial data models, which organize data, spatial models simulate dynamic spatial processes—phenomena that change over time. Examples include the spread of infectious diseases, flood development, or land use changes. Spatial models are crucial for understanding and forecasting the evolution of spatial phenomena, allowing researchers and decision-makers to plan interventions and management strategies effectively.

For further information on spatial data models and spatial process models, refer to the **ArcGIS** documentation for guidance on solving spatial problems and the **Esri** blog for in-depth discussions on spatial analysis. Additionally, R-Spatial.org offers a wealth of resources on spatial data analysis, including tutorials and the latest developments in the field.

12.2 Making a Map

To learn how to make a map we first need spatial data. There are various sources and packages that provide spatial data for different regions and purposes. One such package is `{rnaturalearth}`, this package contains various types of boundaries of countries in the world. For more information type `?rnaturalearth`. In particular, we use the `ne_countries()` function to get the boundaries of Africa, with the option `returnclass = "sf"` to return the data as **simple features**.

```
library(tidyverse)
library(sf)
library(rnaturalearth)

africa <- ne_countries(continent = "Africa",
                       returnclass = "sf")
```

A simple feature object is a type of spatial data that contains the geometry of the spatial features (e.g., points, lines, polygons) and additional attributes such as the name of the country, population, and other information.

This is a simple map of Africa, but we can make it more interesting by adding some colours to the countries. A better resolution of the colored map can be found in the online version of the book.

```
ggplot(data = africa) +
  geom_sf() +
  coord_sf()
# Africa with colours
ggplot(data = africa) +
  geom_sf(aes(fill=name),
          color= "white",
```

```
         linewidth = 1,
         show.legend = F) +
  coord_sf()
```

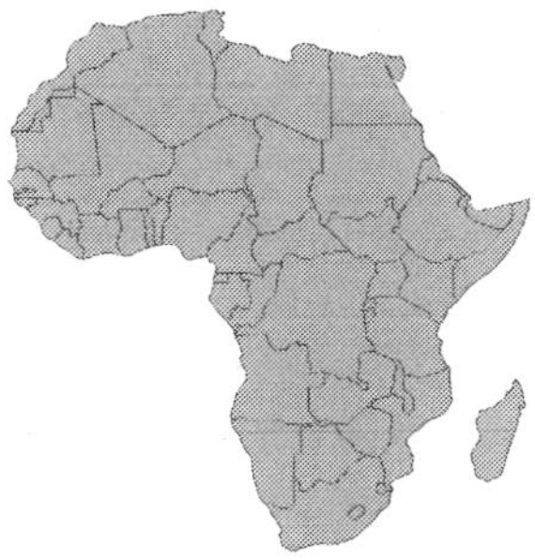

(a) Map of Africa

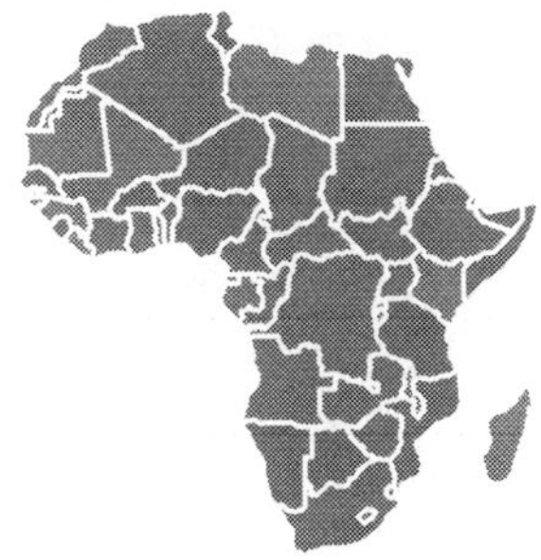

(b) Map of Africa with colors

Figure 12.1 Map of Africa

12.3 Coordinate Reference System (CRS)

A **Coordinate Reference System (CRS)** is a standardised way of defining the spatial location of features on the Earth's surface. It uses a set of coordinates to represent the position of points, lines, and polygons in space. There are different types of CRS, such as **geographic** and **projected** CRS, which are used to represent the Earth's surface in different ways. Geographic CRS (**LatLong**) represents locations on a curved surface using latitude and longitude for global mapping, while projected CRS or **Universal Transverse Mercator (UTM)** projects the curved Earth onto a flat map, using metres for precise mapping. In particular, the UTM system provides the distance in metres from the equator and the central meridian of a specific zone.

We use the `{sf}` package to define and transform CRS. The `st_crs()` function allows you to retrieve the CRS of a spatial object, while the `st_transform()` function allows you to transform the coordinates of a spatial object to a different CRS.

```
africa_crs <- st_crs(africa)
africa_crs
#> Coordinate Reference System:
#>   User input: WGS 84
#>   wkt:
#> GEOGCRS["WGS 84",
#>     DATUM["World Geodetic System 1984",
#>         ELLIPSOID["WGS 84",6378137,298.257223563,
#>             LENGTHUNIT["metre",1]]],
#>     PRIMEM["Greenwich",0,
#>         ANGLEUNIT["degree",0.0174532925199433]],
#>     CS[ellipsoidal,2],
#>         AXIS["latitude",north,
```

```
#>             ORDER[1],
#>             ANGLEUNIT["degree",0.0174532925199433]],
#>         AXIS["longitude",east,
#>             ORDER[2],
#>             ANGLEUNIT["degree",0.0174532925199433]],
#>     ID["EPSG",4326]]
```

For example, the CRS of the Africa map is **WGS 84** or *World Geodetic System 1984* which is a reference system for the Earth's surface that defines origin and orientation of the coordinate axes, called a **datum** (a fact known from direct observation). The **EPSG** is a structured dataset of CRS and Coordinate Transformations, it was originally compiled by the, now defunct, European Petroleum Survey Group[2]. The EPSG code for WGS 84 is 4326.

12.4 Example: Simulation of Infections in Central African Rep.

Synthetic data are created for the Central African Republic. The simulation of the number of infected individuals, their location, and temperature levels are obtained with random numbers generating functions from the `{stats}` package, which is a base package.

The Central African Rep. is a landlocked country in Central Africa, with a population of approximately 5 million people. The country is known for its diverse wildlife and natural resources, and has faced challenges such as political instability and armed conflict.

```
ctr_africa <- africa %>%
  filter(name == "Central African Rep.")
```

12.4.1 Bounding Box

We can use the `st_bbox()` function to retrieve the **bounding box** of the `ctr_africa` object, as a matrix with the minimum and maximum values of the coordinates. A bounding box is a rectangular area defined by two points: the lower-left corner (minimum values of the coordinates) and the upper-right corner (maximum values of the coordinates). It provides a quick way to determine the spatial extent of a region and is often used in spatial analysis to define the boundaries of a study area.

```
bbox <- ctr_africa %>% st_bbox()

bbox
#>     xmin     ymin     xmax     ymax
#> 14.45941  2.26764 27.37423 11.14240
```

12.4.2 Spatial Coordinates

The `st_coordinates()` function allows to extract the coordinates from a geometry vector and release a matrix with 5 columns, where the first two columns are the longitude (X) and latitude (Y), and the other are indexes to group the coordinates into polygons.

[2]https://www.nceas.ucsb.edu/sites/default/files/2020-04/OverviewCoordinateReferenceSystems.pdf

The `as.data.frame()` function converts the matrix to a data frame, and the `dplyr::select()` function selects the longitude and latitude columns. The `summary()` function provides a summary of the data frame, including the mean, median, and quartiles of the longitude and latitude values.

```
ctr_africa_coords <- ctr_africa %>%
  sf::st_coordinates() %>%
  as.data.frame() %>%
  dplyr::select(X, Y)

ctr_africa_coords %>%
  summary()
#>        X                Y
#>  Min.   :14.46   Min.   : 2.268
#>  1st Qu.:16.58   1st Qu.: 4.648
#>  Median :20.96   Median : 5.354
#>  Mean   :20.70   Mean   : 6.294
#>  3rd Qu.:24.26   3rd Qu.: 8.145
#>  Max.   :27.37   Max.   :11.142
```

Synthetic data are created as an image of the spread of infections observed in Central Africa on a specific point in time. Data are generated using random numbers for the number of infected individuals, their location, and temperature levels. The temperature levels consider a min of 20.3 degrees Celsius (69 degrees Fahrenheit), a maximum of 29.2 °C (85 °F), and a daily average of 24.7 °C (76 °F).

The synthetic data are created using the `rbinom()`, `rnorm()`, and `rpois()` functions from the `{stats}` package. Data are generated for 100 locations in Central Africa, with 70% of the locations infected and 30% non-infected. The latitude and longitude values are generated using the `rnorm()` function with mean values of 6.294 and 20.70, respectively. The number of infected individuals is generated using the `rpois()` function with a mean value of 10, and the temperature levels are generated using the `rnorm()` function with a mean value of 25.

Set the number of points:

```
num_points <- 100
```

12.4.3 Data Simulation

```
set.seed(21082024) # set seed for reproducibility
# simulate the presence of infection
# 1 = "infected" and 0 = "non_infected"
longitude <- rnorm(n = num_points, mean = 20.70, sd = 1)
latitude <-  rnorm(n = num_points, mean = 6.294, sd = 1)
presence <- rbinom(100, 1, prob = 0.3)
cases <- ifelse(presence == 1,
                rpois(n = num_points*0.7, lambda = 10), 0)
temperature <- rnorm(n = num_points,
                     mean = 24.7,
                     sd = (29.2 - 20.3) / 4)

# build a dataframe
```

```
df <- data.frame(longitude, latitude,
                 presence, cases, temperature)

head(df)
#>   longitude latitude presence cases temperature
#> 1  21.09134 6.052162        0     0    20.58159
#> 2  22.25082 7.814450        0     0    29.77619
#> 3  21.52356 6.101959        0     0    23.97023
#> 4  19.76787 6.004291        0     0    28.53059
#> 5  21.25535 5.239799        0     0    22.16691
#> 6  20.10175 7.256303        0     0    20.66836
```

The `str()` function allows to inspect the structure of the data frame, showing the type of each column and the first few rows of the data frame.

```
df %>%
  filter(presence == 1) %>%
  head() %>%
  str()
#> 'data.frame':    6 obs. of  5 variables:
#>  $ longitude  : num  18.8 20.3 22.9 20 20.1 ...
#>  $ latitude   : num  4.54 5.09 6.21 8.42 7.63 ...
#>  $ presence   : int  1 1 1 1 1 1
#>  $ cases      : num  13 10 11 13 9 9
#>  $ temperature: num  24 27.3 25.2 25.1 24.2 ...
```

```
ggplot() +
  geom_sf(data = africa) +
  geom_sf(data = ctr_africa, fill = "brown") +
  labs(title = "Map of Africa and Central African Rep.")

ggplot() +
  geom_sf(data = africa) +
  geom_sf(data = ctr_africa,
          fill = alpha("brown", alpha = 0.2)) +
  geom_point(data = df,
             aes(x = longitude, y = latitude,
                 color = factor(presence)),
             shape = ".") +
  labs(title = "Synthetic Data Visualisation",
       color = "Infection Status") +
  theme(legend.position = "top")
```

12.4.4 Correlation between Response and Predictor

The correlation coefficient between the number of infected individuals and the temperature can be calculated using the `cor()` function with the method set to "pearson". This will provide a measure of the strength and direction of the linear relationship between the two variables. A correlation coefficient close to 1 indicates a strong positive linear relationship, while a coefficient close to -1 indicates a strong negative linear relationship. A coefficient close to 0 indicates no significant linear relationship between the variables.

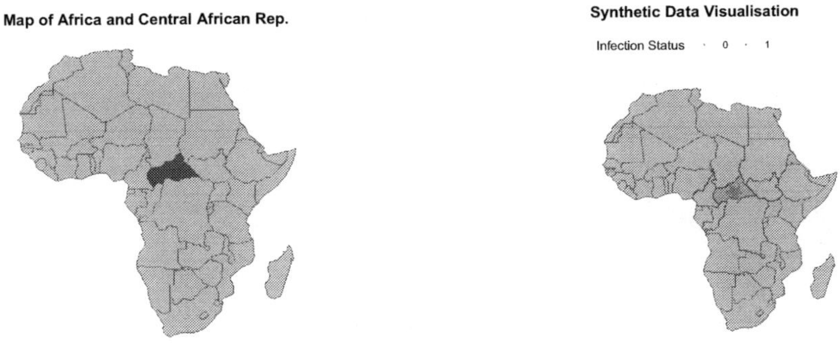

(a) Map of Africa and Central African Rep.

(b) Map of Central African Rep. Simulation of Infections

Figure 12.2 Map of Africa

```
cor(df$cases, df$temperature, method = "pearson")
#> [1] -0.05243272
```

The correlation coefficient is -0.052, suggesting that there is a weak negative linear relationship between the number of infected individuals and the temperature. This indicates that as the temperature increases, the number of infected individuals decreases slightly, but the relationship is not significant.

12.4.5 Histogram and Scatter Plot

To visualise the distribution of the presence of infection in Central Africa, we can create a histogram of the presence variable using the `geom_bar()` function from the `{ggplot2}` package. The histogram shows the frequency of infected and non-infected locations in Central Africa, with the x-axis representing the presence of infection and the y-axis representing the count of locations.

```
ggplot(data = df,
       aes(x = factor(presence))) +
  geom_bar() +
  labs(title = "Histogram of Presence of Infection",
       x = "Presence",
       y = "Count") +
  theme_minimal()

ggplot(data = df %>% filter(presence== 1),
       aes(x = temperature, y = cases)) +
  geom_point() +
  geom_smooth() +
  labs(title = "Infected Individuals based on Temperature",
       x = "Temperature",
       y = "Number of Infected Individuals") +
  theme_minimal()
```

The scatter plot shows the temperature on the x-axis and the number of infected individuals on the y-axis, with each point representing an infected location in Central Africa. The

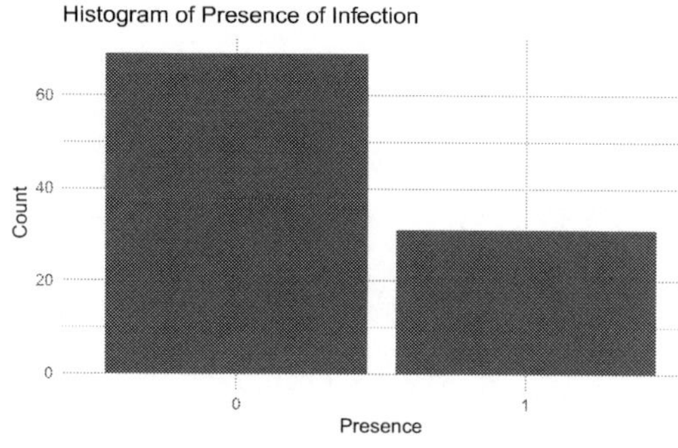

(a) Histogram of Presence of Infection in Central African Rep.

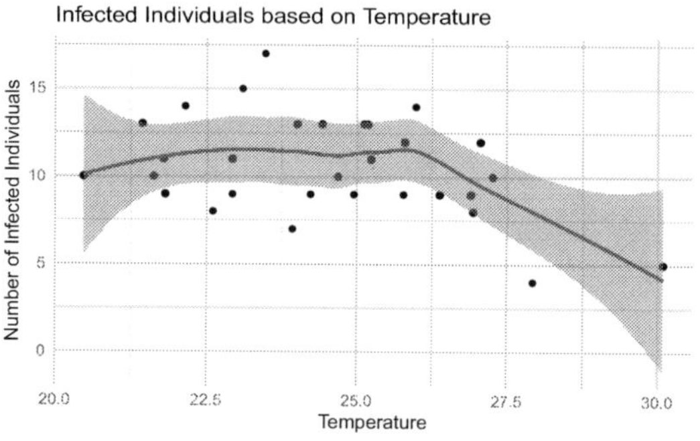

(b) Scatter Plot of Temperature and Infections

Figure 12.3 Histogram of Presence of Infection in Central African Rep.

`geom_point()` function adds the points to the plot, while the `geom_smooth()` function fits a smooth curve to the data, showing the trend between independent and dependent variables, temperature and the number of infected individuals, respectively. The `labs()` function adds titles and labels to the plot, specifying the title, x-axis label, and y-axis label. The `theme_minimal()` function sets the plot theme to a minimal style.

12.4.6 Grid of Points

To create a **grid of points** we transform the `df` data as a simple features object with the `st_as_sf()` function from the `{sf}` package, specifying the longitude and latitude columns as the coordinates and the CRS as 4326[3]. Then, intersect the data with `st_intersection(ctr_africa)` to keep only the points within the country. Finally, select the relevant columns for the analysis.

```
df_sf <- df %>%
  st_as_sf(coords = c("longitude","latitude"),
           # or use crs = 4326
           crs = "+proj=longlat +datum=WGS84") %>%
  st_intersection(ctr_africa) %>%
  st_make_valid()

grid <- df_sf %>%
  st_bbox() %>%
  st_as_sfc() %>%
  st_make_grid(what = "centers",
               cellsize = .2,
               square = F)
```

To generate the grid of points to cover all Central African Republic we can also use the `expand_grid()` function from the `{tidyr}` package, which generates a series of points within specified bounding box, and the point in polygon (`PtInPoly()`) function from the `{DescTools}` package. The `pip` vector contains the information if the point is inside the polygon or not.

[3]More information on the coordinate reference system is here: https://epsg.io/.

```
library(DescTools)
set.seed(240724) # set seed for reproducibility
bbox_grid <- expand_grid(x = seq(from = bbox$xmin,
                                 to = bbox$xmax,
                                 length.out = 100),
                         y = seq(from = bbox$ymin,
                                 to = bbox$ymax,
                                 length.out = 100))

ctr_africa_grid_full <- data.frame(PtInPoly(bbox_grid,
                                            ctr_africa_coords))

ctr_africa_grid_full %>% head()
#>          x        y pip
#> 1 14.45941 2.267640   0
#> 2 14.45941 2.357284   0
#> 3 14.45941 2.446928   0
#> 4 14.45941 2.536572   0
#> 5 14.45941 2.626216   0
#> 6 14.45941 2.715860   0
```

Mapping the grid of points on the map of the Central African Republic, we can visualise the spatial distribution of infected locations.

```
# Window Grid
ggplot() +
  geom_sf(data = ctr_africa)+
  geom_sf(data = grid, shape = ".") +
  geom_sf(data = df_sf %>% filter(presence == 1),
          aes(fill = presence),
          shape = 21, stroke = 0.3) +
  coord_sf() +
  labs(title = "Window Grid") +
  theme(legend.position = "right")

# Central Africa Grid
ggplot(data = ctr_africa_grid_full) +
  geom_point(aes(x, y, color = factor(pip)), shape = ".") +
  geom_sf(data = df_sf %>% filter(presence == 1),
          aes(fill = presence),
          shape = 21, stroke = 0.3,
          show.legend = F,) +
  coord_sf() +
  scale_color_manual(values = c("1" = "grey20", "0" = "grey")) +
  labs(title = "Grid Map",
       color = "PIP") +
  theme(legend.position = "top")
```

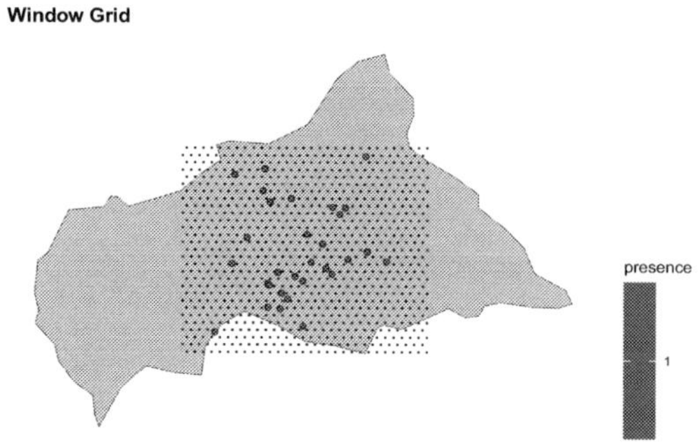

(a) Map of Central African Rep. with a Window Grid

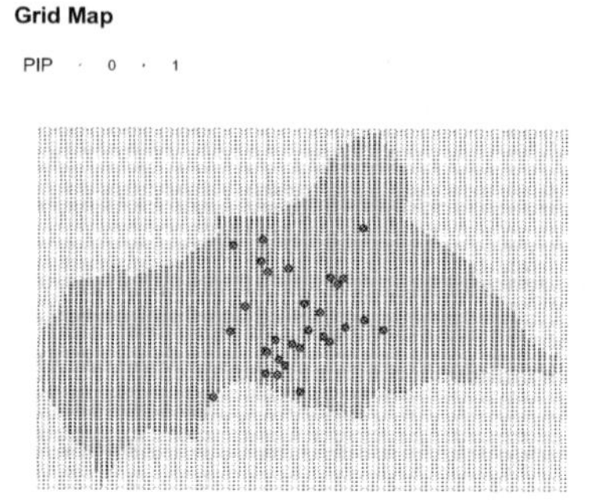

(b) Grid Map of Central African Rep.

Figure 12.4 Map of Central African Rep.

12.4.7 Create a Raster of Temperature

To visualise the temperature data on the map of the Central African Republic we create a raster template. The raster template has the same extent as the simulated infected locations and will be used to **rasterize** the **temperature** data. This means that the temperature data will be converted into a raster format, with each cell in the raster grid representing a specific temperature value. The rasterized temperature data will be visualised as a heatmap on the map, with warmer colours indicating higher temperatures.

The raster template is created using the `rast()` function from the `{terra}` package, specifying the number of rows and columns, the minimum and maximum values for the x and y coordinates, and the coordinate reference system (CRS) of the raster. If you want to know more about the package, type `?terra`.

The raster template is set to have 18 rows and 36 columns, with the x and y coordinates ranging from 11 to 28 and 2 to 12, respectively.

```
library(terra)
raster_template <- terra::rast(nrows = 18, ncols = 36,
                               xmin = 11, xmax = 28,
                               ymin = 2, ymax = 12,
                               crs = st_crs(df_sf)$proj4string)
```

Rasterize the temperature data using the `rasterize()` function to convert the temperature data from the data frame to a raster format based on the raster template. The temperature data are assigned to the raster cells based on the latitude and longitude coordinates.

```
ctr_africa_raster <- rasterize(df_sf,
                                   raster_template,
                                   field = "temperature",
                                   fun = max)
```

Before plotting the rasterized temperature data on the map of the Central African Republic, we need to convert the rasterized data to a data frame format. This will allow us to visualise the temperature data as a heatmap on the map. The rasterized data contains the temperature values for each cell in the raster grid, which are assigned based on the latitude and longitude coordinates of the temperature data.

```
ctr_africa_raster_df <- as.data.frame(ctr_africa_raster,
                                      xy = TRUE)
ctr_africa_raster_df %>% head()
#>            x        y      max
#> 200 20.20833 8.944444 24.09246
#> 203 21.62500 8.944444 21.51325
#> 205 22.56944 8.944444 23.46981
#> 234 19.26389 8.388889 25.77824
#> 235 19.73611 8.388889 25.11388
#> 268 18.31944 7.833333 25.24466
```

```
# Temperature Raster
ggplot() +
  geom_raster(data = ctr_africa_raster_df,
              aes(x = x, y = y, fill = max)) +
  viridis::scale_fill_viridis(name = "Temperature",
                              na.value = "transparent") +
  labs(title = "Rasterized Temperature") +
  theme(legend.position = "right")
```

```
# Central Africa Raster
ggplot() +
  geom_point(data = ctr_africa_grid_full %>% filter(pip == 1),
             aes(x = x, y = y),
             shape = ".") +
  geom_raster(data = ctr_africa_raster_df,
              aes(x = x, y = y, fill = max)) +
  geom_sf(data = df_sf %>% filter(presence == 1),
          aes(size = cases),
          shape = 21, stroke = 0.3) +
  scale_fill_gradient(low = "white", high = "grey30",
                      na.value = "transparent") +
  labs(title = "Max Temperature in Central African Rep.",
       subtitle = "Simulated Values",
       size = "Number of Infections",
       fill = "Max Temperature") +
  theme(legend.position = "right")
```

This plot shows the temperature data as a heatmap on the map of the Central African Republic, with warmer colours indicating higher temperatures. The infected locations are represented as circles with size indicating the number of infected individuals at each location.

12.4.8 The Epicenter of Infection

A central point that represents the spatial distribution of infections in the region is the center of mass. It is a useful metric for understanding the spatial dynamics of disease spread and identifying critical zones for intervention. To calculate the coordinates of the **center of mass**index{Center of mass} for the infections, even called the **epicenter** of the infections, we use the `center_of_mass()` function.

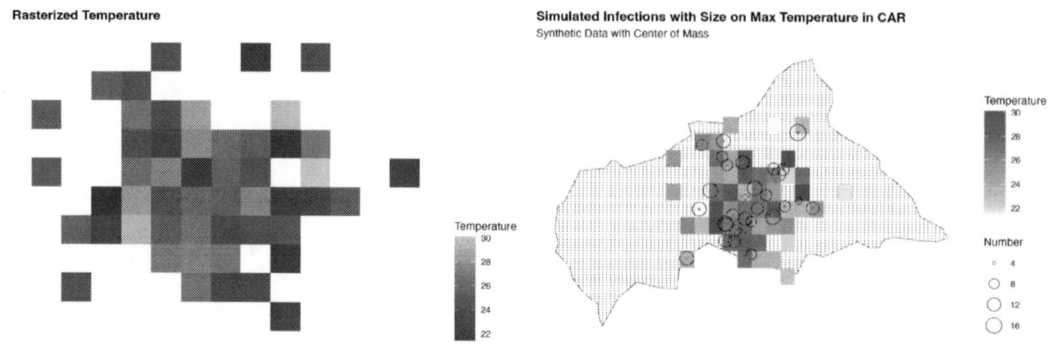

(a) Temperature Raster

(b) Central African Rep. Map of Max Temperature Level

Figure 12.5 Central African Rep. Raster Map of Infections and Max Temperature Level

The center of mass is the average of the latitude and longitude of the infected individuals, weighted by the number of infected individuals at each location.

```
center_of_mass <- function(df) {
  longitude <- sum(df$cases * df$longitude) / sum(df$cases)
  latitude <- sum(df$cases * df$latitude) / sum(df$cases)
  c(longitude, latitude)
  }
```

```
df_com <- tibble(longitude = center_of_mass(df)[1],
                 latitude = center_of_mass(df)[2])
df_com
#> # A tibble: 1 x 2
#>   longitude latitude
#>       <dbl>    <dbl>
#> 1      20.7     6.47
```

Finally, plot the infections on the map of the Central African Republic, with the temperature data represented as a raster layer. The temperature data are displayed as a **heatmap**, with warmer colours indicating higher temperatures. The infections are shown as points on the map, with different colours representing infected and non-infected locations.

Note, here a new package is used, the `{ggnewscale}` package, which is a package that allows you to add multiple colour scales to a single plot. This is useful when you want to visualise different variables with different colour scales in the same plot.

```
# Location of Infections
ggplot() +
  geom_sf(data = df_sf, aes(shape = factor(presence),
                            color = factor(presence))) +
  geom_point(data = df_com,
             aes(x = longitude, y = latitude),
             color = "red", size = 4) +
  scale_colour_manual("Infection Status",
                      values = c("1" = "red", "0" = "blue")) +
```

```
  # combine shape and colour legends
  guides(color = guide_legend(title = "Infection Status"),
         shape = guide_legend(title = "Infection Status")) +
  labs(title = "Simulated Locations in Central African Rep.",
       subtitle = "Synthetic Data with Infections Center of Mass") +
  theme(legend.position = "right")

# Infections Size on Max Temperature
ggplot() +
  geom_point(data = ctr_africa_grid_full %>% filter(pip == 1),
             aes(x = x, y = y), shape = ".") +
  geom_sf(data = ctr_africa, fill = NA) +
  geom_raster(data = ctr_africa_raster_df,
              aes(x = x, y = y, fill = max)) +
  scale_fill_gradient(low = "white", high = "grey30",
                      na.value = "transparent") +
  geom_sf(data = df_sf  %>% filter(presence == 1),
          mapping = aes(group = presence),
          alpha = 0.8, color = "red", size = 0.5) +
  geom_sf(data = df_sf %>% filter(presence == 1),
          aes(size = cases),
          shape = 21, stroke = 0.3) +
  geom_point(data = df_com,
             aes(x = longitude, y = latitude),
             color = "red", size = 4, shape = 13) +
  labs(title = "Simulated Infections with Size on Max Temperature in CAR",
       subtitle = "Synthetic Data with Center of Mass",
       fill = "Temperature",
       size = "Number") +
  theme(legend.position = "right")
```

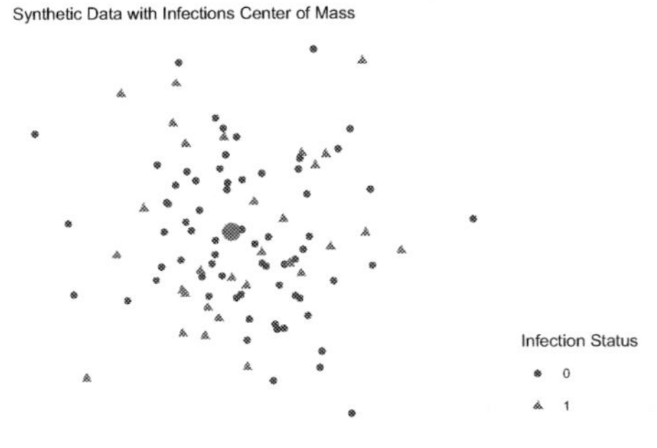

(a) Scatterplot of Simulated Locations

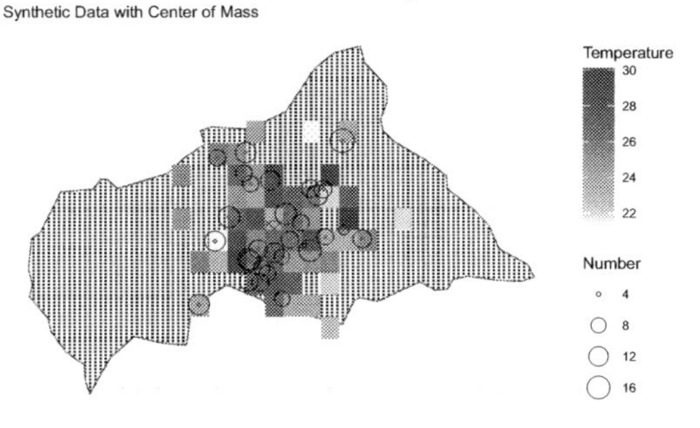

(b) Infected Locations in Central African Rep.

Figure 12.6 Map of Central African Rep.

12.5 Dynamics of Disease Transmission

The spread of infectious diseases, fundamentally depends on the pattern of human contact[4] and the spatial distribution of infected individuals. Understanding the spatial dynamics of disease transmission is crucial for predicting the risk of outbreaks and guiding public health interventions.

To explore the dynamics of disease transmission in Central Africa by simulating the spread of infections we use a type of network characterised by a high degree of clustering and short average path lengths between nodes called **small-world network**. It represents a realistic model of human contact patterns, where individuals are more likely to interact with their neighbours but can also have long-range connections with other individuals. By simulating the spread of infections in a small-world network, we can investigate how the spatial structure of the network influences the transmission dynamics and identify critical nodes for disease control.

We will use the `{igraph}` package to create a small-world network and simulate the spread of infections through the network. The network will consist of nodes representing individuals in Central Africa, with connections between nodes based on a small-world topology. The `sample_smallworld()` function generates a small-world network with the specified parametres: the number of nodes `N`, the average degree `k`, and the rewiring probability `p`. The average degree `k` determines the number of neighbours each node is connected to, while the rewiring probability `p` controls the likelihood of rewiring connections to create long-range connections. By adjusting the parametres `k` and `p`, we can create small-world networks with different topologies and study their impact on disease transmission dynamics.

```
library(igraph)

N <- nrow(df_sf)  # Number of nodes
k <- 3     # Each node connected to k nearest neighbours
p <- 0.1   # Rewiring probability
small_world <- sample_smallworld(dim = 1,
                                 size = N,
                                 nei = k,
                                 p = p)
```

Assign the small_world to a new variable `small_world_dev` and infect 10 random nodes. The status of the nodes is defined as "S" for susceptible and "I" for infectious. The colour of the nodes is assigned based on their infection status, with infectious nodes shown in red and susceptible nodes in gold.

```
V(small_world)$color <- "grey"
# Create a second network for development
small_world_dev <- small_world
# Infect 10 random nodes
V(small_world_dev)$status <- "S"  # Susceptible
infected_nodes <- sample(V(small_world_dev), 10)
V(small_world_dev)$status[infected_nodes] <- "I"  # Infectious
```

[4] Erik M. Volz et al., "Effects of Heterogeneous and Clustered Contact Patterns on Infectious Disease Dynamics," *PLoS Computational Biology* 7, no. 6 (June 2, 2011): e1002042, doi:10.1371/journal.pcbi.1002042.

```
# Assign colours based on infection status
V(small_world_dev)$color <-
        ifelse(V(small_world_dev)$status == "I",
                             "black", "grey80")
```

Plot the graphs:

```
par(mfrow = c(1,2))

set.seed(06082024)
plot(small_world,
     vertex.size = 8,
     vertex.label = NA,
     edge.arrow.size = 0.5,
     edge.width = 0.5)

plot(small_world_dev,
     vertex.size = 8,
     vertex.label = NA,
     edge.arrow.size = 0.5,
     edge.width = 0.5)
```

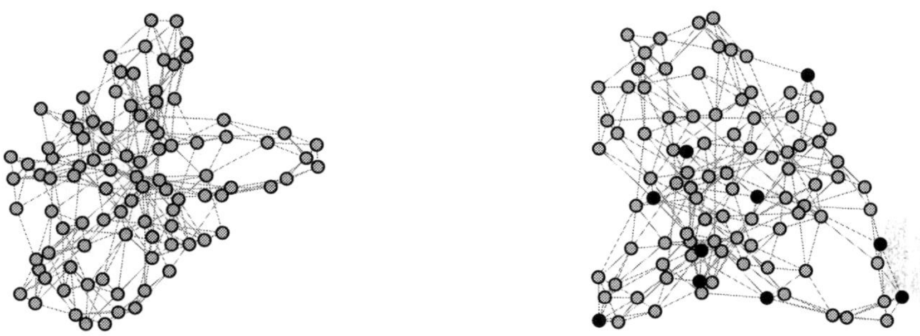

Figure 12.7 Visualization of a Small-World Network: Structure before and after the spread of infections.

We use the Central African Rep. grid of points for prediction, and transform it to a simple features object, with the mean values of the covariates for simplicity.

```
ctr_africa_grid <- ctr_africa_grid_full %>%
  filter(pip == 1)

ctr_africa_grid_sf <- ctr_africa_grid %>%
  st_as_sf(coords = c("x", "y"), crs = 4326) %>%
  st_make_valid() %>%
  mutate(temperature = mean(df$temperature))

infected_sf <- df_sf  %>%
  filter(presence == 1) %>%
  st_make_valid()
```

Visualise the grid of points and the observed infections on the map of the Central African Republic. To understand the spatial distribution of infections and the covariates for prediction, we use the small-world network made above, to simulate the connections between individuals. Assign the attributes to the nodes of the small-world network based on the synthetic data (`df_sf`). The attributes include the type of individual (infected or non-infected), the latitude and longitude coordinates, and the number of infected individuals. The edges of the network represent the connections between nodes.

```
coords <- st_coordinates(df_sf$geometry)
# Assign attributes to nodes
V(small_world)$presence <- df_sf$presence
V(small_world)$longitude <- coords[,1]
V(small_world)$latitude <- coords[,2]
V(small_world)$cases <- df_sf$cases
```

```
edges <- igraph::as_data_frame(small_world, what = "edges")

nodes <- coords %>%
     as_tibble() %>%
     rename(longitude = X, latitude = Y)%>%
     mutate(id = 1:nrow(.))

edges <- edges %>%
  left_join(nodes, by = c("from" = "id")) %>%
  rename(lat_from = latitude,
         lon_from = longitude) %>%
  left_join(nodes, by = c("to" = "id")) %>%
  rename(lat_to = latitude,
         lon_to = longitude)
```

```
ggplot() +
  geom_sf(data = ctr_africa_grid_sf,
          shape = 21, stroke = 0.5,
          fill = NA, size = 0.5, color = "grey") +
  geom_sf(data = infected_sf,
          aes(size = cases),
          shape = 21, stroke = 0.2, color="black") +
  scale_color_continuous(name = "Observed",
                         low = "white", high = "red") +
  labs(title = "Observed Infections")  +
  theme(legend.position = "right")

ggplot() +
  geom_sf(data = ctr_africa, fill = NA) +
  geom_sf(data = ctr_africa_grid_sf,
          shape = 21, stroke = 0.5,
          fill = NA, size = 0.5, color = "grey") +
  geom_segment(data = edges,
               aes(x = lon_from, y = lat_from,
                   xend = lon_to, yend = lat_to),
               color = "grey20", alpha = 0.2, linewidth = 0.2) +
  geom_sf(data = df_sf,
```

```
             aes(shape = factor(presence),
                 color = factor(presence)),
          size = 0.5) +
  geom_sf(data = infected_sf,
          aes(size = cases),
          shape = 21, stroke = 0.2, color="black") +
  guides(color = "none") +
  scale_color_manual(values = c("0" = "grey20", "1" = "red")) +
  labs(title = "Small-World Network with Infection Status",
       x = "Longitude", y = "Latitude", shape = "Presence") +
  theme(legend.position = "right")
```

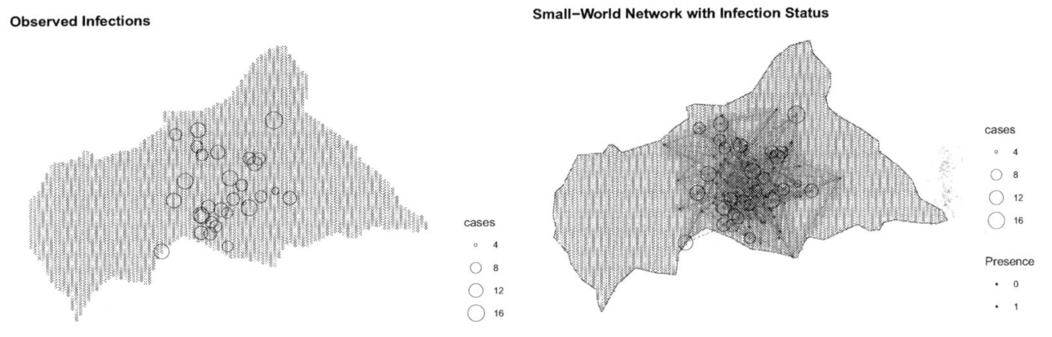

(a) Observed Size of Infections

(b) Map of Infection Status and Small-World Network

Figure 12.8 Map of Central African Rep.

The clustering of close-proximity contacts that occurs within individuals is an important factor in the spread of diseases and subject of many mathematical models.

12.5.1 The Euclidean Distance

To estimate the likelihood of transmission between individuals based on their spatial proximity the **Euclidean** distance is used. It is calculated as the square root of the sum of the squares of the differences between corresponding coordinates of the two points.

The Euclidean distance formula:

$$d_{i,j} = \sqrt{(x_i - x_j)^2 + (y_i - y_j)^2} \tag{12.1}$$

Where: (x_i, y_i) are the coordinates (e.g., latitude and longitude) of the first point (A), e.g., infected individual, and (x_j, y_j) are the coordinates of the second point (B), e.g., susceptible individual or location.

It calculates the straight-line distance between two points in a two-dimensional space, which can be applied to model the spatial spread of infectious diseases based on the proximity of individuals or locations.

To calculate the Euclidean distance we make a function that considers the distance between the center of mass and the infection coordinates.

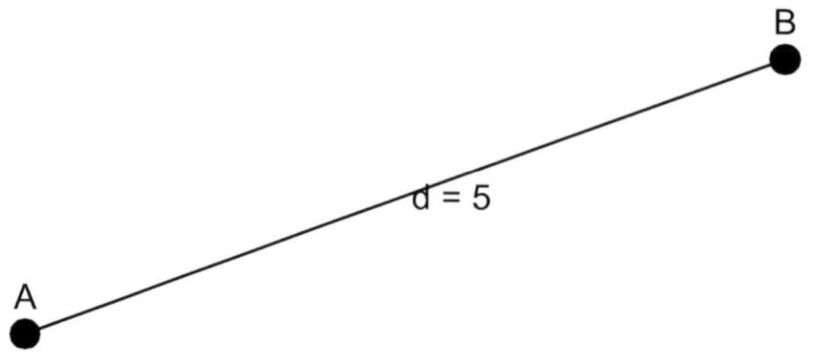

Figure 12.9 Representation of Euclidean Distance between Points A and B

```
# helper function for calculating euclidean distance metric
euclidean_distance <- function(longitude, latitude,
                               long_com, lat_com) {
  long_distances <- (longitude - long_com[1])^2
  lat_distances <- (latitude - lat_com[1])^2
  return((long_distances + lat_distances) * 0.5)
}
```

There are other type of distance metrics that can be used, such as the **Manhattan** distance, which calculates the sum of the absolute differences between the coordinates of two points, the **Mahlanobis** distance, which considers the correlation between the variables, and the **Chebyshev** distance, which calculates the maximum difference between the coordinates of two points.

12.5.2 Spatial Autocorrelation

Spatial autocorrelation refers to the principle that spatial data points close to each other are more likely to have similar values than those further apart. By analysing the spatial distribution of cases, areas with high spatial autocorrelation indicated clusters where infections spread is particularly intense.

Using tools like **Moran's I** and its variants, infection hotspots can be detected by identifying areas where high case rates cluster together. To check the presence of spatial autocorrelation the **Global Moran's law** is used:

$$I = \frac{N \sum_{i=1}^{N} \sum_{j=1}^{N} w_{ij}(x_i - \bar{x})(x_j - \bar{x})}{W \sum_{i=1}^{N} (x_i - \bar{x})^2} \tag{12.2}$$

Where x_i and x_j are the values of the variable of interest at location i and j, $\bar{x}$ is the mean value and N indicates the number of spatial units, and w_{ij} are the spatial weight between locations.

I measures the degree to which infection is clustered, dispersed or randomly distributed, with values ranging from -1 indicating perfect dispersion to +1 indicating perfect spatial clustering. A value of 0 indicates no spatial autocorrelation, suggesting a random spatial pattern.

We use the {spdep} package, which provide `dnearneigh()`, `nb2listw()`, and `moran.test()` functions for calculating the neighbourhood contiguity by distance, the spatial weights for neighbours lists, and finally the Moran's I test for spatial autocorrelation, respectively.

```
library(spdep)
library(sp)

coordinates(df) <- ~longitude + latitude
# Define neighbours (using a distance threshold, for example)
# Neighbours within a distance of 2 units
nb <- dnearneigh(coordinates(df), 0, 2)

# Create spatial weights
lw <- nb2listw(nb, style="W")

# Calculate Moran's I for infections
moran_result <- moran.test(df$cases, lw)
moran_result
#>
#>  Moran I test under randomisation
#>
#> data:  df$cases
#> weights: lw
#>
#> Moran I statistic standard deviate = -0.18432, p-value = 0.5731
#> alternative hypothesis: greater
#> sample estimates:
#> Moran I statistic       Expectation          Variance
#>      -0.0126043530     -0.0101010101      0.0001844513
```

The result of the Moran's I test of -0.013 shows a slight negative spatial autocorrelation, indicating that the location of infected individuals is slightly dispersed across the region. This suggests that the spatial distribution of infections is not significantly clustered or dispersed, but rather randomly distributed. The p-value of 0.5731 indicates that the observed Moran's I value is not statistically significant, suggesting that the spatial distribution of infections is consistent with a random spatial pattern. And we know it is as we have simulated the data.

12.5.3 Spatial Proximity with Kriging

Although the Moran's I test is useful for understanding the overall spatial pattern of infections, it does not provide detailed information on the spatial distribution of cases across the region. To estimate the spatial distribution of infections and predict the risk of outbreaks, we can use spatial interpolation techniques such as **Kriging**.[5]

This method is used to estimate the spatial distribution of cases by creating a raster of the predicted spatial distribution of infections. It creates a continuous surface that estimates the risk of infection across the entire study area by interpolating the number of infected individuals across a region.

[5] "Kriging," July 18, 2024, https://en.wikipedia.org/w/index.php?title=Kriging&oldid=1235203584.

For example, the application of Kriging was used to predict the spatial distribution of Dengue outbreaks in regions like Khyber Pakhtunkhwa, Pakistan.[6] Similarly, during the COVID-19 pandemic, **Empirical Bayesian Kriging (EBK)**[7] was used to estimate the spatial distribution of COVID-19 cases in sub-Saharan Africa. This approach combined time series data of confirmed cases with socio-demographic indicators to create detailed spatial risk maps, aiding in understanding and controlling the outbreak.

Particularly useful for **visualising the spatial dynamics** of disease spread, while considering the impact of environmental factors such as temperature, or humidity on disease transmission; Kriging requires an estimation of the variance of points at locations.

For estimating the variance, a **variogram model** is fit to the observed data. The variogram is a function of the distance `h` that describes the degree of spatial dependence of a spatial random field or stochastic process. It takes consideration of the spatial auto-correlation of the data. This means, for instance, the number of cases observed in one location are supposed to be correlated with the number of cases observed in nearby locations. This also considers the environmental variables that interact with the disease transmission.

The variogram model formula:

$$\gamma(h) = \frac{1}{2N(h)} \sum_{i=1}^{N(h)} (Z(x_i) - Z(x_i + h))^2 \tag{12.3}$$

Where: $\gamma(h)$ is the semivariance, $N(h)$ is the number of pairs of points separated by a distance h, $Z(x_i)$ is the value of the variable at location x_i, and $Z(x_i + h)$ is the value of the variable at location $x_i + h$.

We use the `{gstat}` package to perform Kriging with `variogram()`[8],[9] `fit.variogram()`, and `gstat()` functions to perform **Universal Kriging**, a kriging method that allows to incorporate an external drift, such as temperature. The predictions are visualised on the grid of points generated earlier, with warmer colours indicating higher predicted values.

```
library(gstat)
```

```
v <-  variogram(object = cases ~  temperature, data = df_sf)

v_model <- fit.variogram(v, model = vgm("Sph"))

plot(v, model = v_model)
```

[6]Hammad Ahmad et al., "Spatial Modeling of Dengue Prevalence and Kriging Prediction of Dengue Outbreak in Khyber Pakhtunkhwa (Pakistan) Using Presence Only Data," *Stochastic Environmental Research and Risk Assessment* 34, no. 7 (July 1, 2020): 1023–36, doi:10.1007/s00477-020-01818-9.

[7]Amobi Andrew Onovo et al., "Using Supervised Machine Learning and Empirical Bayesian Kriging to Reveal Correlates and Patterns of COVID-19 Disease Outbreak in Sub-Saharan Africa: Exploratory Data Analysis," n.d., doi:10.1101/2020.04.27.20082057.

[8]Edzer J Pebesma, "Multivariable Geostatistics in s: The Gstat Package," *Computers & Geosciences* 30, no. 7 (August 1, 2004): 683–91, doi:10.1016/j.cageo.2004.03.012.

[9]Hans Wackernagel, "Linear Regression and Simple Kriging," ed. Hans Wackernagel (Berlin, Heidelberg: Springer, 2003), 15–26, doi:10.1007/978-3-662-05294-5_3.

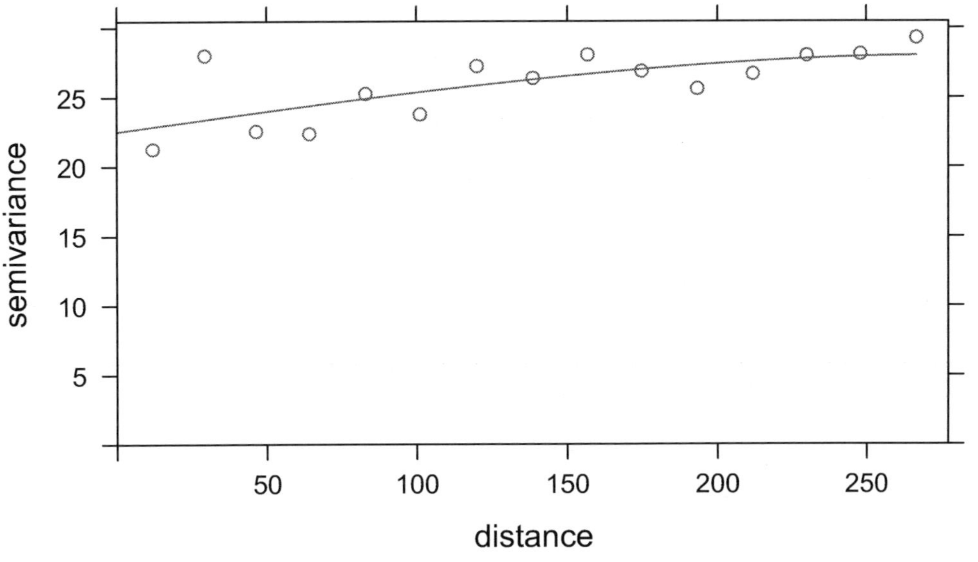

Figure 12.10 Variogram of Infections and Temperature

Or, just use the `kbfit()` function,[10] which tries different initial values and models to find the best fit for the variogram, the function can be used directly from the book package `hmsidwR::kbfit()`.

Then, the Kriging technique is applied by using the `gstat::gstat()` function,[11] to predict the number of infected individuals at unobserved locations, based on the best variogram model.

Kriging Model Formula:

$$Z(u) = \sum_{i=1}^{n} \lambda_i Z(x_i) \tag{12.4}$$

Where: $Z(u)$ is the predicted value at location u, λ_i is the weight assigned to each observed value $Z(x_i)$, and n is the number of observed values.

The predictions are visualised on the grid of points generated earlier, with warmer colours indicating higher predicted values. The predictions are stored in the `kpred` object, which contains the predicted values and the variance of the predictions.

```
# Perform Kriging
k <- gstat::gstat(formula = presence ~ temperature,
                  data = df_sf,
                  model = v_model)

kpred <- predict(k, newdata = ctr_africa_grid_sf)
```

[10]"Kriging Best Fit: Kbfit - Fit Variogram Models and Kriging Models to Spatial Data and Select the Best Model Based on the Metrics Values — Kbfit," n.d., https://fgazzelloni.github.io/hmsidwR/reference/kbfit.html.

[11]Paula Moraga, *Chapter 14 Kriging | Spatial Statistics for Data Science: Theory and Practice with R*, n.d., https://www.paulamoraga.com/book-spatial/kriging.html?q=kri#kriging.

```
#> [using universal kriging]

data.frame(geo = kpred$geometry,
           var = kpred$var1.var,
           pred = kpred$var1.pred) %>%
  head()
#>                     geometry      var      pred
#> 1 POINT (14.58986 4.688027) 29.18857 0.3473599
#> 2 POINT (14.58986 4.777671) 29.18857 0.3473599
#> 3 POINT (14.58986 4.867316) 29.18857 0.3473599
#> 4  POINT (14.58986 4.95696) 29.18857 0.3473599
#> 5 POINT (14.58986 5.046603) 29.18857 0.3473599
#> 6 POINT (14.58986 5.136248) 29.18857 0.3473599
```

Visualise predictions:

```
ggplot() +
  geom_sf(data = kpred,
          aes(fill = var1.pred),
          shape=21, stroke=0.5) +
  geom_sf(data = infected_sf) +
  scale_fill_viridis_c() +
  labs(title = "Kriging Prediction in Central African Rep.") +
  theme(legend.position = "right")

ggplot() +
  geom_sf(data = kpred,
          aes(fill = var1.var),
          shape=21, stroke=0.5) +
  geom_sf(data = infected_sf) +
  scale_fill_viridis_c() +
  labs(title = "Kriging Variance in Central African Rep.") +
  theme(legend.position = "right")
```

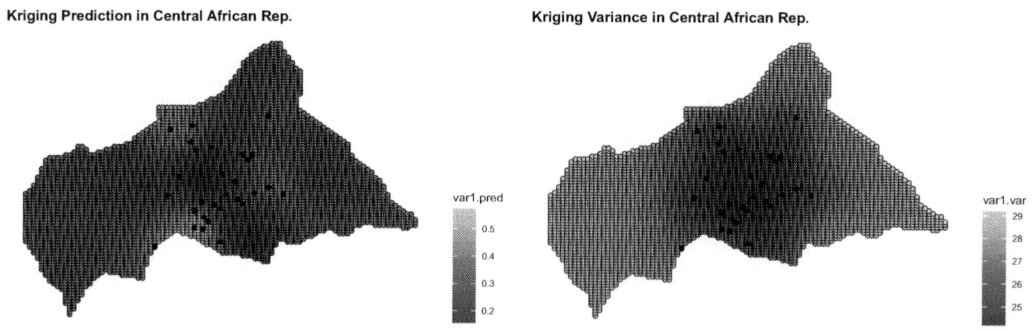

(a) Kriging Prediction in Central African Rep. **(b)** Kriging Variance in Central African Rep.

Figure 12.11 Kriging Map of Central African Rep.

12.6 Mapping Risk of Infections

To map the risk of infections in Central Africa, we can combine the Kriging predictions with the spatial distribution of infections and the small-world network. The Kriging predictions provide an estimate of the risk of infections across the region, while the spatial distribution of infections and the small-world network represent the spatial dynamics of disease transmission.

The risk of infections is visualised on the map of Central African Republic, with warmer colours indicating higher predicted values. The spatial distribution of infections is shown as points on the map, with different colours representing infected and non-infected locations. The small-world network is overlaid on the map, showing the connections between nodes and the spatial dynamics of disease transmission.

This is a different way to visualise the Kriging predictions, first a data frame is created with the coordinates and the predicted values, and then the predictions plotted on the map of Central African Republic. The predictions are shown as a **raster layer**.

```
kriging_df <- kpred %>%
  sf::st_coordinates() %>%
  cbind(as.data.frame(kpred) %>% select(var1.pred)) %>%
  rename(longitude = X, latitude = Y)
```

```
ggplot() +
  geom_sf(data = ctr_africa, fill = "grey") +
  geom_raster(data =  kriging_df,
              aes(x = longitude, y = latitude,
                  fill = var1.pred)) +
  scale_fill_viridis_c() +
  geom_segment(data = edges,
               aes(x = lon_from, y = lat_from,
                   xend = lon_to, yend = lat_to),
               color = "grey", alpha = 0.2, linewidth = 0.2) +
  geom_sf(data = df_sf %>% filter(presence == 1),
          aes(size = cases),
          # show.legend = F,
          shape = 21, stroke = 0.2) +
  geom_sf(data = df_sf,
        aes(color = factor(presence)),
        shape = ".") +
  scale_color_manual(values = c("0" = "grey", "1" = "red")) +
  guides(size = guide_legend(order = 1),
         color = guide_legend(order = 2),
         fill = guide_colorbar(order = 3)) +
  labs(title = "Kriging Prediction of Infections Size on Max Temperature",
       fill = "Prediction of Infections",
       size = "Infections Size",
       color = "Presence") +
  ggthemes::theme_map() +
  theme(legend.position = "bottom",
        legend.box = "vertical",
```

```
        legend.key.size = unit(0.5, "cm"),
        legend.title = element_text(size = 8),
        legend.text = element_text(size = 6))
```

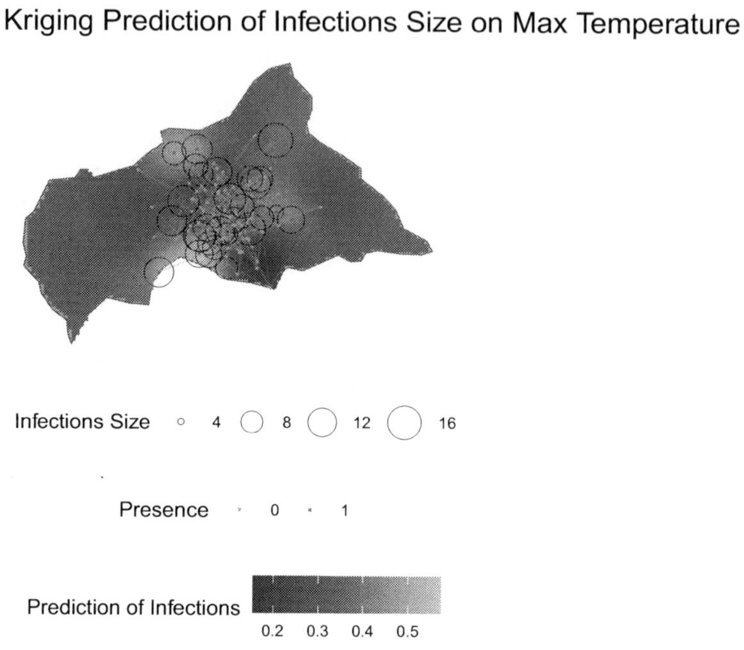

Figure 12.12 Kriging Prediction of Infections Size on Max Temperature

Finally, the last plot is made with the `spplot()` function from the `{sp}` package, which creates a **spatial plot** of the Kriging predictions. The predictions are visualised as a **heatmap** on the map of the Central African Republic, with warmer colours indicating higher predicted values. The plot provides a detailed view of the spatial distribution of infections and the risk of outbreaks across the region.

```
kriging_sp <- kriging_df
coordinates(kriging_sp) <- ~longitude+latitude
spplot(kriging_sp, "var1.pred", main = "Kriging Prediction of Infections")
```

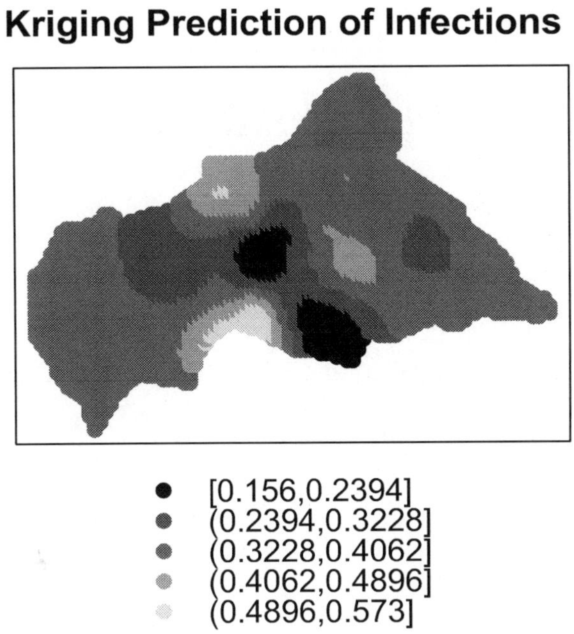

Figure 12.13 Kriging Prediction of Infections with a Spplot

12.7 Summary

In this chapter, we have explored the spatial dynamics of disease transmission in Central Africa using a combination of spatial analysis techniques and visualisation tools. We have simulated the spatial distribution of infections, created a grid of points to cover the region, and visualised the spatial distribution of infections on the map of Central African Republic. We have used a small-world network to model the spatial connections between individuals and simulated the spread of infections through the network. We have shown how the Euclidean distance between points is calculated, to estimate the likelihood of transmission based on spatial proximity and performed spatial autocorrelation analysis to understand the spatial pattern of infections. We have used Kriging to estimate the spatial distribution of infections and predict the risk of outbreaks across the region. The results provide valuable insights into the spatial dynamics of disease transmission and the spatial distribution of infections in Central Africa, which can inform public health interventions and guide efforts to control the spread of infectious diseases.

13

Advanced Data Visualisation Techniques

Learning Objectives

- Learn advanced data visualisation techniques
- Create contour plots to visualise interaction effects
- Create a pyramid plot to visualise population distribution

In this chapter, we will learn how to create advanced data visualisation techniques using `ggplot2`. We will create contour plots to visualise interaction effects and pyramid plots to visualise population distribution.

13.1 Example: Detecting Interaction Effects with Contour Plots

Interaction effects can cause predictors to act together on the response variable, leading to additional variation in the response. Interaction effects occur when the combined effect of two or more predictors is different from what would be expected if the impact of each predictor were considered alone. For instance, in the case of **cardiovascular disease (CVD)** risk prediction, the interaction between age and cholesterol levels can have a significant impact on the risk of developing heart disease. In addition, if smoke is added to the model, the effect of cholesterol levels on CVD risk may change depending on whether the individual is a smoker or non-smoker. So, smoke is said to interact with cholesterol levels in predicting CVD risk, as well as age, but in what way?

$$y = \beta_0 + \beta_1 x_1 + \beta_2 x_2 + \beta_3 x_3 + \epsilon \tag{13.1}$$

where y is the risk of developing heart disease, β_0 is the intercept, β_1 and β_2 are the coefficients for the predictors x_1 and x_2, respectively, and β_3 is the coefficient for the **interaction term** $x_1 * x_2$. The error term ϵ accounts for the variability in the response variable that is not explained by the predictors.

There are four type of interactions:

1. additive is when $\beta_3 \approx 0$
2. antagonistic is when $\beta_3 < 0$
3. synergistic is when $\beta_3 > 0$
4. atypical is when $\beta_3 \neq 0$

In order to simulate the interaction effects for each type of interaction, we cannot just simulate random values for y, we need to simulate different levels of interactions between

DOI: 10.1201/9781032625935-13

predictors setting up the values for the coefficients β_0, β_1, β_2, and β_3, and the predictors x_1 and x_2 and the error term ϵ.

Load the necessary libraries and set the seed for reproducibility.

```
library(tidyverse)
set.seed(123)
```

Simulate the data ready for different interaction effects.

```
beta0<- rep(0,200)
beta1<- rep(1,200)
beta2<- rep(1,200)
```

Then, simulate the predictors x_1 and x_2 and the error term ϵ for 200 observations.

```
x1<- runif(200, min = 0, max = 1)
x2 <- runif(200, min = 0, max = 1)
e <- rnorm(200)
```

Then for each of the three cases we simulate a β_3 based on antagonism, no interaction, or synergism with values -10, 0, and 10 respectively.

Case 1: Antagonism

```
beta3 <- rep(-10,200)
```

Assemble the values for the coefficients and predictors into the equation, to obtaining the response variable y. This will be our synthetic "observed" data.

```
y1 = beta0 + beta1*x1 + beta2*x2 + beta3*(x1*x2) + e
```

Apply a linear model to the observed data to predict the response variable y based on interaction between x_1 and x_2.

```
observed1 <- tibble(y1, x1, x2)

mod1 <- lm(y1 ~ x1*x2, data = observed1)

observed1$z <- predict(mod1, observed1)
```

Then create a grid of values for x_1 and x_2 to predict the response variable y based on the interaction between x_1 and x_2.

```
grid <- with(observed1,
             interp::interp(x = x1, y = x2, z))
griddf <- subset(data.frame(x = rep(grid$x, nrow(grid$z)),
                            y = rep(grid$y,
                                    each = ncol(grid$z)),
                            z = as.numeric(grid$z)),!is.na(z))
```

```
p1 <- ggplot(griddf, aes(x, y, z = z)) +
  geom_contour(aes(colour = after_stat(level),
                   linetype = factor(after_stat(level))),
                   linewidth = 2) +
  scale_color_viridis_c()+
  guides(linetype = "none")+
```

```
  labs(title="Antagonism",
       color="Prediction", x = "x1", y = "x2")+
  theme(legend.position = "top")
```

Case 2: Additive (no interaction)

```
beta3 <- rep(0,200)
```

```
y2 = beta0 + beta1*x1 + beta2*x2 + beta3*(x1*x2) + e

observed2 <- tibble(y2, x1, x2)

mod2 <- lm(y2 ~ x1*x2, data = observed2)
observed2$z <- predict(mod2, observed2)

grid <- with(observed2, interp::interp(x = x1, y = x2, z))
griddf <- subset(data.frame(x = rep(grid$x, nrow(grid$z)),
                            y = rep(grid$y,
                                    each = ncol(grid$z)),
                            z = as.numeric(grid$z)),!is.na(z))
```

```
p2 <- ggplot(griddf, aes(x, y, z = z)) +
  geom_contour(aes(colour = after_stat(level),
                   linetype = factor(after_stat(level))),
                   linewidth = 2) +
  scale_color_viridis_c()+
  guides(linetype = "none")+
  labs(title="Antagonism",
       color="Prediction", x = "x1", y = "x2")+
  theme(legend.position = "top")
```

Case 3: Synergism

```
beta3<- rep(10,200)
```

```
y3 = beta0 + beta1*x1 + beta2*x2 + beta3*(x1*x2) + e

observed3 <- tibble(y3, x1, x2)

mod3 <- lm(y3 ~ x1 * x2 , data = observed3)
observed3$z <- predict(mod3, observed3)

grid <- with(observed3, interp::interp(x=x1,y=x2,z))
griddf <- subset(data.frame(x = rep(grid$x, nrow(grid$z)),
                            y = rep(grid$y, each = ncol(grid$z)),
                            z = as.numeric(grid$z)),!is.na(z))
```

```
p3 <- ggplot(griddf, aes(x, y, z = z)) +
  geom_contour(aes(colour = after_stat(level),
                   linetype = factor(after_stat(level))),
                   linewidth = 2) +
  scale_color_viridis_c()+
  guides(linetype = "none")+
```

```
  labs(title="Antagonism",
       color="Prediction", x = "x1", y = "x2")+
  theme(legend.position = "top")
```

```
library(patchwork)
p1|p2|p3
```

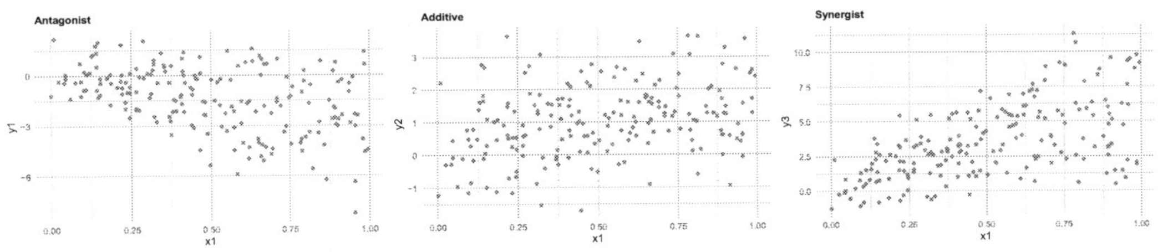

(a) Scatterplot for Antagonistic

(b) Scatterplot for Additive

(c) Scatterplot for Synergistic

Figure 13.1 Scatterplots

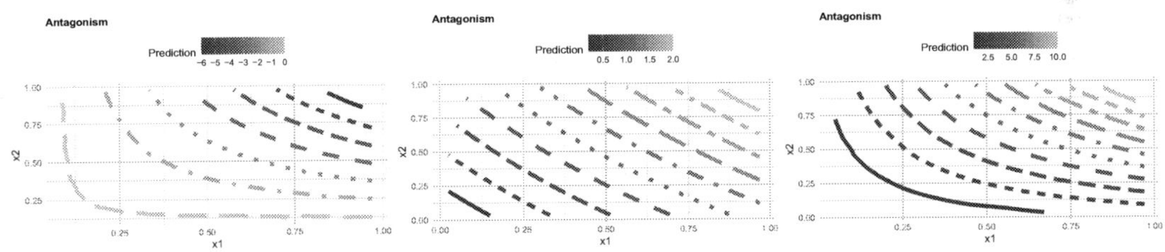

(a) Contour plot for Antagonistic

(b) Contour plot for Additive

(c) Contour plot for Synergistic

Figure 13.2 Contour Plots

13.2 Example: Pyramid Plot

A pyramid plot is a type of bar chart that displays the distribution of a population by age. We use the data from the `{wpp2022}` package, `data(package = "wpp2022")` which is a collection of population datasets, with population estimates. Data are from the United Nations World Population Prospects 2022.

```
library(wpp2022)
```

The data contains the following columns:

```
# load the data on the population
data(popAge1dt)
popAge1dt %>% head()
#>    country_code   name  year   age        popM       popF       pop
#>           <int> <char> <int> <int>       <num>      <num>     <num>
#> 1:          900  World  1949     0 41312.32 39439.29 80751.61
#> 2:          900  World  1949     1 35761.05 34274.35 70035.40
```

```
#> 3:          900  World  1949        2 33514.72 32065.08 65579.81
#> 4:          900  World  1949        3 31076.46 29780.73 60857.19
#> 5:          900  World  1949        4 28786.66 27647.06 56433.72
#> 6:          900  World  1949        5 28082.09 26882.94 54965.03
```

Check all Countries in the dataset with `View()`:

```
popAge1dt %>% count(name) %>% View
```

Data are then aggregated to show the total population for all ages by year. Here, in particular, we show the use of `geomtextpath::geom_textline()` to add a label to the World line plot. `{geomtextpath}` is a nice R-package which allows you to add text along a path.

```
all_ages <- popAge1dt %>%
  group_by(year, name) %>%
  reframe(tot_pop=sum(pop))

all_ages %>%
  filter(!name == "World")%>%
  ggplot(aes(x = year, y = tot_pop, group = name)) +
  geom_line(color= "grey", linewidth =0.2) +
  geomtextpath::geom_textline(data = all_ages %>% filter(name == "World"),
                              aes(label=name),
                              color = "red", linewidth = 1) +
  labs(title = "United Nations World Population Prospects [1949 - 2021]",
       x = "Year", y = "Population in thousands",
       caption = "Data Source: UN World Pop 2022| Graphic: @fgazzelloni")
```

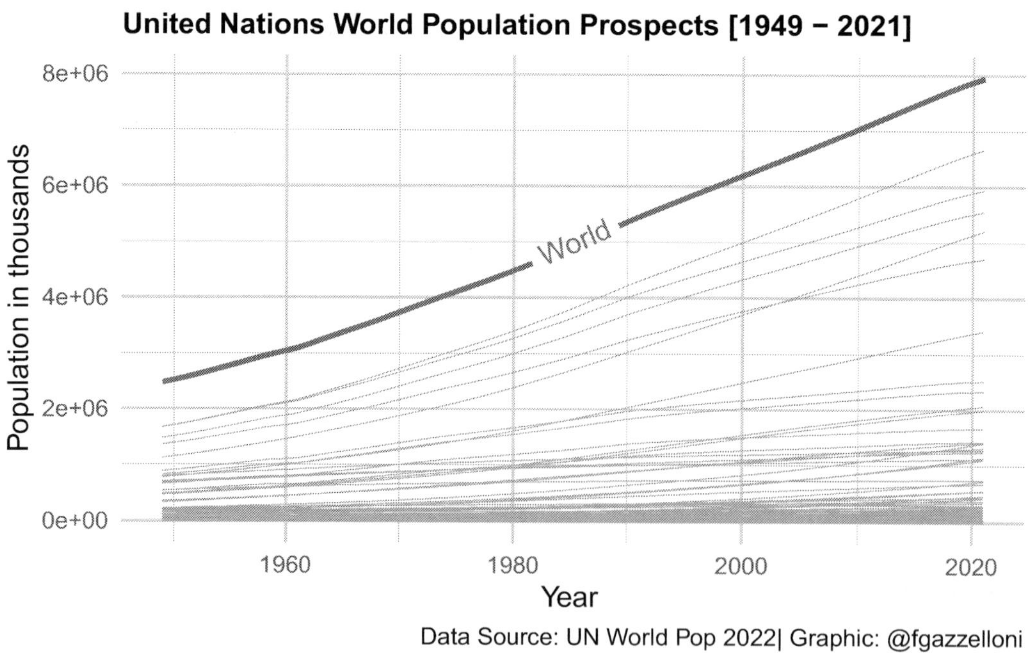

Figure 13.3 Population for all ages from 1949 to 2021

Data are then transformed to a long format to create a pyramid plot. We select the columns `name`, `year`, `age`, `popF`, and `popM` and pivot the data to a long format using the `pivot_longer()` function. We then create a new column `value` that contains positive values for male population and negative values for females.

```
data <- popAge1dt %>%
  select(name, year, age, popF, popM) %>%
  pivot_longer(cols = c(popM, popF),
               names_to = "sex",
               values_to = "population") %>%
  mutate(value = ifelse(sex == "popF",
                        as.integer(population * -1),
                        as.integer(population)))

data %>% head()
#> # A tibble: 6 x 6
#>   name   year   age sex   population  value
#>   <chr> <int> <int> <chr>      <dbl>  <int>
#> 1 World  1949     0 popM      41312.  41312
#> 2 World  1949     0 popF      39439. -39439
#> 3 World  1949     1 popM      35761.  35761
#> 4 World  1949     1 popF      34274. -34274
#> 5 World  1949     2 popM      33515.  33514
#> 6 World  1949     2 popF      32065. -32065
```

Then, we can create pyramid plots that show the distribution of the population by age for **High-income countries**, **Lower-middle-income countries**, and **Low-income countries**, and put them in one chunk with the option `layout-ncol: 3`.

```
data %>%
  filter(name == "High-income countries") %>%
  ggplot(aes(x = age, y = value, fill = sex)) +
  geom_bar(stat = "identity") +
  scale_fill_manual(values = c("#CC6666", "#9999CC")) +
  coord_flip() +
  labs(title = "United Nations World Population Prospects 2022",
       subtitle = "High-income countries",
       x= "Age", y = "Population in thousands", fill = "",
       caption = "Data Source: UN World Pop | Graphic: @fgazzelloni") +
  theme_minimal() +
  theme(plot.title = element_text(face = "bold",
                                  hjust = 0.5),
        plot.subtitle = element_text(hjust = 0.5),
        axis.text = element_text(size = 10))

data %>%
  filter(name == "Lower-middle-income countries") %>%
  ggplot(aes(x = age, y = value, fill = sex)) +
  geom_bar(stat = "identity") +
  scale_fill_manual(values = c("#CC6666", "#9999CC")) +
  coord_flip() +
  labs(title = "United Nations World Population Prospects 2022",
       subtitle = "Lower-middle-income countries",
```

```
       x= "Age", y = "Population in thousands", fill = "",
       caption = "Data Source: UN World Pop | Graphic: @fgazzelloni") +
  theme_minimal() +
  theme(plot.title = element_text(face = "bold",
                                  hjust = 0.5),
        plot.subtitle = element_text(hjust = 0.5),
        axis.text = element_text(size = 10))

data %>%
  filter(name == "Low-income countries") %>%
  ggplot(aes(x = age, y = value, fill = sex)) +
  geom_bar(stat = "identity") +
  scale_fill_manual(values = c("#CC6666", "#9999CC")) +
  coord_flip() +
  labs(title = "United Nations World Population Prospects 2022",
       subtitle = "Low-income countries",
       x= "Age", y = "Population in thousands", fill = "",
       caption = "Data Source: UN World Pop | Graphic: @fgazzelloni") +
  theme_minimal() +
  theme(plot.title = element_text(face = "bold",
                                  hjust = 0.5),
        plot.subtitle = element_text(hjust = 0.5),
        axis.text = element_text(size = 10))
```

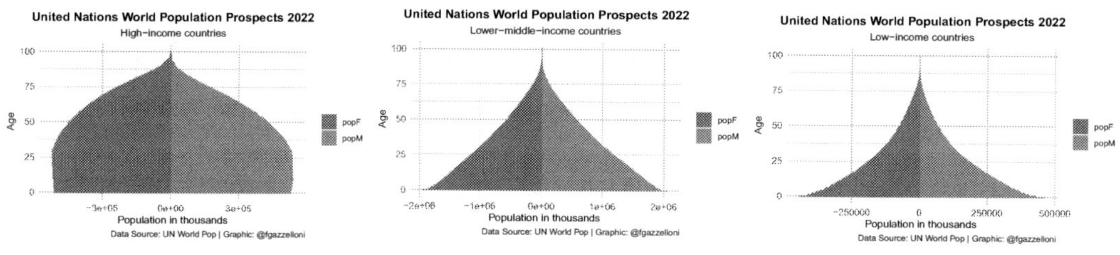

(a) High-income countries **(b)** Lower-middle-income countries **(c)** Low-income countries

Figure 13.4 Pyramid Plots

```
pyramid <-
  data %>%
  filter(name == "World") %>%
  ggplot(aes(x = age, y = value, fill = sex)) +
  geom_bar(stat = "identity") +
  scale_fill_manual(values = c("#CC6666", "#9999CC")) +
  coord_flip() +
  labs(title = "UN Pop 2022 - {closest_state}",
       x= "Age", y = "Population in thousands", fill = "",
       caption = "Data Source: UN World Pop | Graphic: @fgazzelloni") +
       theme_minimal() +
       theme(plot.title = element_text(face = "bold",
                                        hjust = 0.5),
             axis.text = element_text(size = 10))
```

```
library(gganimate)
pyramid_gif <- pyramid +
  transition_states(year,
                    transition_length = 1,
                    state_length = 2) +
  enter_fade() +
  exit_fade() +
  ease_aes("cubic-in-out")

animate(pyramid_gif,
        fps = 72, duration = 6,
        width = 1200, height = 1400, res = 180,
        renderer = gifski_renderer("images/12_unp_pyramid.gif"))
```

Part IV

Infectious Diseases

14

Introduction to Infectious Diseases

Learning Objectives

- Learn about the dynamics of infectious diseases and their impact on human health
- Understand the role of mathematical models in predicting infectious disease outbreaks
- Explore the components of infectious disease models and their implications

"Several infectious diseases are emerging and threatening human health worldwide. The burden of infectious diseases is undeniably a global issue, causing millions of deaths annually."[1]

The advent of machine learning (ML) has revolutionised the field of **infectious disease research** by providing robust tools for predicting outbreaks and understanding the dynamics of spread. In this chapter, we will enhance our understanding of these diseases and look at the effects on Disability-Adjusted Life Years (DALYs) by applying **machine learning** and **data visualisation** techniques learned in previous chapters (Chapter 6 and Chapter 10). To further improve the knowledge of the impact of infectious diseases on global health, we will explore how integrating ML models can improve the accuracy of disease burden estimations and provide valuable insights into the impact of infectious diseases on public health.

14.1 Infectious Diseases the Invisible Enemies

Emerging infectious diseases are a global concern, causing millions of deaths annually. Understanding their behaviour and predicting outbreaks is fundamental not only for public health but also for advancing prediction techniques that can be applied in other fields.

Microorganisms, including **bacteria** and **viruses**, adapt and evolve at a rate much faster than humans. For example, the generation time for bacteria can be as short as 20–30 minutes, while viruses can replicate in even shorter time frames. This rapid adaptation allows **pathogens** to evolve quickly, developing resistance to treatments and evading the **host**'s immune system.

Infectious diseases follow a multi-stage progression that begins when the infective agent, whether **viral**, **bacterial**, or **parasitic**, begins to thrive and multiply throughout the body[2] and the process of infection starts. The rate at which the pathogen proliferates varies significantly depending on the type of organism involved. Each infectious disease has a

[1] Omar Enzo Santangelo et al., "Machine Learning and Prediction of Infectious Diseases: A Systematic Review," *Machine Learning and Knowledge Extraction* 5, no. 1 (March 2023): 175–98, doi:10.3390/make5010013.

[2] Broemeling, *Bayesian Analysis of Infectious Diseases*.

DOI: 10.1201/9781032625935-14

unique **incubation period**, which is the interval between the initial establishment of the pathogen in the host and the onset of symptoms.

The incubation period can range from a few hours to several months, influenced by factors such as the pathogen's growth rate, the host's immune response, and the route of transmission. For example, the incubation period for the **influenza virus** is typically 1 to 4 days, whereas for diseases like **hepatitis B**, it can be as long as 6 months. Understanding the incubation period helps in identifying the time frame for potential exposure.

Several factors influence an individual's susceptibility to infection, including:

- Infection dose (quantity of invading germs)
- Virulence (the ability of the organism to cause disease)
- Immune status (the condition of the body's immune system)
- Transmission route (contact with the source of infection for contagious diseases)

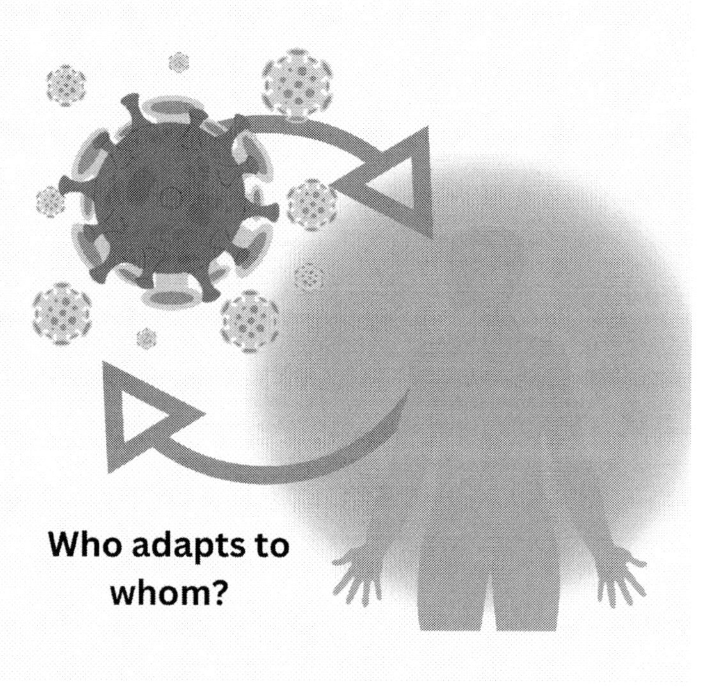

Figure 14.1 Pathogens and humans have co-evolved over centuries, each adapting in response to the other. This ongoing adaptation shapes the future of health and disease.

Viruses, word derived from the Latin word for **"poisonous substance"**, are intracellular parasites that can only replicate within living host cells. Their sizes range from 20 to 400 nm in diameter and can only be observed with an electron microscope. Outside of a living cell, a virus is a dormant particle of various shapes. Once inside a cell, it replicates, often killing the cell or altering its functions.

The following seven diseases are all caused by an infectious agent such as virus or bacteria, generally cause acute symptoms, ranging from mild to severe, and require prompt medical attention to prevent complications and further spread:

1. Acute Respiratory Infection (ARI)

2. COVID-19
3. Dengue
4. Influenza/Influenza-Like Illness (ILI)
5. Malaria
6. West Nile Virus
7. Zika

These diseases are transmitted through various means and can be grouped by **transmission methods**:

- **Vector-Borne**: Dengue, Malaria, West Nile Virus, and Zika are primarily spread through mosquito bites.
- **Respiratory Droplets**: ARI, COVID-19, and Influenza/ILI are transmitted via respiratory droplets when infected individuals cough or sneeze.

14.2 Mathematical Models for Infectious Diseases

The application of mathematical models to infectious diseases dates back over a century, with significant contributions from pioneers such as *Kermack* and *McKendrick*, who established the foundations of the subject.[3] Their work introduced the concept of categorising individuals based on their epidemiological status: **susceptible**, **infected**, and **recovered**.

14.2.1 The SIR Model

One of the simplest and most fundamental epidemiological models, the **SIR model**, to which we had a quick look in the previous chapters (Chapter 6 and Chapter 7), is based on these three compartments and uses a system of differential equations to describe how individuals move between these compartments based on **infection rate** and the **recovery rate**. These parameters help predict the epidemic's progression, showing how the number of susceptible individuals decreases as the number of infected individuals increases, eventually leading to recovery and a decline in new infections, as shown in Equation 6.1.

More complex models, includes:

- **SEIR Model**: This model introduces an exposed (E) compartment, which represents individuals who have been infected but are not yet infectious. This compartmentalization is particularly useful for diseases with significant incubation periods (e.g., COVID-19). Practical applications are in Section 6.3.2 and Section 15.3 .
- **SIS Model**: In this model, individuals who recover from infection do not gain lasting immunity, meaning they return to the susceptible class and can become reinfected.
- **MSIR Model**: In some diseases, such as measles, maternal antibodies provide temporary immunity to newborns. The M (maternal immunity) compartment is used in such cases.

[3] M. J. Keeling and L. Danon, "Mathematical Modelling of Infectious Diseases," *British Medical Bulletin* 92, no. 1 (December 1, 2009): 33–42, doi:10.1093/bmb/ldp038.

14.3 Components of Infectious Disease Models

1. **Infection Rate**: This parameter, often denoted as β (beta), controls how quickly the susceptible population becomes infected. It depends on factors such as contact rate and the probability of transmission per contact. It is the rate at which individuals move from the susceptible compartment to the infected compartment. The infection rate is proportional to the product of susceptible and infected individuals.[4]

$$\beta = \text{Contact Rate} \times \text{Probability of Transmission per Contact} \tag{14.1}$$

2. **Recovery Rate**: Denoted by γ (gamma), this defines the rate at which infected individuals recover and either gain immunity or become susceptible again (depending on the model). The average duration of infection is the reciprocal of the recovery rate.

$$\gamma = \frac{1}{\text{Average Duration of Infection}} \tag{14.2}$$

3. **Incubation Period**: In models like SEIR, the incubation period is the average time that exposed individuals take before they become infectious. This is a critical factor in diseases like COVID-19 and Ebola. The incubation period is the reciprocal of the rate at which individuals move from the exposed compartment to the infected compartment. σ is the rate at which individuals move from the exposed compartment to the infected compartment.

$$\text{Incubation Period} = \frac{1}{\sigma} \tag{14.3}$$

4. **Transmission Rate**: The transmission rate often depends on how a disease spreads—whether it's through respiratory droplets, direct contact, vectors like mosquitoes, or other means. Transmission rates are also influenced by human behaviours, such as hygiene practices and social distancing measures. The transmission rate is the product of the probability of transmission per contact and the number of contacts. β is the probability of transmission per contact, and the number of contacts is the average number of people an infected individual comes into contact with.

$$\text{Transmission Rate} = \beta \times \text{Number of Contacts} \tag{14.4}$$

5. **Reproduction Ratio (R_0)**: A key metric that indicates the **average number of secondary cases generated by one infectious individual in a fully susceptible population** is the **basic reproduction ratio (R_0)**. This value is calculated using the formula in Equation 14.5. β is the transmission rate and γ is

[4] Theodore Kolokolnikov and David Iron, "Law of Mass Action and Saturation in SIR Model with Application to Coronavirus Modelling," *Infectious Disease Modelling* 6 (November 16, 2020): 91–97, doi:10.1016/j.idm.2020.11.002.

the recovery rate. As the ratio of the transmission rate to the recovery rate, R_0 provides a measure of the disease's ability to spread.

$$R_0 = \frac{\beta}{\gamma} \tag{14.5}$$

In summary, the SIR model is a simple yet powerful tool for understanding the dynamics of infectious diseases. By tracking the movement of individuals between susceptible, infected, and recovered compartments, the model can predict the course of an epidemic and help public health officials make informed decisions about disease control measures. The value of R_0 determines the epidemic **threshold**:

$$\text{If } R_0 \begin{cases} > 1 = \text{Epidemic} \\ < 1 = \text{End of Infection Transmission} \end{cases} \tag{14.6}$$

To accounts for changes in the population's immunity, the **effective reproduction number** (R_{eff}) is calculated on a susceptible population which is not completely susceptible, and value of R_{eff} results less than $R0$ due to the presence of immune individuals in the population.

Another critical concept in infectious disease is the **herd immunity**, which refers to the indirect protection from infectious diseases that occurs when a large percentage of a population becomes immune to the infection, either through vaccination or previous infections. The herd immunity is reached when the effective reproduction number is less than 1, and the disease stops spreading.

The SIR model shows the dynamics of an epidemic by looking at how it grows and eventually declines. Initially, the number of cases rises exponentially, leading to a peak, but as the susceptible population start reducing in number due to various factors, the growth rate slows with subsequent decline.

14.4 Advancements and Extensions

Mathematical modelling has evolved to include more complex factors such as age structure, stochasticity, and spatial dynamics. Age-structured models, for example, consider how different age groups interact and contribute to the spread of diseases, which is particularly important for diseases like measles or COVID-19. Stochastic models account for random events that can influence the course of an epidemic, such as the introduction of the disease into a new population.

The use of machine learning algorithms such as **decision trees**, **random forests**, **support vector machines**, and **deep-learning networks** such as **Long Short-Term Memory (LSTM)** models, effectively improve the identification of patterns and trends that may not be obvious with mechanistic models. These models are able to improve prediction accuracy working smoothly with large datasets.

Combining models and data sources enhances prediction accuracy, various models and techniques can be applied to reduce bias and the risk of overfitting. For instance, **ensemble learning** combines the predictions of multiple models to improve accuracy. In this context, we will explore how machine learning can predict infectious disease outbreaks and their impacts on human health, ultimately aiming to reduce the burden of disease.

Another significant aspect to consider is the emerging use of **transfer learning**, which involves applying knowledge gained from one predictive task to another. This approach is especially useful when data are limited and models need to be adapted. Although relatively under-explored in infectious disease research, transfer learning holds significant promise for improving predictions in areas with scarce data. By leveraging information from related tasks, this technique can enhance model performance, leading to more accurate and reliable predictions in public health scenarios.[5]

14.5 The Impact on DALYs

To understand the magnitude of infectious diseases impacts on DALYs, we can simply consider the DALYs rate of change. The percentage change in total DALYs and DALYs due to infectious diseases, in general or for a specific infective virus such as COVID19, allows us to assess the impact on the overall burden of disease. In the case of COVID19 for example, the percentage change in DALYs due to COVID19 can explain how this virus affected global health and produced excess mortality and morbidity.

$$\text{Percent change in DALYs} = \frac{\text{DALYs due to Infectious Diseases}}{\text{Total DALYs}} \times 100 \qquad (14.7)$$

Where the $DALYs = \sum_{i=1}^{n}(YLD_i + YLL_i)$, YLD and YLL are the years lived with disability and the years of life lost respectively.

This percentage change provides a measure of the impact of infectious diseases on the overall burden of disease. The DALYs due to infectious diseases can be calculated as the sum of the DALYs for each disease, and the total DALYs can be calculated as the sum of the DALYs for all diseases. The percentage change in DALYs due to infectious diseases can then be calculated as the ratio of the DALYs due to infectious diseases to the total DALYs, multiplied by 100.

Furthermore, the use of machine learning models used to predict the variation of number of DALYs due to infectious diseases over time can be a valuable tool to understand the impact of infectious diseases on global health. Two approaches can be valued:

1. DALYs as a function of the **socio-demographic index (SDI)**: A composite index of the average income per person, educational attainment, and total fertility rate. The model function can be expressed as:

   $$DALY_{id} = f(SDI) + \epsilon \qquad (14.8)$$

   where is the number of $DALYs$ is the response variable, SDI the socio-demographic index acting as predictor, $f(.)$ is the function that relates the number of DALYs to the socio-demographic index, and ϵ is the error term.

2. DALYs as a function of the **human development index (HDI)**: A composite index of life expectancy, education, and per capita income indicators. The model function can be expressed as:

   $$DALY_{id} = f(HDI) + \epsilon \qquad (14.9)$$

[5] Roster, Connaughton, and Rodrigues, "Forecasting New Diseases in Low-Data Settings Using Transfer Learning".

where is the number of $DALYs$ is the response variable, HDI the human development index where is the number of $DALYs$ is the response variable, HDI the socio-demographic index acting as predictor, $f(.)$ is the function that relates the number of DALYs to the socio-demographic index, and ϵ is the error term. Big data analytics with machine learning analysis are used to classify the patterns of global disease burden by human development index (HDI) to have a better understanding of DALYs caused by infectious diseases such as COVID19 given different levels of HDI.

This can help us to understand the trends and patterns of infectious diseases and their impact on global health.

15

COVID-19 Outbreaks

Learning Objectives

- Understand the key characteristics and impact of COVID-19
- Explore how COVID-19 spreads through populations and environments
- Learn to map and visualize COVID-19 outbreaks using spatial data

In this chapter, we explore the dynamics of **COVID-19** disease outbreaks in more detail. We examine the results of various model's applications that simulate the spread of the virus.

15.1 Epidemiology

COVID-19, short for **"Coronavirus Disease 2019,"** is an infectious disease caused by the novel coronavirus SARS-CoV-2, a type of virus that is part of the **Coronaviridae**[1] family of viruses that can cause illness in animals and humans alike. The disease was first identified in December 2019 in Wuhan, Hubei province, China, and has since then spread globally, leading to a **pandemic.**[2]

The origin of the virus is still under investigation,[3] but it is believed to have **zoonotic**[4] origins, with **bats** being the most likely reservoir. The virus has also been linked to **pangolins,**[5] mammals that are illegally trafficked for their scales and meat. The virus is thought to have jumped from animals to humans, possibly through a wet market in Wuhan where live animals were sold.

Zoonotic diseases are a critical area of study in public health and epidemiology due to their significant impact on human populations and the potential for pandemics. As discussed by **MD Laura H. Kahn** in **One Health and the Politics of COVID-19,**[6] the pandemic's origins and spread highlight the critical need for a holistic understanding of health systems that integrates human, animal, and environmental health. Zoonotic viruses can be transmitted from animals to humans through direct contact, consumption of contaminated food or water, or exposure to infected animal products. These viruses can cause a range of diseases, from

[1] "Coronaviridae - Wikipedia," n.d., https://en.wikipedia.org/wiki/Coronaviridae.

[2] "Pandemic - Wikipedia," n.d., https://en.wikipedia.org/wiki/Pandemic.

[3] "WHO-Convened Global Study of Origins of SARS-CoV-2: China Part," n.d., https://www.who.int/publications/i/item/who-convened-global-study-of-origins-of-sars-cov-2-china-part.

[4] "Zoonosis - Wikipedia," n.d., https://en.wikipedia.org/wiki/Zoonosis.

[5] Xing-Yao Huang et al., "A Pangolin-Origin SARS-CoV-2-Related Coronavirus: Infectivity, Pathogenicity, and Cross-Protection by Preexisting Immunity," *Cell Discovery* 9, no. 1 (June 17, 2023): 1–13, doi:10.1038/s41421-023-00557-9.

[6] M. D. Laura H. Kahn, *One Health and the Politics of COVID-19* (Johns Hopkins University Press, 2024), doi:10.56021/9781421449326.

DOI: 10.1201/9781032625935-15

mild illnesses to severe respiratory infections, and can have devastating effects on public health and economies.

Examples of Zoonotic Viruses:

1. Influenza (Flu) Viruses: Avian (bird) flu and swine (pig) flu.
2. Coronavirus: SARS, MERS, and COVID-19 from fruit bats, pangolins.
3. Ebola Virus: Likely originated from fruit bats.
4. HIV/AIDS: Believed to have originated from non-human primates (chimpanzees).
5. Rabies: Spread from infected animals like dogs, bats, and raccoons.

On January 30, 2020, The **World Health Organization (WHO)** declared the **COVID-19 Outbreak** a *Public Health Emergency of International Concern*, and a worldwide investigation started to understand more about the virus and its effects on humans. This challenge involved the unprecedented identification of this type of virus, requiring thorough testing and confirmation of the incubation period, recovery rate, and infection rate through the collection of cases globally.

The virus spreads primarily through respiratory droplets. Symptoms can include loss of taste and smell, fatigue, muscle aches, and gastrointestinal issues, with fever, cough, and shortness of breath. Severe cases can lead to **pneumonia**, **acute respiratory distress syndrome (ARDS)**, and **death**. The emergency was primarily due to the high number of deaths occurring without a known pharmacological intervention to contain it.

Various preventive measures were established, but the presence of asymptomatic and symptomatic cases created challenges in identifying the incubation time, leading governments to impose restrictions through lockdowns of entire cities and regions in affected countries. These measures restricted movement and activities to curb the virus's transmission.

Some notable examples of lockdown measures include:

- **China**: The initial epicentre in Wuhan experienced strict lockdowns, with entire cities quarantined and movement heavily restricted. These measures were effective in reducing the initial spread of the virus.
- **Italy**: One of the first European countries severely impacted, Italy imposed nationwide lockdowns in March 2020, closing schools, businesses, and restricting travel.
- **United States**: Lockdown measures varied by state, with significant restrictions during the early waves of the pandemic. These included stay-at-home orders, business closures, and mask mandates.
- **India**: Implemented one of the world's largest lockdowns in March 2020, affecting millions of people and including strict travel bans and business closures.
- **Australia**: Used localised lockdowns effectively, particularly in cities like Melbourne, which saw extended periods of strict restrictions.
- **United Kingdom**: Imposed several lockdowns, including a strict nationwide lockdown in early 2021, along with tiered restrictions based on regional infection rates.

The pandemic has led to widespread healthcare challenges, economic disruptions, and significant changes to daily life, including social distancing measures, lockdowns, and travel restrictions.

Since its identification, COVID-19 has caused multiple outbreaks globally. The incubation period ranges from 2 to 14 days, during which an infected person may be asymptomatic but still contagious. As of May 2024, there have been over 775 million confirmed cases and more than seven million deaths worldwide. The impact of the pandemic has varied across regions, influenced by factors such as virus variants, public health responses, and vaccination rates.

Public Health COVID-19 Prevention Measures:

- **Diagnostic Tests**: PCR (polymerase chain reaction) tests and rapid antigen tests are used to detect active infections, while antibody tests determine past infections.
- **Treatment**: While there is no specific antiviral treatment for COVID-19, supportive care, including oxygen therapy and mechanical ventilation, is used for severe cases. Some antiviral medications and therapies have been repurposed or developed specifically for COVID-19.
- **Vaccination**: Vaccines have been developed and distributed globally to prevent COVID-19. These vaccines, including mRNA vaccines (Pfizer-BioNTech and Moderna), viral vector vaccines (AstraZeneca and Johnson & Johnson), and inactivated virus vaccines (Sinovac and Sinopharm), have shown high efficacy in preventing severe disease and reducing transmission.

COVID-19 has had a profound impact on global health, economies, and daily life. Efforts to combat the pandemic have involved unprecedented levels of international cooperation, scientific research, and public health initiatives. Ongoing vaccination campaigns and adherence to public health guidelines are critical in controlling the spread of the virus and preventing further outbreaks. However, vaccine hesitancy and resistance, driven by concerns about the speed of development and potential long-term effects, remain significant challenges in achieving widespread vaccination coverage.

15.2 Mapping COVID-19 Outbreaks

Mapping COVID-19 outbreaks helps identify infection hotspots, track the virus's spread, and inform public health interventions. Geographic Information Systems (GIS) and spatial analysis techniques can visualise and analyse COVID-19 data, such as the number of cases, deaths, and recoveries, at local, regional, and global levels.

15.3 Example: Modelling the Spread of COVID-19

Spatiotemporal modelling of COVID-19 outbreaks can provide valuable insights into the pandemic's dynamics and help guide public health responses. In this example, we'll use the **Susceptible-Exposed-Infected-Recovered (SEIR)** model to simulate the spread of COVID-19 infections, as we saw in Section 6.3.2. A **Bayesian machine learning approach** is used to predict the spread of the virus over time and across different regions. Bayesian methods handle uncertainties and allow for the integration of prior information into the model.

15.3.1 SEIR Model

First, we use the **SEIR model** function to simulate the spread of the disease. The model compartments are: the number of susceptible (S), the exposed (E), the infected (I), and R represents the number of recovered individuals. The parameters of the model are the transmission rate (β) and the recovery rate (γ), (t_{exp}) the latent period, and (N) is the total population.

```
library(deSolve)
library(tidyverse)
# Define parameters
N <- 1e6 # Total population
beta <- 0.5 # Transmission rate
gamma <- 0.1 # Recovery rate
t_exp <- 5 # Latent period - or incubation period

# Initial conditions
init <- c(S = N - 1, E = 1, I = 0, R = 0)

# Define the SEIR model
seir_model <- function(t, y, parameters) {
  with(as.list(y), {
    dS <- -beta * S * I / N
    dE <- beta * S * I / N - (1 / t_exp) * E
    dI <- (1 / t_exp) * E - gamma * I
    dR <- gamma * I
    return(list(c(dS, dE, dI, dR)))
  })
}
```

As seen previously, we'll use the `ode()` function from the `{deSolve}` package to solve the ordinary differential equations (ODEs) and simulate the spread of the virus over a period of 365 days:

```
times <- seq(0, 365, by = 1)
result <- ode(y = init, times = times, func = seir_model)
result %>% head()
#>      time        S         E         I           R
#> [1,]    0 999999.0 1.0000000 0.0000000 0.000000000
#> [2,]    1 999999.0 0.8614244 0.1750967 0.009130285
#> [3,]    2 999998.8 0.8186971 0.3169955 0.033923201
#> [4,]    3 999998.6 0.8440094 0.4441703 0.072045032
#> [5,]    4 999998.4 0.9214811 0.5692891 0.122692748
#> [6,]    5 999998.1 1.0429872 0.7015882 0.186144186
```

```
ggplot(as.data.frame(result), aes(time, I, color = "Infected")) +
  geom_line() +
  geom_line(aes(time, R, color = "Recovered")) +
  geom_line(aes(time, S, color = "Susceptible")) +
  geom_line(aes(time, E, color = "Exposed")) +
  scale_color_discrete(name = "Compartment") +
  labs(x = "Time (days)", y = "Number of individuals")
```

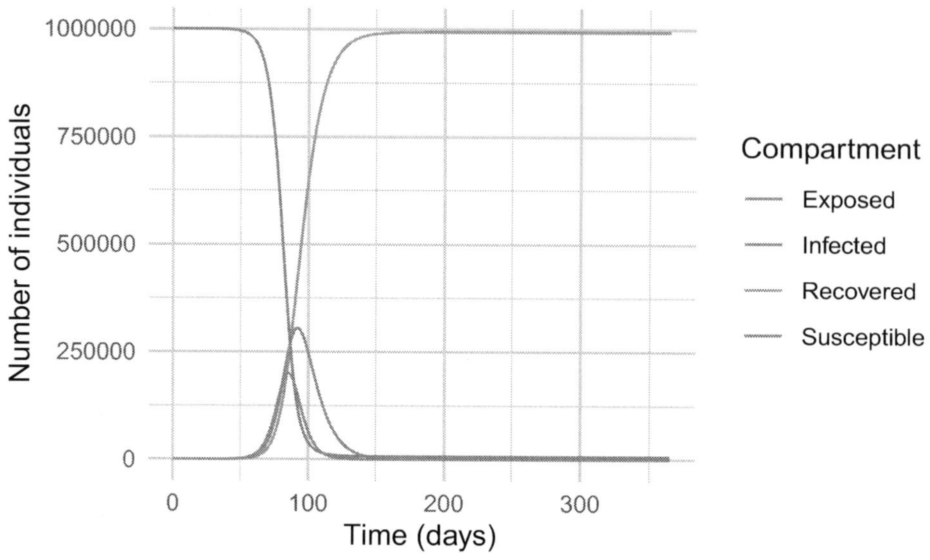

Figure 15.1 Simulation of the SEIR model for COVID-19

In reality, the spread of a virus is much more complex and influenced by many factors such as human behaviour, government policies, healthcare systems, vaccination campaigns, and human contact.

15.3.2 Bayesian Analysis

The use of **Bayesian analysis** in modelling infectious diseases offers several advantages in understanding and predicting the dynamics of the spread. We implement a Bayesian regression model for COVID-19 cases using the `{brms}` package, which is an interface of **Stan** for Bayesian analysis. The source for **Stan** is available at https://mc-stan.org/.

The application of Bayesian analysis allows us to estimate the regression coefficients for the lag-1 and lag-7 cases, which can help predict the number of infected individuals over time, with the flexibility to incorporate prior knowledge and uncertainties into the model.

The model is specified as follows:

$$I_t \sim \text{Normal}(\beta \times I_{t-1} + \gamma \times I_{t-7}, \sigma)$$

where I_t is the number of infected individuals at time t, β is the regression coefficient for the lag-1 cases, γ is the regression coefficient for the lag-7 cases, and σ is the error term. The model assumes that the number of infected individuals at time t is normally distributed around the predicted value based on the number of cases at times $t-1$ and $t-7$.

We can specify the prior distributions for β and γ using expert knowledge and available data. For example, we might specify a gamma distribution with a mean of 0.1 and a standard deviation of 0.05 for β, and a gamma distribution with a mean of 0.05 and a standard deviation of 0.02 for γ.

```
result <- as.data.frame(result)
```

```
cv19_data <- result %>%
  mutate(date = as.Date(time, origin = "2022-01-01"),
         day_of_week = wday(date, label = TRUE),
         week_of_year = week(date),
         month = month(date),
         lag_1_cases = lag(I, 1),
         lag_7_cases = lag(I, 7)) %>%
  drop_na()
```

```
cv19_data %>% head(n = 3) %>% glimpse()
#> Rows: 3
#> Columns: 11
#> $ time         <dbl> 7, 8, 9
#> $ S            <dbl> 999997.2, 999996.7, 999996.0
#> $ E            <dbl> 1.409890, 1.659350, 1.959605
#> $ I            <dbl> 1.016210, 1.211223, 1.439964
#> $ R            <dbl> 0.3565260, 0.4676444, 0.5998941
#> $ date         <date> 2022-01-08, 2022-01-09, 2022-01-10
#> $ day_of_week  <ord> Sat, Sun, Mon
#> $ week_of_year <dbl> 2, 2, 2
#> $ month        <dbl> 1, 1, 1
#> $ lag_1_cases  <dbl> 0.8484115, 1.0162103, 1.2112229
#> $ lag_7_cases  <dbl> 0.0000000, 0.1750967, 0.3169955
```

In this example we do not split the data into training and testing sets, but in a real-world scenario, it is essential to validate the model's performance on unseen data. Our data are made of 359 observations and 11 variables.

```
cv19_data %>% dim()
#> [1] 359  11
```

The `brm()` function from the `{brms}` package, fits the Bayesian regression model to the data by specifying the outcome variable `I` (number of infected individuals) and the predictors `day_of_week`, `week_of_year`, `month`, `lag_1_cases`, and `lag_7_cases`. We use a Gaussian likelihood function and specify prior distributions for the regression coefficients and the error term. The **Stan algorithm** is used to sample from the posterior distribution of the model parameters. In particular, we use a **normal prior distribution** with a mean of 0 and standard deviation of 10 for the regression coefficients and a **Cauchy prior distribution** with a scale of 5 for the error term.

The decision to use a normal and a Cauchy prior is based on the properties of the data and the model assumptions. In this case, we assume that the regression coefficients are normally distributed around 0 with a standard deviation of 10, and the error term is distributed according to a Cauchy distribution with a scale of 5.

The model is run for 2000 iterations with a `warmup` of 1000 iterations and 4 chains. The reason for the warmup is to allow the **Markov Chain Monte Carlo (MCMC) algorithm** to converge to the posterior distribution. The chains are run in parallel to explore the parameter space and estimate the posterior distribution of the model parameters.

```
library(brms)
```

```
# Define the Bayesian regression model
bayesian_model <- brm(
  I ~ day_of_week + week_of_year + month + lag_1_cases + lag_7_cases,
  data = cv19_data,
  family = gaussian(),
  prior = c(set_prior("normal(0, 10)", class = "b"),
            set_prior("cauchy(0, 5)", class = "sigma")),
  iter = 2000,
  warmup = 1000,
  chains = 4,
  seed = 42
  )
```

The `bayesian_model` object contains the fitted model, including the posterior samples of the model parameters. We can inspect the summary of the model to assess the convergence of the chains, the posterior distribution of the parameters, and the model fit statistics.

```
summary(bayesian_model)$fixed %>%
  rownames_to_column(var = "parameter") %>%
  head(n = 3) %>%
  glimpse()
#> Rows: 3
#> Columns: 8
#> $ parameter  <chr> "Intercept", "day_of_week.L", "day_of_week.Q"
#> $ Estimate   <dbl> 866.78250835, -0.04239118, -0.16213817
#> $ Est.Error  <dbl> 145.09866, 10.17293, 10.07890
#> $ `l-95% CI` <dbl> 576.67263, -19.85932, -19.61945
#> $ `u-95% CI` <dbl> 1137.71086, 20.30390, 19.72001
#> $ Rhat       <dbl> 1.000109, 1.000764, 1.000761
#> $ Bulk_ESS   <dbl> 5660.295, 5486.962, 5309.553
#> $ Tail_ESS   <dbl> 3204.207, 2641.086, 2846.849
```

The model output tells us about the convergence of the chains, the posterior distribution of the parameters, and the model fit statistics. We can see the mean, median, and 95% credible intervals for the regression coefficients, as well as the standard deviation of the error term. The `Rhat` statistic measures the convergence of the chains, with values close to 1 indicating convergence. The `n_eff` statistic measures the effective sample size of the chains, with higher values indicating more reliable estimates. The `looic` statistic is the leave-one-out cross-validation information criterion, which measures the model's predictive performance.

Or access the formula used in the model:

```
bayesian_model$formula
#> I ~ day_of_week + week_of_year + month + lag_1_cases + lag_7_cases
```

After fitting the model, we can plot the model diagnostics to assess its performance with the `plot()` function. The diagnostics include trace plots of the chains, density plots of the posterior distributions, and the `Gelman-Rubin statistic`, which measures the convergence of the chains. The Gelman-Rubin statistic should be close to 1 for the model to have converged.

```
# Plot the model diagnostics
plot(bayesian_model)
```

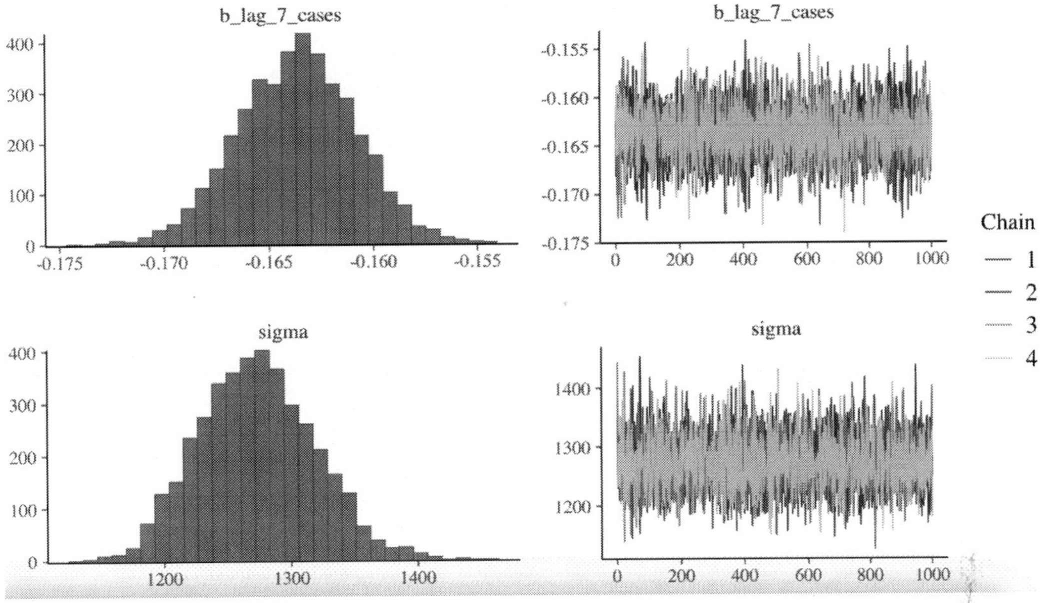

Figure 15.2 Bayesian Model diagnostics

Then, finally we can make predictions using the fitted model and visualise the actual vs. predicted COVID-19 cases over time. The `predictions` object is type matrix/array.

```
predictions <- predict(bayesian_model, newdata = cv19_data)
predictions %>% head()
#>       Estimate Est.Error      Q2.5    Q97.5
#> [1,] 779.2025  1263.317 -1657.152 3299.250
#> [2,] 837.3495  1270.743 -1627.192 3305.897
#> [3,] 813.2604  1283.773 -1696.402 3337.646
#> [4,] 877.0629  1271.697 -1580.855 3388.625
#> [5,] 823.5526  1294.345 -1754.888 3282.143
#> [6,] 820.5984  1277.846 -1770.321 3205.060
```

Create a new data frame with the actual and predicted values for COVID-19 cases, and then plot the actual vs. predicted values over time.

```
predictions <- as_tibble(predictions)
cv19_data_pred <- cv19_data %>%
  mutate(predicted_cases = predictions$Estimate)

# Plot actual vs. predicted values
ggplot(data = cv19_data_pred,
       aes(x = I, y = predicted_cases)) +
  geom_point() +
  geom_abline() +
  labs(title = "Actual vs. Predicted COVID-19 Cases",
       x = "Date", y = "Cases", color = "Legend")

ggplot(data = cv19_data_pred, aes(x = date)) +
```

```
  geom_point(aes(y = I,
                 color = "Actual")) +
  geom_line(aes(y = predicted_cases,
                color = "Predicted")) +
  labs(title = "Actual vs. Predicted COVID-19 Cases",
       x = "Date", y = "Cases", color = "Legend")
```

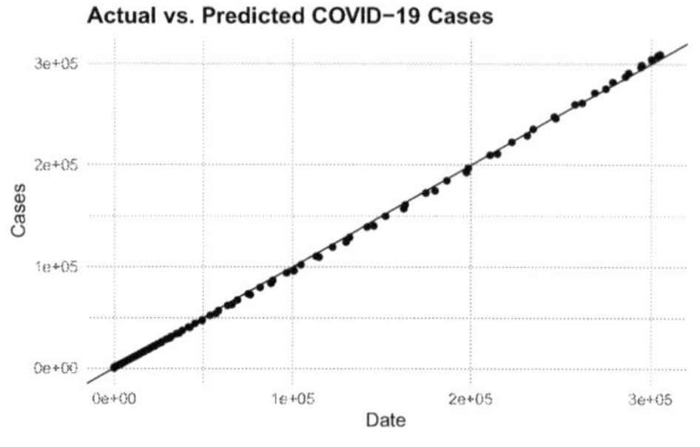

Figure 15.3 Actual vs. Predicted COVID-19 Cases

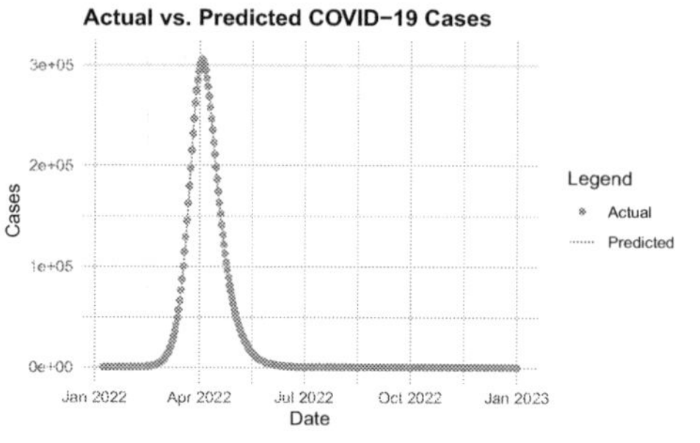

Figure 15.4 Actual vs. Predicted COVID-19 Cases

15.3.3 Ensemble Modelling - Combining Multiple Models

We have been able to simulate the spread of COVID-19 using the SEIR and predict the spread using the Bayesian regression model. However, combining the predictions of multiple models can provide more accurate and robust forecasts. This technique is known as **ensemble modelling**.

Ensemble modelling combines the predictions of multiple models to improve the overall accuracy and robustness of predictions. This technique is particularly useful in infectious disease modelling to account for uncertainties and variability in data, providing more reliable estimates of disease spread.

This method combines the strengths of different models to produce more accurate and stable predictions by averaging the results of individual models or using more sophisticated techniques such as **stacking** or **boosting**.

For example, ensemble models have been used to predict confirmed COVID-19 cases and provide short-term forecasts by integrating multiple model types. Other methods combine sub-epidemic models over various forecasting periods to enhance prediction accuracy.[7]

In this example, we use the `{tidymodels}` meta-package and other key packages such as `{modeltimes}`, and `{stacks}` to combine different types of models. We will use: Decision Tree, Random Forest, K-Nearest Neighbours (KNN), and Support Vector Machines (SVM) models to combine and predict the spread of COVID-19 cases.

```
library(tidymodels)
library(modeltime)
library(stacks)
```

[7] Gerardo Chowell et al., "An Ensemble n-Sub-Epidemic Modeling Framework for Short-Term Forecasting Epidemic Trajectories: Application to the COVID-19 Pandemic in the USA," *PLOS Computational Biology* 18, no. 10 (October 6, 2022): e1010602, doi:10.1371/journal.pcbi.1010602.

We start by splitting the data into training and testing sets using the `initial_split()` function from the `{rsample}` package. The training set will be used to train the models, while the testing set will be used to evaluate the models' performance.

```
set.seed(10011)
# Split the data into training and testing sets
cv_split <- initial_split(cv19_data, prop = 0.8)
cv_train <- training(cv_split)
cv_test <- testing(cv_split)
```

Create a `vfold_cv()` object for cross-validation with 10 folds. This object will be used to evaluate the models' performance during training.

```
set.seed(1001)
cv_folds <- vfold_cv(cv_train, v = 10)
```

We also define a recipe to preprocess the data, including log transformation and dummy encoding of categorical variables. The recipe is then used to create a workflow that combines the preprocessing steps with the model specifications.

```
cv_recipe <- recipe(I ~ ., data = cv_train) %>%
  step_scale(all_numeric(), -all_outcomes()) %>%
  step_dummy(all_nominal(), -all_outcomes())
```

To check the output of the recipe transformation: `cv_recipe %>% prep() %>% juice()`

Define the models' specifications with the parameters to tune, and the engine to use:

```
# Decision Tree
cart <- decision_tree(cost_complexity = tune(),
                      tree_depth = tune(),
                      min_n = tune()) %>%
  set_engine("rpart") %>%
  set_mode("regression")

# Random Forest
rand_forest <- rand_forest(mtry = tune(),
                           min_n = tune()) %>%
  set_engine('ranger') %>%
  set_mode('regression')

# K-Nearest Neighbors (KNN)
knn <- nearest_neighbor(neighbors = tune()) %>%
  set_engine("kknn") %>%
  set_mode("regression")

# Support Vector Machine (SVM)
svm <- svm_rbf(cost = tune(),
               rbf_sigma = tune()) %>%
  set_engine("kernlab") %>%
  set_mode("regression")
```

Then, create a `workflow_set()` that combines the predictions of different models:

```
cv_wkf <- workflow_set(
  preproc = list(id = cv_recipe),
  models = list(Decision_tree = cart,
                Random_Forest = rand_forest,
                Knn = knn,
                SVM = svm))

cv_wkf
#> # A workflow set/tibble: 4 x 4
#>   wflow_id         info              option     result
#>   <chr>            <list>            <list>     <list>
#> 1 id_Decision_tree <tibble [1 x 4]> <opts[0]> <list [0]>
#> 2 id_Random_Forest <tibble [1 x 4]> <opts[0]> <list [0]>
#> 3 id_Knn           <tibble [1 x 4]> <opts[0]> <list [0]>
#> 4 id_SVM           <tibble [1 x 4]> <opts[0]> <list [0]>
```

Create a `workflow_map()` to fit the models to the training data. We use the `{finetune}` package to use the `tune_race_anova` function to tune the hyperparameters of the models. The `race_ctrl` object specifies the control parameters for the tuning process, such as the number of resamples and the grid size. The `parallel_over` argument allows the tuning process to run in parallel over multiple cores for faster computation.

```
# Fit the models to the training data
library(finetune)
set.seed(112233)
race_ctrl <-
  control_race(save_pred = TRUE,
               parallel_over = "everything",
               save_workflow = TRUE)

race_results <- cv_wkf %>%
  workflow_map("tune_race_anova",
               seed = 1503,
               resamples = cv_folds,
               grid = 3,
               control = race_ctrl)

race_results
#> # A workflow set/tibble: 4 x 4
#>   wflow_id         info              option     result
#>   <chr>            <list>            <list>     <list>
#> 1 id_Decision_tree <tibble [1 x 4]> <opts[3]> <race[+]>
#> 2 id_Random_Forest <tibble [1 x 4]> <opts[3]> <race[+]>
#> 3 id_Knn           <tibble [1 x 4]> <opts[3]> <race[+]>
#> 4 id_SVM           <tibble [1 x 4]> <opts[3]> <race[+]>
```

Then we collect the metrics for the models to evaluate their performance. We filter the results for the root mean squared error (`rmse`) and arrange them in ascending order to identify the best-performing model.

```
rmse <- collect_metrics(race_results) %>%
  filter(.metric == "rmse") %>%
```

```
  select(wflow_id, .config, mean) %>%
  arrange(mean)

rmse
#> # A tibble: 5 x 3
#>   wflow_id          .config                mean
#>   <chr>             <chr>                 <dbl>
#> 1 id_Random_Forest Preprocessor1_Model2  5595.
#> 2 id_SVM            Preprocessor1_Model1  7642.
#> 3 id_Decision_tree Preprocessor1_Model2  8057.
#> 4 id_Knn            Preprocessor1_Model3 14034.
#> 5 id_Knn            Preprocessor1_Model2 14817.
```

Plot the root mean squared error (`rmse`) values for the models to visualise their performance.

```
rmse %>%
  ggplot(aes(x = fct_reorder(wflow_id, mean), y = mean)) +
  geom_col(fill = "navy") +
  labs(title = "Root Mean Squared Error (RMSE) for Models",
       x = "Model", y = "RMSE")
```

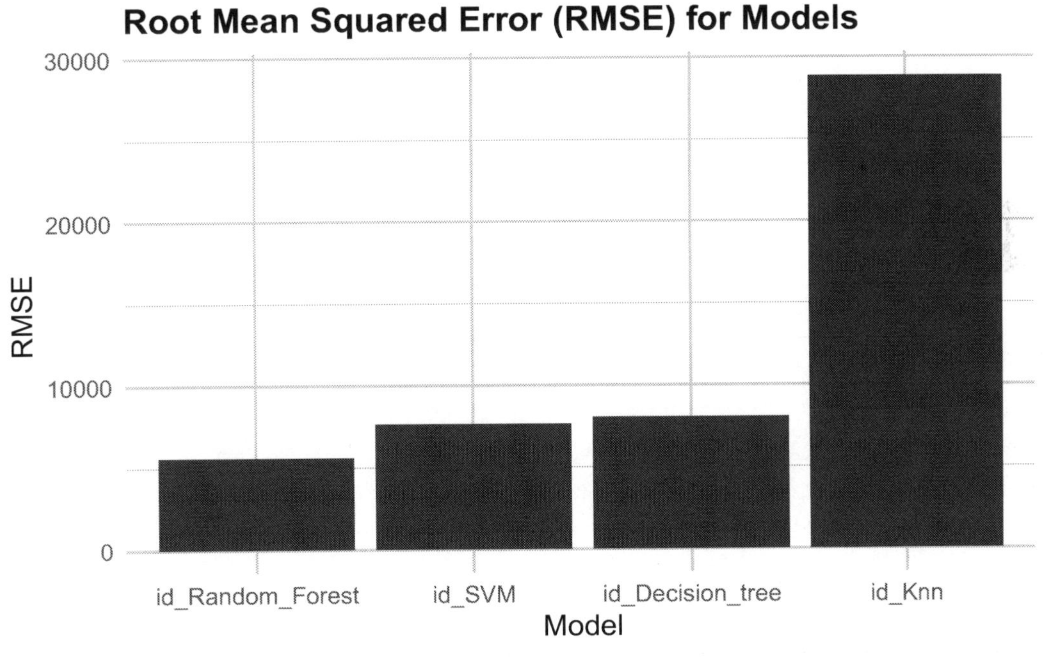

Figure 15.5 Root Mean Squared Error (RMSE) for Models

The results of the race show that the Random Forest model has the lowest `rmse` value, indicating better performance compared to the other models.

Extract the model's estimations:

```
race_results %>%
  collect_predictions() %>%
  ggplot(aes(x = I, y = .pred,
             group= model,
             shape= model,
             color = model)) +
  geom_point() +
  geom_abline()
```

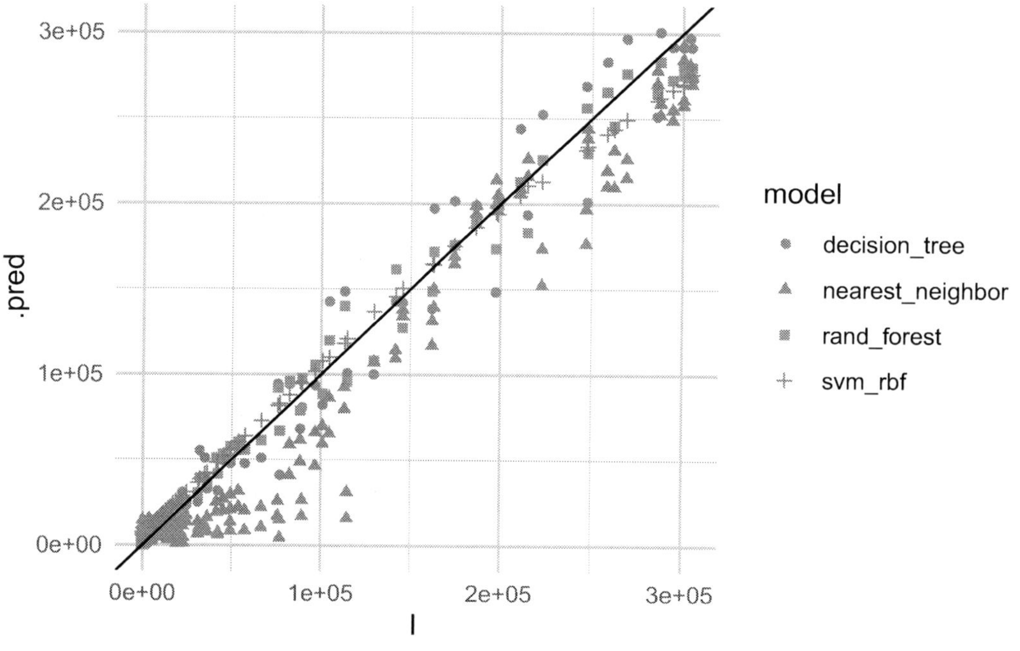

Figure 15.6 Actual vs. Predicted COVID-19 Cases

The plot shows the actual vs. predicted values for COVID-19 cases using the different models. The Random Forest model appears to have the best fit to the data, closely following the 45-degree line, indicating accurate predictions.

So, let's see how combined predictions look like:

```
race_results %>%
  collect_predictions() %>%
  group_by(I) %>%
  summarise(mean_pred = mean(.pred)) %>%
  ggplot(aes(x = I, y = mean_pred)) +
  geom_point() +
  geom_abline()
```

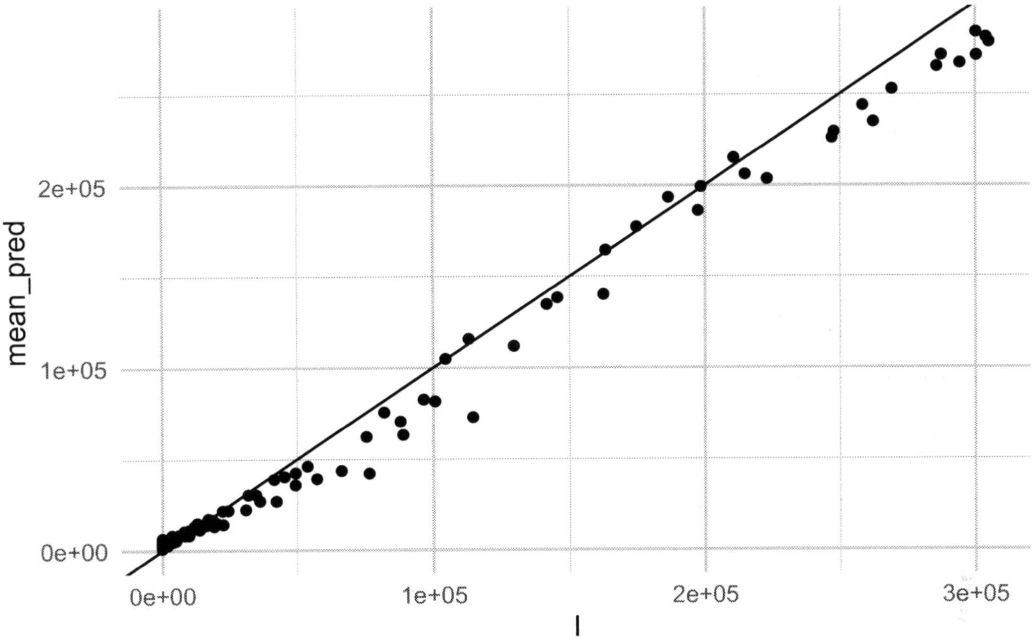

Figure 15.7 Ensemble Predictions of COVID-19 Cases

Finally, we can combine the predictions of the models using the `{stacks}` package to create an ensemble model. The `stack()` function combines the predictions of the models using a meta-learner, such as a linear regression model, to produce a final prediction.

```
cv_stack <- stacks() %>%
  add_candidates(race_results)
cv_stack
#> # A data stack with 4 model definitions and 5 candidate members:
#> #   id_Decision_tree: 1 model configuration
#> #   id_Random_Forest: 1 model configuration
#> #   id_Knn: 2 model configurations
#> #   id_SVM: 1 model configuration
#> # Outcome: I (numeric)
```

Blend the predictions of the models:

```
set.seed(2001)
cv_ens <- blend_predictions(cv_stack)
cv_ens
#> # A tibble: 3 x 3
#>   member                type              weight
#>   <chr>                 <chr>              <dbl>
#> 1 id_SVM_1_1            svm_rbf            0.751
#> 2 id_Random_Forest_1_2 rand_forest        0.190
#> 3 id_Knn_1_3            nearest_neighbor   0.147
```

```
autoplot(cv_ens, "weights")
```

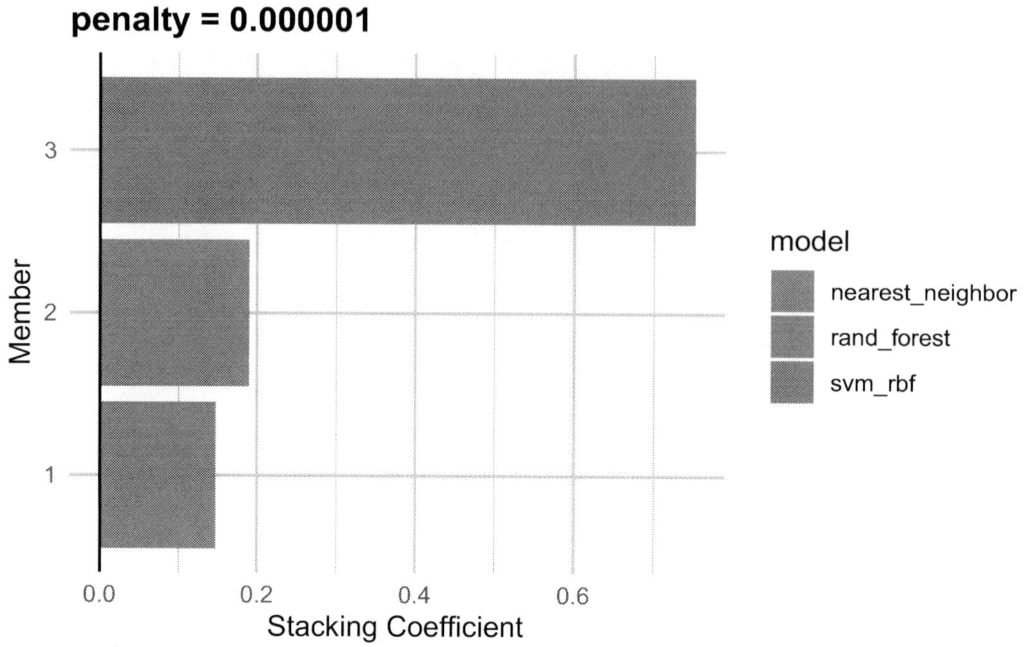

Figure 15.8 Ensemble Model Weights

```
fit_cv_ens <- fit_members(cv_ens)
fit_cv_ens
#> # A tibble: 3 x 3
#>   member                  type               weight
#>   <chr>                   <chr>               <dbl>
#> 1 id_SVM_1_1              svm_rbf             0.751
#> 2 id_Random_Forest_1_2 rand_forest            0.190
#> 3 id_Knn_1_3              nearest_neighbor    0.147
```

```
cv_ens_test_pred <-
  predict(fit_cv_ens, new_data = cv_test) %>%
  bind_cols(cv_test)
```

```
cv_ens_test_pred %>%
  ggplot(aes(x = I, y = .pred)) +
  geom_point(alpha=0.5) +
  geom_abline()
```

In summary, integrating machine learning models and advanced statistical techniques such as Bayesian analysis and ensemble modelling can significantly enhance our ability to predict and understand the spread of infectious diseases like COVID-19. These models provide critical insights that can inform public health responses and help mitigate the impact of pandemics.

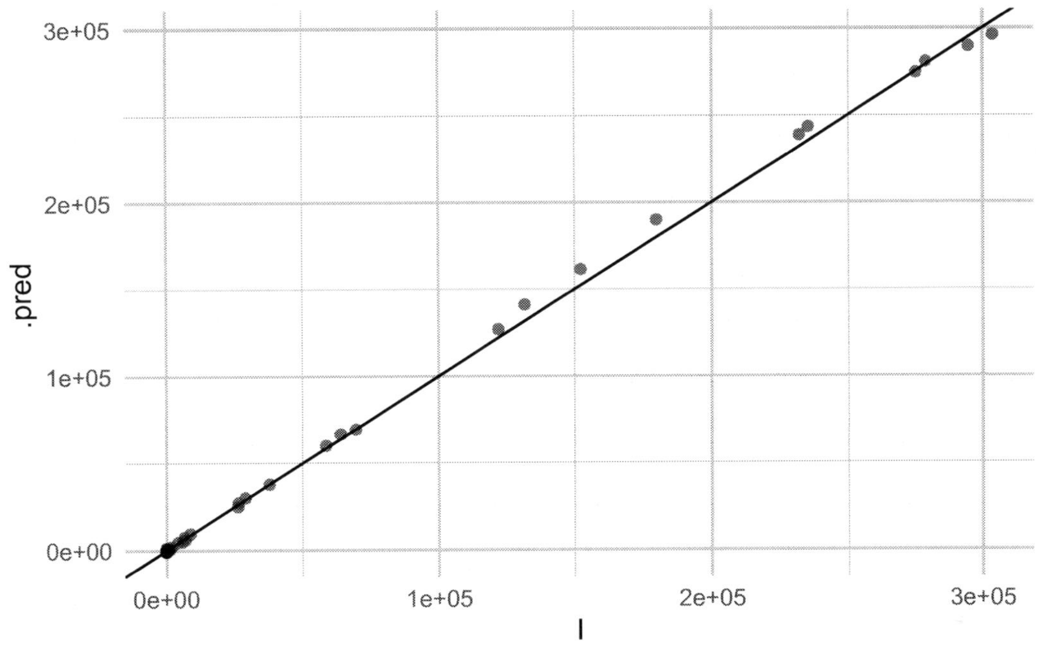

Figure 15.9 Ensemble Predictions of COVID-19 Cases

15.4 COVID-19 and DALYs

The influence of COVID-19 on global health can be measured using the DALYs. We use the data from the JHU official GitHub repository **CSSEGISandData**[8] to calculate the DALYs for COVID-19. The data includes the number of confirmed cases, deaths, and recovered cases for each country and region. We will calculate the DALYs for the US, China, United Kingdom, and Canada.

Data are loaded from the repository with the `read.csv()` function, and need a bit of adjustment before can be used.

```
tidyverse_conflicts()
```

Here we use the `pivot_longer()` to combine all cases by day in one column, and see the first rows:

```
cases1 <- cases %>%
  pivot_longer(cols = starts_with("X"),
               names_to = "date",
               values_to = "cases") %>%
  mutate(date = gsub("X", "", date),
         date = as.Date(date, format = "%m.%d.%y")) %>%
  janitor::clean_names()
```

[8]https://github.com/CSSEGISandData/COVID-19

```
cases1 %>% head()
#> # A tibble: 6 x 6
#>   province_state country_region   lat  long date       cases
#>   <chr>          <chr>          <dbl> <dbl> <date>     <int>
#> 1 ""             Afghanistan     33.9  67.7 2020-01-22     0
#> 2 ""             Afghanistan     33.9  67.7 2020-01-23     0
#> 3 ""             Afghanistan     33.9  67.7 2020-01-24     0
#> 4 ""             Afghanistan     33.9  67.7 2020-01-25     0
#> 5 ""             Afghanistan     33.9  67.7 2020-01-26     0
#> 6 ""             Afghanistan     33.9  67.7 2020-01-27     0
```

The same is done with deaths:

```
deaths1 <- deaths %>%
  pivot_longer(cols = starts_with("X"),
               names_to = "date",
               values_to = "deaths") %>%
  mutate(date = gsub("X", "", date),
         date = as.Date(date, format = "%m.%d.%y")) %>%
  janitor::clean_names()

deaths1 %>% head()
#> # A tibble: 6 x 6
#>   province_state country_region   lat  long date       deaths
#>   <chr>          <chr>          <dbl> <dbl> <date>      <int>
#> 1 ""             Afghanistan     33.9  67.7 2020-01-22      0
#> 2 ""             Afghanistan     33.9  67.7 2020-01-23      0
#> 3 ""             Afghanistan     33.9  67.7 2020-01-24      0
#> 4 ""             Afghanistan     33.9  67.7 2020-01-25      0
#> 5 ""             Afghanistan     33.9  67.7 2020-01-26      0
#> 6 ""             Afghanistan     33.9  67.7 2020-01-27      0
```

Then, the next step is to join the two sets by province, country, lat, long, and date. Sum the number of cases and deaths and calculate the case fatality ratio (CFR) as deaths divided by cases.

```
COVID19 <- cases1 %>%
  left_join(deaths1,
            by = c("province_state",
                   "country_region",
                   "lat", "long", "date")) %>%
  mutate(cases = ifelse(is.na(cases), 0, cases),
         deaths = ifelse(is.na(deaths), 0, deaths)) %>%
  group_by(country_region, date) %>%
  mutate(cases = sum(cases),
         deaths = sum(deaths),
         cfr = round(deaths / cases, 3)) %>%
  filter(cases > 0) %>%
  arrange(country_region, date)

COVID19 %>%
  select(country_region, date, cases, deaths, cfr) %>%
```

```
  arrange(desc(date)) %>%
  head()
#> # A tibble: 6 x 5
#> # Groups:   country_region, date [6]
#>   country_region date        cases deaths   cfr
#>   <chr>          <date>      <int>  <int> <dbl>
#> 1 Afghanistan    2023-03-09 209451   7896 0.038
#> 2 Albania        2023-03-09 334457   3598 0.011
#> 3 Algeria        2023-03-09 271496   6881 0.025
#> 4 Andorra        2023-03-09  47890    165 0.003
#> 5 Angola         2023-03-09 105288   1933 0.018
#> 6 Antarctica     2023-03-09     11      0 0
```

Now that the `COVID19` set is human readable we can select our countries: US, China, United Kingdom, and Canada.

```
COVID19_4countries <- COVID19 %>%
  filter(country_region %in%
    c("US", "China", "United Kingdom", "Canada"))

COVID19_4countries %>%
  select(- lat, -long) %>%
  head()
#> # A tibble: 6 x 6
#> # Groups:   country_region, date [1]
#>   province_state   country_region date       cases deaths   cfr
#>   <chr>            <chr>          <date>     <int>  <int> <dbl>
#> 1 Alberta          Canada         2020-01-23     2      0     0
#> 2 British Columbia Canada         2020-01-23     2      0     0
#> 3 Diamond Princess Canada         2020-01-23     2      0     0
#> 4 Grand Princess   Canada         2020-01-23     2      0     0
#> 5 Manitoba         Canada         2020-01-23     2      0     0
#> 6 New Brunswick    Canada         2020-01-23     2      0     0
```

Here we can see how COVID19 cases and deaths distributed along the years with a simple line plot:

```
COVID19 %>%
  ggplot(aes(x = date, y = cases,
             group = country_region)) +
  geom_line(color = "grey",
            linewidth = 0.2) +
  geomtextpath::geom_textline(
    data = COVID19_4countries,
    aes(label = country_region),
    show.legend = F) +
  scale_y_log10() +
  labs(title = "COVID-19 Cases by Country",
       x = "Date",
       y = "Cases")

COVID19 %>%
```

```
ggplot(aes(x = date, y = deaths,
           group = country_region)) +
geom_line(color = "grey",
          linewidth = 0.2) +
geomtextpath::geom_textline(
  data = COVID19_4countries,
  aes(label = country_region),
      show.legend = F) +
scale_y_log10() +
labs(title = "COVID-19 Deaths by Country",
     x = "Date",
     y = "Deaths")
```

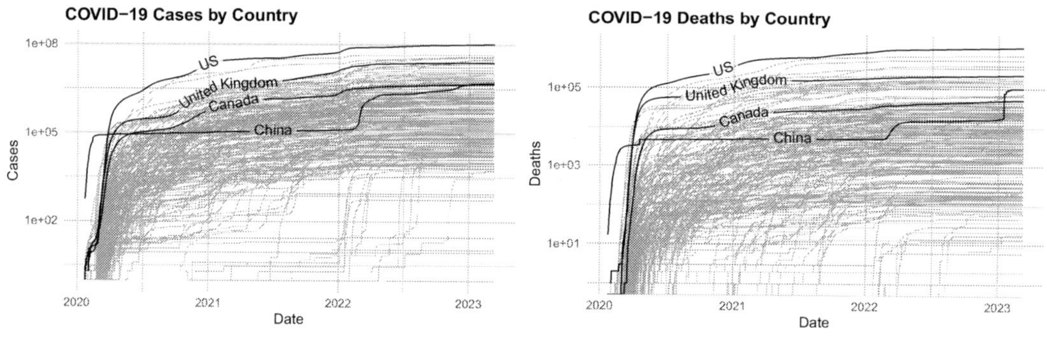

(a) COVID-19 Cases by Country **(b)** COVID-19 Deaths by Country

Figure 15.10 COVID-19 Cases and Deaths by Country

Now, to visualise the total number of cases and deaths by selected countries on a map, we use the `map_data()` function to retrieve the world geographic coordinates, and calculate the centroids by grouping by `country_region`.

```
worldmap <- map_data("world") %>%
  filter(!region == "Antarctica")

centroids <- COVID19 %>%
  group_by(country_region, lat, long) %>%
  reframe(tot_cases = sum(cases),
          tot_deaths = sum(deaths),
          avg_cfr = round(mean(cfr), 3)) %>%
  distinct()
```

```
ggplot() +
  geom_polygon(data = worldmap,
               aes(x = long, y = lat, group = group),
               fill = "grey",
               color = "white") +
  geom_point(data = centroids,
             aes(x = long, y = lat,
             size = tot_cases,
             color = avg_cfr),
```

```
            alpha = 0.5) +
  scale_size_continuous(name = "Total cases (M)",
                        labels = scales::unit_format(unit = "M",
                                                     scale = 1e-6)) +
  scale_color_viridis_c(name = "Average CFR (log scale)",
                        trans = "log",
                        labels = scales::label_number(accuracy = 0.001)) +
  guides(color = guide_colorbar(order = 1),
         size = guide_legend(order = 2)) +
  coord_quickmap() +
  labs(title = "COVID-19 Cases by Country",
       caption = "Data Source: JHU CSSEGISandData/COVID-19
       \nCircle size: total cases, Color: average CFR",
      size= "Total cases (M)",
      color= "Avg CFR (log scale)",
      x = "", y = "") +
  theme(axis.text = element_blank(),
        plot.subtitle = element_text(size = 8),
        legend.key.size = unit(0.5, "cm"),
        legend.text = element_text(size = 8),
        legend.title = element_text(size = 9))
```

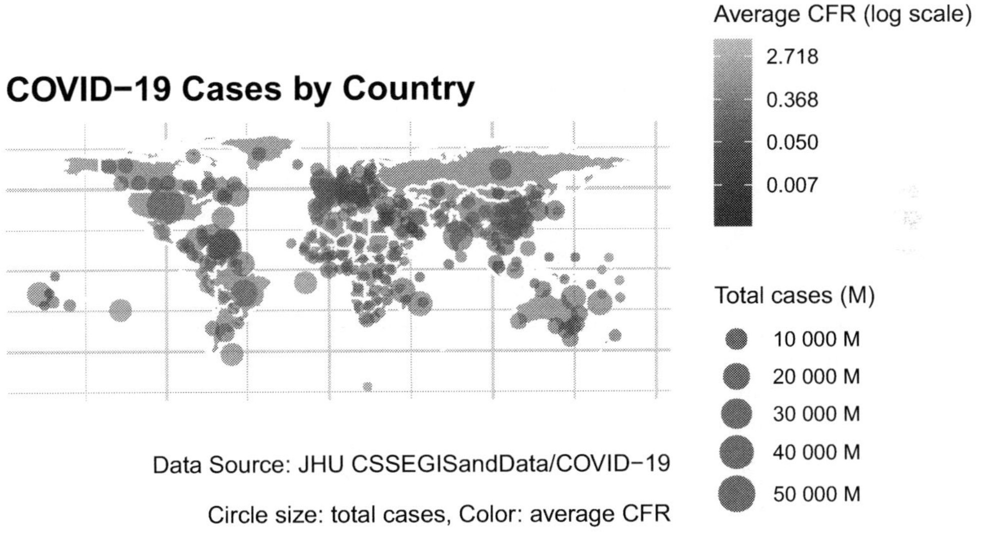

Figure 15.11 COVID-19 Cases by Country

The same graph is made with selected countries only.

```
ggplot() +
  geom_polygon(data = worldmap,
               aes(x = long, y = lat, group = group),
               fill = "grey",
               color = "white") +
  geom_point(data = centroids %>%
```

```
           filter(country_region %in%
           c("US", "China","United Kingdom", "Canada")),
           aes(x = long, y = lat,
               size = tot_cases,
               color = avg_cfr),
               alpha = 0.5) +
  scale_size_continuous(name = "Total cases (M)",
                        labels = scales::unit_format(unit = "M",
                                                     scale = 1e-6)) +
  scale_color_viridis_c(name = "Average CFR (log scale)",
                        trans = "log",
                        labels = scales::label_number(accuracy = 0.001)) +
  guides(color = guide_colorbar(order = 1),
         size = guide_legend(order = 2)) +
  coord_quickmap() +
  labs(title = "COVID-19 Cases by Country",
       caption = "Data Source: JHU CSSEGISandData/COVID-19
       \nCircle size: total cases, Color: average CFR",
       subtitle = "US, China, United Kingdom, Canada",
      size= "Total cases (M)",
      color= "Avg CFR (log scale)",
      x = "", y = "") +
  theme(axis.text = element_blank(),
        plot.subtitle = element_text(size = 8),
        legend.key.size = unit(0.5, "cm"),
        legend.text = element_text(size = 8),
        legend.title = element_text(size = 9))
```

The difference in the number of cases and deaths between the US and China is striking. The US has the highest number of cases and deaths, while China has the lowest number of cases and deaths. The United Kingdom and Canada have a similar number of cases and deaths, but the United Kingdom has a higher **case fatality rate (CFR)** than Canada.

Let's now calculate the DALYs for COVID-19, starting with the YLLs. We know that the simplified formula for YLLs is the number of deaths multiplied by the standard life expectancy at the age of death. The standard life expectancy for these countries varies, but we can use the global average of 72.6 years.

Also, we group the date by 4 months cycles to calculate the YLLs.

```
COVID19_yll_4months <- COVID19_4countries %>%
  mutate(month = as.numeric(format(date, "%m")),
         year = as.numeric(format(date, "%Y")),
         month_cycle = case_when(month %in% 1:4 ~ "Jan-Apr",
                                 month %in% 5:8 ~ "May-Aug",
                                 month %in% 9:12 ~ "Sep-Dec")) %>%
  group_by(country_region, year, month_cycle) %>%
  summarise(cases = sum(cases),
            deaths = sum(deaths),
            cfr = round(deaths / cases, 3)) %>%
  mutate(ylls = deaths * 72.6) %>%
  arrange(year, month_cycle, ylls)
```

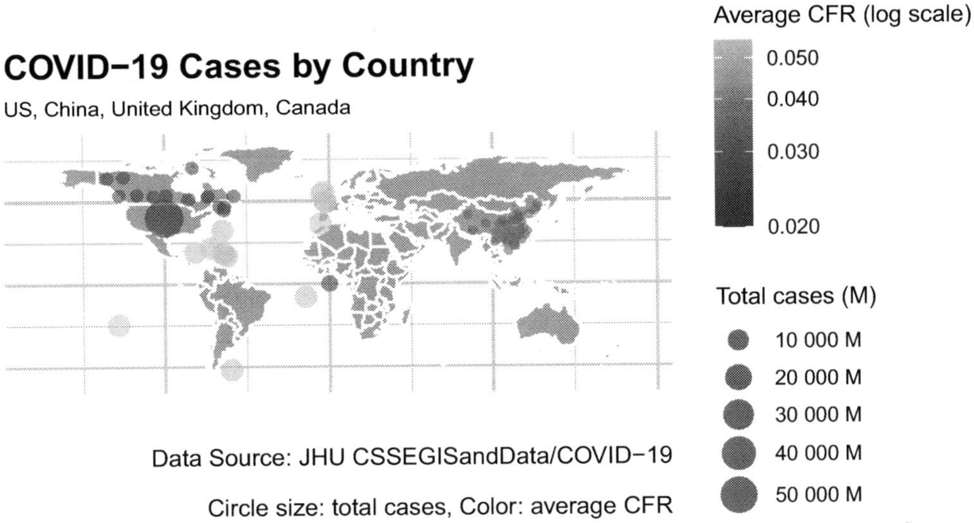

Figure 15.12 COVID-19 Cases by Selected Countries

```
COVID19_yll_4months %>%
  select(year, month_cycle, ylls) %>%
  head()
#> # A tibble: 6 x 4
#> # Groups:   country_region, year [4]
#>   country_region  year month_cycle        ylls
#>   <chr>          <dbl> <chr>             <dbl>
#> 1 Canada          2020 Jan-Apr       62225750.
#> 2 US              2020 Jan-Apr       80674499.
#> 3 China           2020 Jan-Apr      655246654.
#> 4 United Kingdom  2020 Jan-Apr      800881092
#> 5 US              2020 May-Aug     1158612365.
#> 6 Canada          2020 May-Aug     1165061568
```

And then plot the YLLs by country and month cycle, with the y axis representing the YLLs formatted in millions.

```
COVID19_yll_4months %>%
  ggplot() +
  geom_col(aes(x = month_cycle, y = ylls,
               fill = country_region)) +
  scale_y_continuous(
        labels = scales::unit_format(unit = "M",
                                     scale = 1e-6)) +
  scale_fill_grey(start = 0.2, end = 0.8) +
  labs(title = "YLLs by Country and Month Cycle",
```

```
      fill = "Country",
      x = "4-Month cycle",
      y = "YLLs") +
  facet_wrap(~year) +
  theme(axis.text.x = element_text(angle = 45, hjust = 1))
```

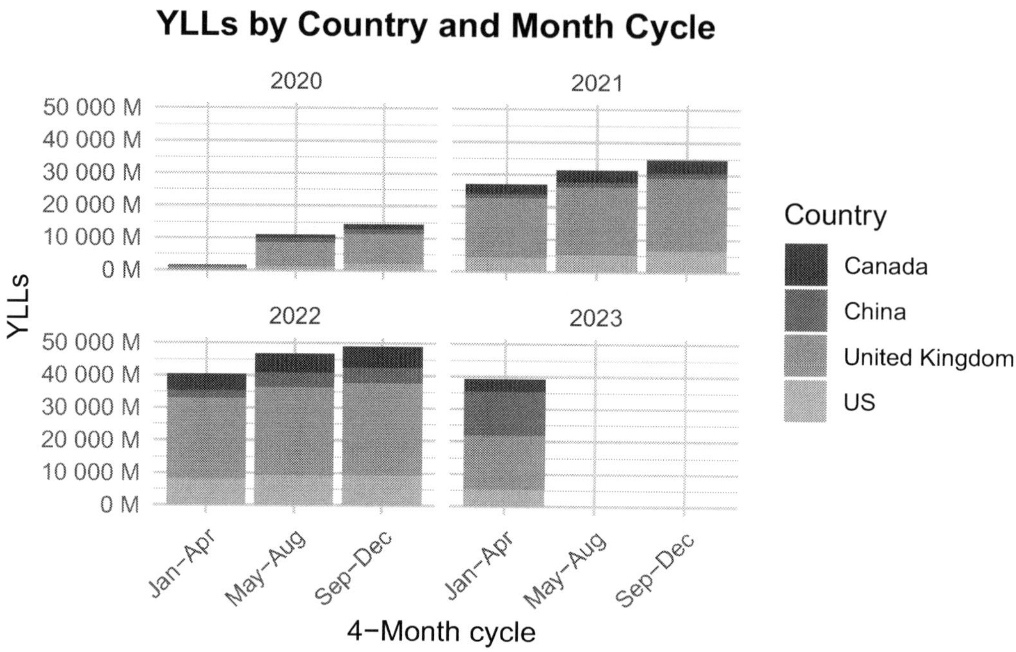

Figure 15.13 YLLs by Country and Month Cycle

The majority of YLLs are in the United Kingdom, followed by the US, Canada, and China. The YLLs are highest in the first 4-month cycle (Jan-Apr) and decrease in the following cycles.

Let's now calculate the YLDs for COVID-19. The YLDs are calculated by multiplying the number of cases by the disability weight. The Disability Weight applied is that for low respiratory diseases which is 0.133. As of 2020, the Global Burden of Disease Study 2019 estimated that the DALYs for lower respiratory diseases was 1,000,000. We can use the **{hmsidwR}** package to get the disability weight for lower respiratory diseases.

```
hmsidwR::disweights %>%
  filter(str_detect(sequela, "lower respiratory")) %>%
  select(sequela, dw)
#> # A tibble: 4 x 2
#>   sequela                                    dw
#>   <chr>                                   <dbl>
#> 1 Moderate lower respiratory infections 0.051
#> 2 Severe lower respiratory infections   0.133
#> 3 Moderate lower respiratory infections 0.0506
#> 4 Severe lower respiratory infections   0.133
```

We know that the simplified formula for YLDs is the prevalence of the disease multiplied by the disability weight. To calculate the prevalence, we need the population of each country. For this task we use the `{wpp2022}` package, which provides the population data from the 2022 revision of the **United Nations World Population Prospects (WPP 2022)**. It includes both historical estimates and projections of demographic indicators such as population counts and fertility rates, accommodating the challenges brought on by events like the COVID-19 pandemic and transitioning from five-year to one-year data intervals.

```
library(wpp2022)
# data(package = "wpp2022")
```

```
data(pop1dt)
pop_4countries <- pop1dt %>%
  filter(
    year %in% c(2020, 2021),
    name %in% c(
      "United States of America",
      "China",
      "United Kingdom",
      "Canada")) %>%
  mutate(name = ifelse(name == "United States of America", "US", name)) %>%
  select(name, year, pop) %>%
  arrange(year, name)

pop_4countries %>% head()
#>                name  year         pop
#>              <char> <int>       <num>
#> 1:           Canada  2020    38019.18
#> 2:            China  2020  1425861.54
#> 3:               US  2020   336495.77
#> 4:   United Kingdom  2020    67167.77
#> 5:           Canada  2021    38290.85
#> 6:            China  2021  1425925.39
```

Calculate the prevalence of COVID-19 cases per 1,000,000 people.

$$prevalence = \frac{cases}{population} * 1,000,000$$

```
COVID19_dalys <- COVID19_yll_4months %>%
  full_join(pop_4countries,
            by = c("country_region" = "name", "year")) %>%
  mutate(prevalence = cases / pop * 1000000,
         dw = 0.133,
         ylds = prevalence * dw,
         dalys = ylls + ylds) %>%
  arrange(year, month_cycle, prevalence) %>%
  select(country_region, year,
         month_cycle, ylls, ylds, dalys)


COVID19_dalys %>%
```

```
  head()
#> # A tibble: 6 x 6
#> # Groups:   country_region, year [4]
#>   country_region  year month_cycle        ylls       ylds      dalys
#>   <chr>          <dbl> <chr>             <dbl>      <dbl>      <dbl>
#> 1 US              2020 Jan-Apr       80674499.   8342075.   89016575.
#> 2 China           2020 Jan-Apr      655246654.  21433596.  676680249.
#> 3 Canada          2020 Jan-Apr       62225750.  60966727.  123192477.
#> 4 United Kingdom  2020 Jan-Apr      800881092  107263600.  908144692.
#> 5 China           2020 May-Aug     1434752563.  34879873. 1469632436.
#> 6 US              2020 May-Aug     1158612365. 153456778. 1312069143.
```

If we calculate the YLDs with the incidence instead of prevalence, we get the same results, because the incidence is the number of new cases in a given period, while the prevalence is the number of existing cases in a given period. So, we should consider the cumulative number of cases to calculate the prevalence. In order to calculate the cumulative number of cases, we need to group the data by year and month cycle.

And then plot the YLDs by country and month cycle, with the y axis representing the YLDs formatted in millions.

```
COVID19_dalys %>%
  filter(year %in% c(2020, 2021)) %>%
  ggplot() +
  geom_col(aes(x = month_cycle, y = ylds,
               fill = country_region)) +
  scale_y_continuous(
          labels = scales::unit_format(unit = "M",
                                       scale = 1e-6)) +
  scale_fill_grey(start = 0.2, end = 0.8) +
  labs(title = "YLDs by Country and Month Cycle",
       fill = "Country",
       x = "4-Month Cycle", y = "YLDs") +
  facet_wrap(~year) +
  theme(axis.text.x = element_text(angle = 45, hjust = 1))
```

We can see that the YLDs are highest in the United Kingdom, followed by the US, Canada, and China. The YLDs are highest in the first 4-month cycle (Jan-Apr) and decrease in the following cycles.

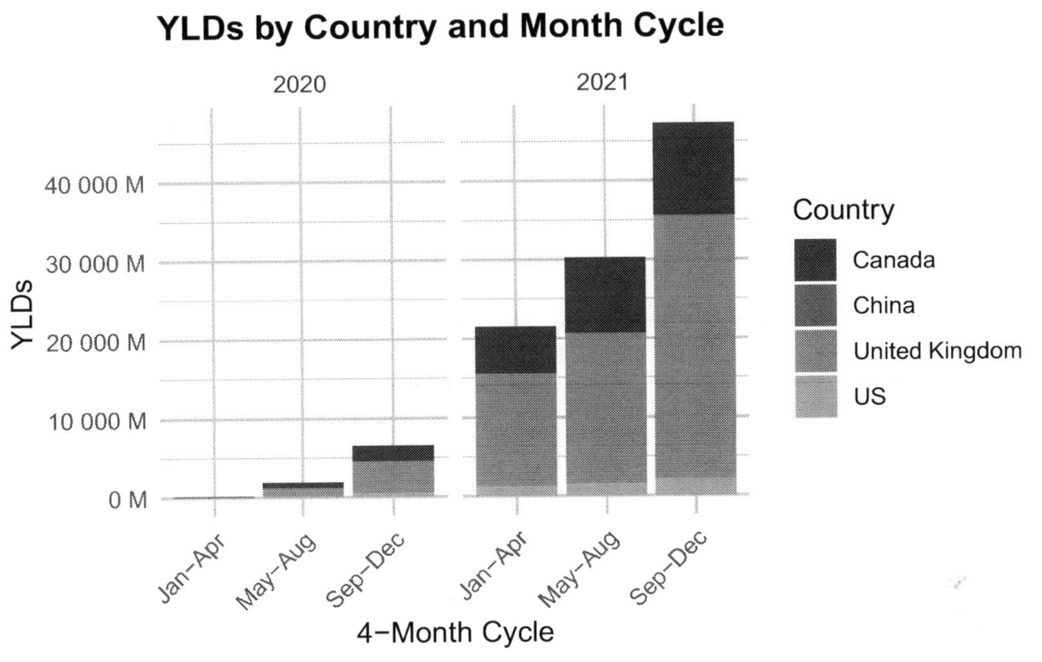

Figure 15.14 YLDs by Country and Month Cycle

Finally, let's plot the DALYs by country and month cycle, with the y axis representing the DALYs formatted in millions.

```
COVID19_dalys %>%
  filter(year %in% c(2020, 2021)) %>%
  ggplot() +
  geom_col(aes(x = month_cycle, y = dalys,
               fill = country_region)) +
  scale_y_continuous(
            labels = scales::unit_format(unit = "M",
                                         scale = 1e-6)) +
  scale_fill_grey(start = 0.2, end = 0.8) +
  labs(title = "DALYs by Country and Month Cycle",
       fill = "Country",
       x = "4-Month Cycle", y = "DALYs") +
  facet_wrap(~year) +
  theme(axis.text.x = element_text(angle = 45, hjust = 1))
```

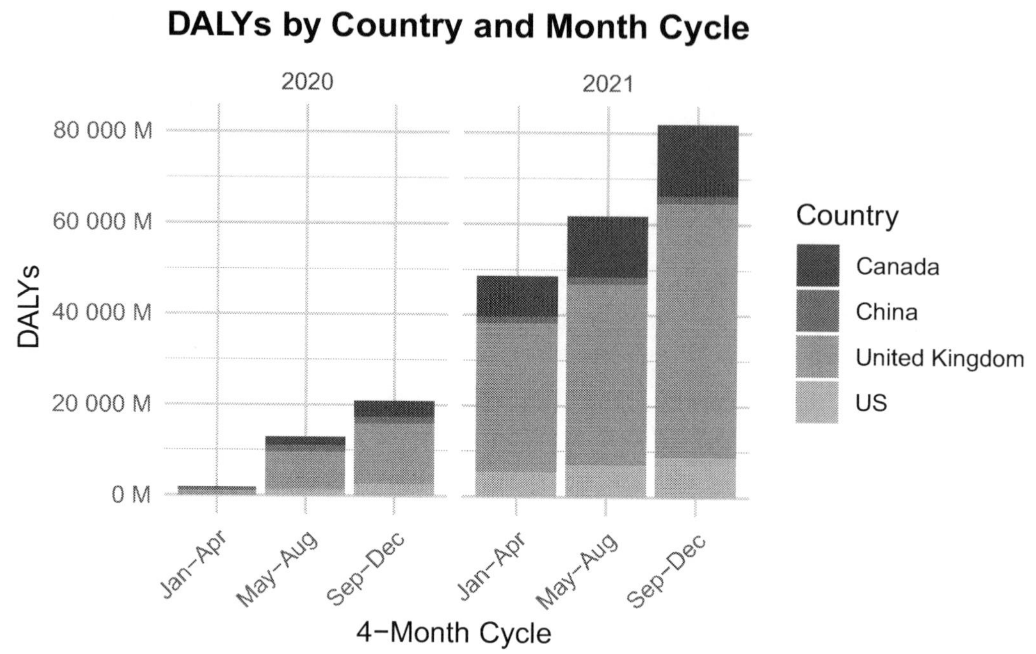

Figure 15.15 DALYs by Country and Month Cycle

15.5 Summary

This chapter examined the COVID-19 pandemic, covering its origin, spread, and global impact. We explored the epidemiology of the virus, including its zoonotic origins, symptoms, and transmission methods.

Key preventive measures such as diagnostic testing, treatments, and vaccination efforts were discussed, emphasizing strategies to control the pandemic.

We also analysed COVID-19 modelling, using: - The SEIR model to simulate virus transmission, - Bayesian analysis for infection rate predictions, and - Ensemble modelling (Decision Tree, Random Forest, KNN, SVM) to enhance forecast accuracy.

Additionally, we highlighted the use of GIS mapping to track and visualize outbreaks and assessed COVID-19's health burden through Disability-Adjusted Life Years (DALYs) using JHU GitHub data.

16

The Case of Malaria

Learning Objectives

- Understand the key characteristics and impact of Malaria
- Explore how Malaria spreads through populations and environments
- Learn to map and visualize Malaria outbreaks using spatial data

In this chapter, we explore the dynamics of Malaria transmission in more detail. We examine the results of various model's applications that simulate the spread of the virus.

16.1 Epidemiology

Malaria is a mosquito-borne infectious disease that affects humans and other animals. It is caused by parasitic protozoans belonging to the Plasmodium type. The disease is **transmitted through the bites of Anopheles mosquitoes**. The symptoms of malaria typically include fever, fatigue, vomiting, and headaches. If left untreated, malaria can be fatal. Malaria is a major public health concern in many tropical and subtropical regions, particularly in Africa.

Malaria transmission dynamics are influenced by various factors, including the prevalence of infected individuals, the density of mosquito vectors, and environmental conditions. The transmission of malaria occurs when an infected mosquito bites a human host, injecting the Plasmodium parasites into the bloodstream. The parasites then multiply within the host's red blood cells, leading to the characteristic symptoms of malaria. The parasites can be transmitted back to mosquitoes when they feed on infected individuals, completing the transmission cycle.

16.2 Mapping Malaria Outbreaks

Mapping malaria outbreaks is essential for locating high-risk areas and guiding effective public health interventions. Geographic Information Systems (GIS) enable the visualisation of malaria's spatial distribution, revealing transmission patterns and hotspots. The analysis of malaria cases, alongside environmental factors, such as temperature, humidity, and vegetation cover, allows the identification of conditions that facilitate transmission and support the development of targeted control strategies.

DOI: 10.1201/9781032625935-16

In this example, we will use the `malariaAtlas` package to download malaria data for Nigeria and visualise the distribution of malaria cases in the country. We will plot the malaria hotspots on a map of Nigeria to identify regions with the highest incidence of the disease.

```
# Load necessary libraries
library(malariaAtlas)
library(tidyverse)
library(sf)
library(rnaturalearth)
```

```
tidyverse_conflicts()
```

To download malaria data we can use the `getPR()` function, it releases the data from the Malaria Atlas Project API. The function requires the country and species of Plasmodium to be specified. In this example, we will download data for Nigeria and the *Plasmodium falciparum species.*

```
nigeria_data <- getPR(country = "Nigeria",
                      species = "Pf")
```

```
#> [1] NA NA
#> [1] 27  2
```

Data contains cases for 23 years spanning from 1985 to 2018. We can extract the relevant information (year_start (of the survey), longitude, latitude, and number of positive cases) and convert the data to a spatial object using the `st_as_sf()` function from the `sf` package.

```
nigeria_data <- nigeria_data %>%
  arrange(year_start) %>%
  select(year_start,longitude,latitude,positive) %>%
  filter(!is.na(longitude) & !is.na(year_start))

nigeria_data_sf <- nigeria_data %>%
  st_as_sf(coords = c("longitude", "latitude"),
           crs = 4326)

head(nigeria_data_sf)
#> Simple feature collection with 6 features and 2 fields
#> Geometry type: POINT
#> Dimension:     XY
#> Bounding box:  xmin: 3.05 ymin: 6.316 xmax: 12.76 ymax: 11.1578
#> Geodetic CRS:  WGS 84
#>   year_start positive              geometry
#> 1       1985      113   POINT (3.132 6.501)
#> 2       1985      760   POINT (3.283 6.667)
#> 3       1987        7    POINT (3.05 7.167)
#> 4       1988      433 POINT (12.76 11.1578)
#> 5       1988      363 POINT (10.632 7.2333)
#> 6       1988      181   POINT (7.549 6.316)
```

To get the administrative boundaries of Nigeria we use the `{rnaturlaearth}` package:

```
nigeria_sf <- ne_countries(country = "Nigeria",
                           returnclass = "sf")
```

And finally plot the malaria hotspots on a map of Nigeria to visualise the distribution of malaria cases in the country.

```
# Plot Malaria Hotspots with expanded spatial data range
ggplot() +
  geom_sf(data = nigeria_sf,
          fill = "gray90",
          color = "white")+
geom_sf(data = nigeria_data_sf,
        aes(size=positive, color = positive),
        alpha=0.5)+
  scale_color_viridis_c(option = "plasma", name = "Malaria Cases") +
  guides(size = "none") +
  labs(title = "Malaria Hotspots in Nigeria",
       subtitle = "1985-2018",
       caption = "Source: Malaria Atlas Project | @fgazzelloni") +
  theme(legend.position = "right")
```

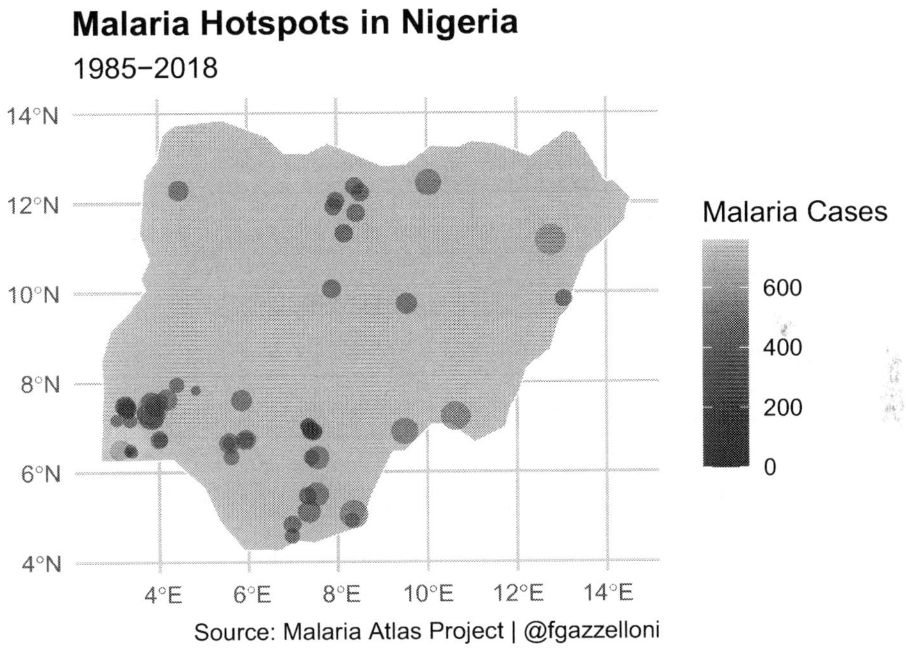

Figure 16.1 The map shows the distribution of malaria cases in Nigeria, with the size and color of the points representing the number of positive cases. The map highlights regions with a high incidence of malaria, providing valuable information for public health interventions.

Spatial data on climate, population density, and mosquito habitats are instrumental in predicting high-risk areas for malaria, aiding preventive measures like bed net distribution and indoor residual spraying. In Tanzania, for example, spatial models identified villages with the highest malaria incidence, allowing the government and NGOs to prioritize these areas for intervention.[1] This targeted approach enhances the cost-effectiveness of malaria

[1]Majige Selemani et al., "Assessing the Effects of Mosquito Nets on Malaria Mortality Using a Space

control programs, reducing the disease burden by directing resources to areas with the greatest need.

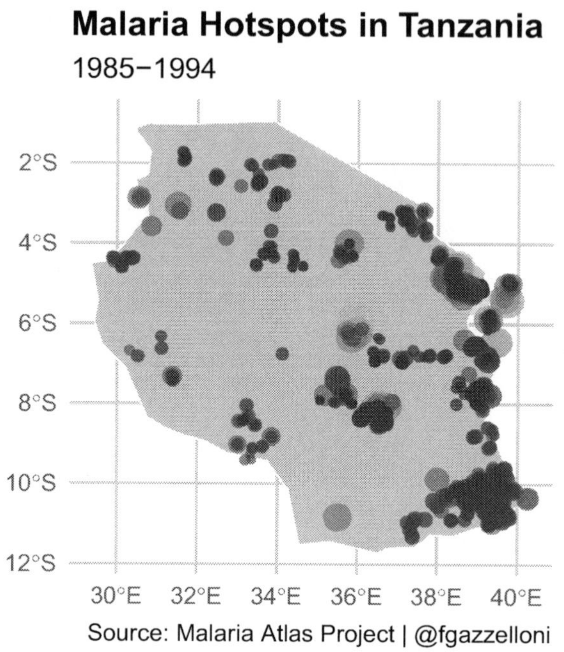

Figure 16.2 The map shows the distribution of malaria cases in Tanzania, with the size and color of the points representing the number of positive cases. The map highlights regions with a high incidence of malaria, providing valuable information for public health interventions.

16.3 Example: Simulating Malaria Transmission Dynamics

In this example, we will use data for Malaria positive cases in Nigeria from the **Malaria Atlas Project** to evaluate the transmission dynamics using a simple mathematical model. We will use machine learning to predict future trends.

To illustrate the modelling and prediction process we will use the `{caret}` package, which provides a unified interface for training and evaluating machine learning models. We will train a Random Forest model to predict future trends in malaria transmission based on historical data.

```
nigeria_cases <- nigeria_data %>%
  group_by(year_start) %>%
  reframe(positive = sum(positive)) %>%
  rename(year = year_start) %>%
  drop_na() %>%
  select(year, positive)
```

Time Model: A Case Study of Rufiji and Ifakara Health and Demographic Surveillance System Sites in Rural Tanzania," *Malaria Journal* 15, no. 1 (May 4, 2016): 257, doi:10.1186/s12936-016-1311-9.

```
head(nigeria_cases)
#> # A tibble: 6 x 2
#>    year positive
#>   <int>    <dbl>
#> 1  1985      873
#> 2  1987        7
#> 3  1988     1276
#> 4  1989      134
#> 5  1990      352
#> 6  1992       92
```

Visualize the dynamics of malaria transmission in Nigeria using a line plot to show the number of infected cases over time.

```
nigeria_cases %>%
  ggplot() +
  geom_line(aes(x = year, y = positive),
            color = "navy",
            linetype = "solid") +
  labs(title = "Malaria Transmission Dynamics in Nigeria",
       subtitle = "23 years spanning from 1985 to 2018",
       x = "Time(Year)",
       y = "Number of Infected Cases") +
  theme_minimal()
```

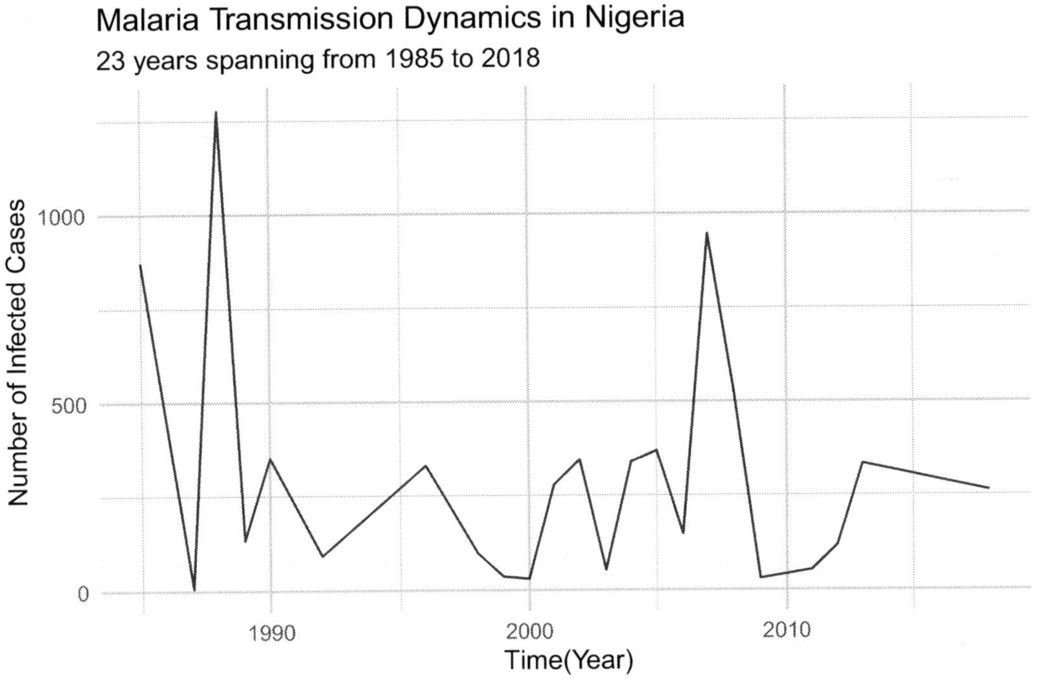

Figure 16.3 The plot shows the dynamics of malaria transmission in Nigeria from 1985 to 2018. The blue line represents the number of infected cases over time, highlighting the fluctuations in malaria incidence during this period.

16.3.1 Modelling with caret

To train a machine learning model to predict future trends in malaria transmission, we will be using 80% of the original data to train the model and 20% to test it. Then, we will evaluate its performance using the Root Mean Squared Error (RMSE).

The `{caret}` package provides a unified interface for training and evaluating machine learning models in R (Chapter 8). It supports a wide range of algorithms and provides tools for hyperparameter tuning, cross-validation, and model evaluation.

```
# Load libraries and check for conflicts
library(caret)
conflicted::conflicts_prefer(dplyr::lag)
```

16.3.1.1 Feature Engineering

Create lagged variables to capture the temporal dynamics of malaria transmission. For time series forecasting, it's helpful to create variables, which represent past values of the target variable. This allows the model to learn trends from previous values.

```
# Create lagged features (e.g., previous year's cases)
nigeria_cases <- nigeria_cases %>%
  arrange(year) %>%
  mutate(lag_1 = lag(positive, 1),
         lag_2 = lag(positive, 2),
         lag_3 = lag(positive, 3)) %>%
  drop_na()

head(nigeria_cases)
#> # A tibble: 6 x 5
#>    year positive lag_1 lag_2 lag_3
#>   <int>    <dbl> <dbl> <dbl> <dbl>
#> 1  1989      134  1276     7   873
#> 2  1990      352   134  1276     7
#> 3  1992       92   352   134  1276
#> 4  1996      331    92   352   134
#> 5  1998       98   331    92   352
#> 6  1999       36    98   331    92
```

Create partition for training and testing data using the `createDataPartition()` function from the `caret` package.

```
set.seed(123)
train_index <- createDataPartition(nigeria_cases$positive,
                                   p = 0.8, list = FALSE)
train <- nigeria_cases[train_index, ]
test <- nigeria_cases[-train_index, ]
```

16.3.1.2 Model Selection and Training (Parameter Calibration)

Define the machine learning model specific for investigating Malaria dynamics. In this case, we will use the time and number of lagged cases to predict the number of infected cases.

We will use the `train()` function from the `{caret}` package to train the model. A suitable model would be? List the models that can be used for this task:

- Random Forest ("rf")
- Gradient Boosting ("gbm")
- Support Vector Machines ("svm")
- Neural Networks ("nnet") - etc.

In the `method` argument, specify the model to be used (e.g., "rf" for Random Forest). The `trControl` argument specifies the cross-validation method for hyperparameter tuning, and the `tuneGrid` argument defines the hyperparameter grid for tuning.

```
# Define the training control with 5-fold cross-validation
train_control <- trainControl(method = "cv",
                              number = 5)

# Define a tuning grid for mtry
# (number of variables sampled at each split)
tuning_grid <- expand.grid(mtry = c(1, 2, 3))

# Train the Random Forest model
set.seed(123)
rf_model <- train(
  positive ~ lag_1 + lag_2 + lag_3,
  data = train,
  method = "rf",
  trControl = train_control,
  tuneGrid = tuning_grid,
  ntree = 500)  # Number of trees
```

The parameter calibration (hyperparameter tuning) is performed by the `train` function automatically using cross-validation to select the optimal hyperparameters for the model.

16.3.1.3 Model Evaluation

Testing the model on observed data will show how the model performs in estimating the number of infected cases.

```
# Predict on the test data
nigeria_cases$pred <- predict(rf_model,
                              newdata = nigeria_cases)
```

```
nigeria_cases %>%
 ggplot(aes(x = year, y = positive)) +
  geom_line(color = "navy", linetype = "solid") +
  geom_line(aes(y = pred),
            color = "darkred", linetype = "dashed") +
  labs(title = "Malaria Positive Cases in Nigeria",
       subtitle = "Observed vs Predicted - Random Forest",
       x = "Year",
       y = "Number of Positive Cases") +
  theme_minimal()
```

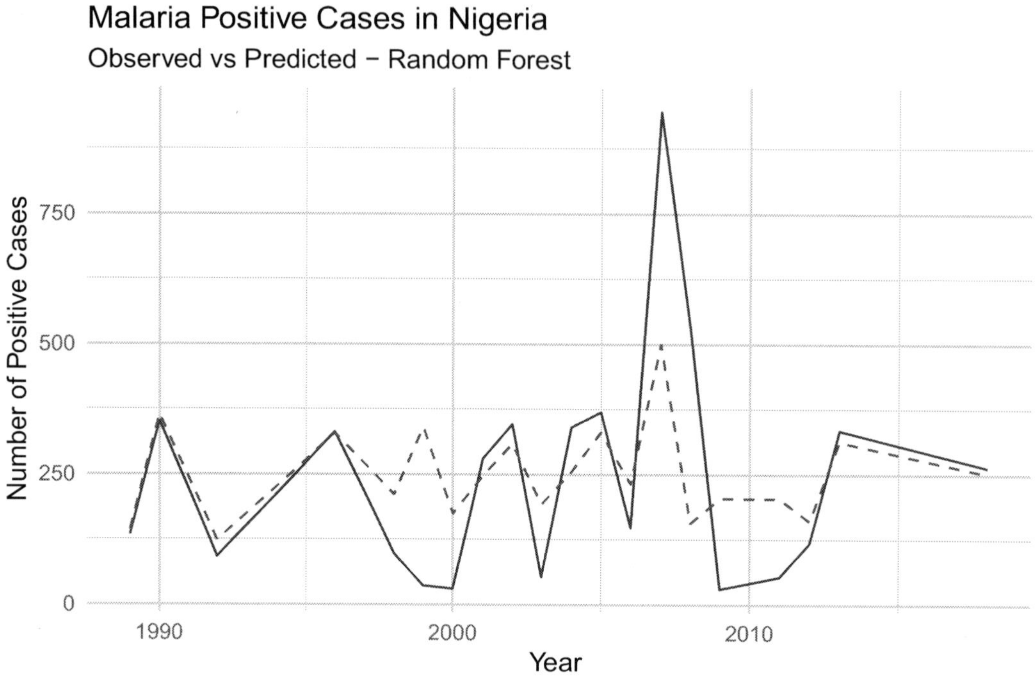

Figure 16.4 The plot shows the observed vs predicted malaria positive cases in Nigeria made with a Random Forest model. The blue line represents the observed cases, while the red line represents the predicted cases. The model's predictions are not closely aligned with the observed values, indicating potential limitations in capturing the dynamics of malaria transmission.

To evaluate the model's ability in predicting future trends, we predict the number of infected cases on the test data and calculate the Root Mean Squared Error (RMSE). Test data are a subset of the original data that were not used for training the model and provide an independent evaluation of the model's performance.

```
# Predict on the test data
test$pred <- predict(rf_model,
                    newdata = test)

# View predictions alongside actual values
head(test[, c("year", "positive", "pred")])
#> # A tibble: 4 x 3
#>    year positive  pred
#>   <int>    <dbl> <dbl>
#> 1  1999       36  340.
#> 2  2004      340  255.
#> 3  2006      148  232.
#> 4  2008      528  157.
```

Visualize the predicted vs actual infected cases using a line plot to compare the model's predictions with the actual data.

```
# Reshape data for plotting
plot_data_rf <- test %>%
  select(year, positive, pred) %>%
  rename(Observed = positive, Predicted = pred) %>%
  pivot_longer(cols = c("Observed", "Predicted"),
               names_to = "Type", values_to = "Cases")

plot_data_rf %>% head()
#> # A tibble: 6 x 3
#>    year Type      Cases
#>   <int> <chr>     <dbl>
#> 1  1999 Observed    36
#> 2  1999 Predicted  340.
#> 3  2004 Observed   340
#> 4  2004 Predicted  255.
#> 5  2006 Observed   148
#> 6  2006 Predicted  232.
```

```
# Plot observed vs predicted cases
ggplot(plot_data_rf, aes(x = year, y = Cases,
                         color = Type, linetype = Type)) +
  geom_line(size = 1) +
  geom_point(size = 2) +
  scale_color_manual(values = c("navy", "darkred")) +
  labs(title = "Malaria Positive Cases in Nigeria",
       subtitle = "Observed vs Predicted - Random Forest",
       x = "Year",
       y = "Number of Positive Cases") +
  theme_minimal() +
  theme(legend.position = "top")
```

Evaluate the model's performance using RMSE:

```
# Calculate RMSE
rmse <- sqrt(mean((test$positive - test$pred)^2))
cat("RMSE:", rmse, "\n")
#> RMSE: 247.3936
```

A Root Mean Squared Error (RMSE) of 247.3936 indicates the average difference between the predicted and actual values of infected cases. Lower RMSE values indicate better model performance.

The output shows that the model's predictions are not closely aligned with the observed values, the predicted trend seems to be relatively flat or declining, while the observed cases show significant fluctuations. This mismatch suggests that the current model setup may not be effectively capturing the dynamics of malaria transmission in this dataset.

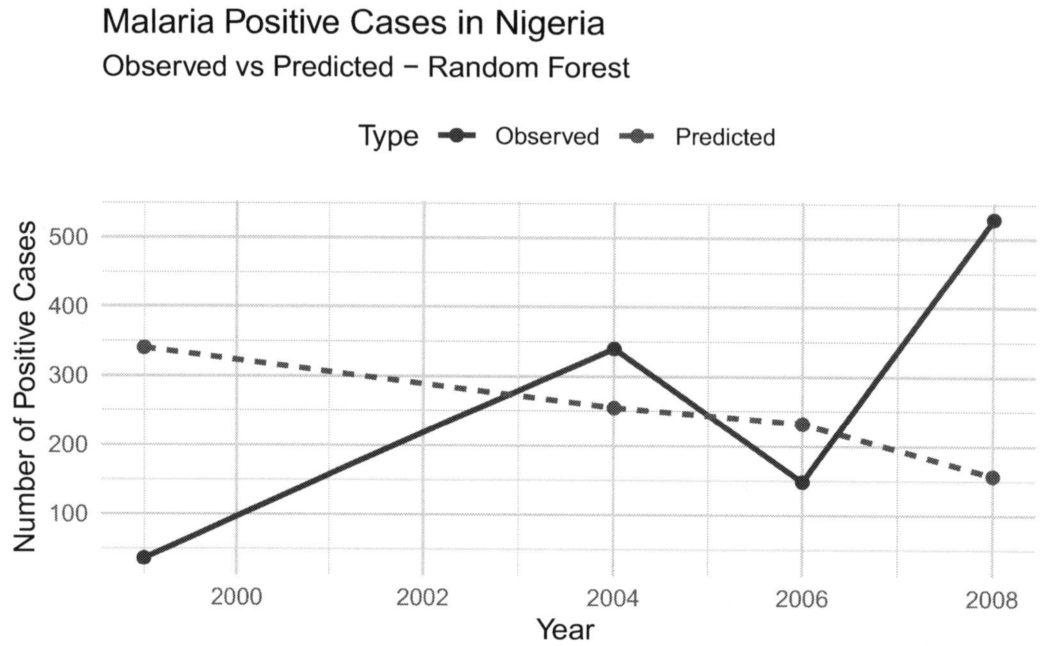

Figure 16.5 The plot shows the observed vs predicted malaria positive cases in Nigeria made with a Random Forest model. The blue line represents the observed cases, while the red line represents the predicted cases. The model's predictions are not closely aligned with the observed values, indicating potential limitations in capturing the dynamics of malaria transmission.

16.4 Model Refinement

To improve the model's performance, we can refine the model by adjusting parameters such as 'mtry' in Random Forest. For example, increase the number of folds in cross-validation, adjust the tuning grid, or add additional features to improve the model's performance.

```
# Increase the number of folds in cross-validation
train_control <- trainControl(method = "cv",
                              number = 10)

# Scaling data in caret
rf_model2 <- train(
  positive ~ year + lag_1 + lag_2 + lag_3,
  data = train,
  method = "rf",
  trControl = train_control,
  tuneGrid = expand.grid(mtry = 2:4),
  preProcess = c("center", "scale"))
```

Predict future trends using the trained adjusted Random Forest model on the test data.

```
# Predict on the test data
test$pred_rf2 <- predict(rf_model2,
                         newdata = test)
```

Visualize the predicted vs actual infected cases using a line plot to compare the adjusted Random Forest model's predictions with the actual data.

```
# Reshape data for plotting
plot_data_xgb <- test %>%
  select(year, positive, pred_rf2) %>%
  rename(Observed = positive, Predicted = pred_rf2) %>%
  pivot_longer(cols = c("Observed", "Predicted"),
               names_to = "Type", values_to = "Cases")

plot_data_xgb %>% head()
#> # A tibble: 6 x 3
#>    year Type      Cases
#>   <int> <chr>     <dbl>
#> 1  1999 Observed    36
#> 2  1999 Predicted  326.
#> 3  2004 Observed   340
#> 4  2004 Predicted  257.
#> 5  2006 Observed   148
#> 6  2006 Predicted  247.
```

```
# Plot observed vs predicted cases
ggplot(plot_data_xgb, aes(x = year, y = Cases,
                          color = Type, linetype = Type)) +
  geom_line(size = 1) +
  geom_point(size = 2) +
  scale_color_manual(values = c("navy", "darkred")) +
  labs(title = "Malaria Cases in Nigeria",
       subtitle = "Observed vs Predicted - Adjusted Random Forest (XGBoost)",
       x = "Year",
       y = "Number of Positive Cases") +
  theme_minimal() +
  theme(legend.position = "top")
```

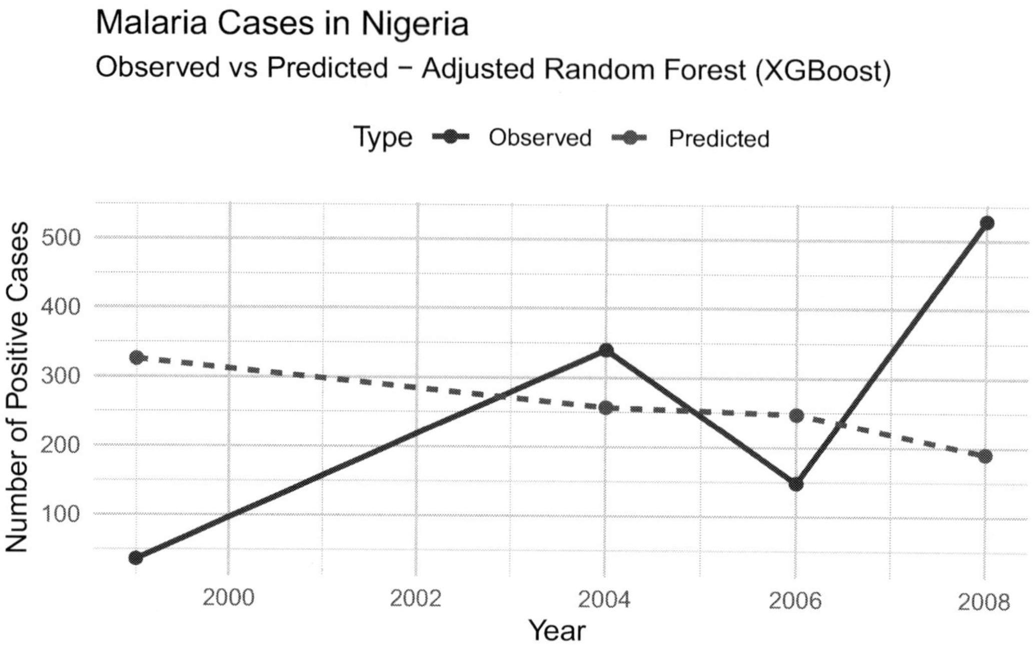

Figure 16.6 The plot shows the observed vs predicted malaria positive cases in Nigeria made with an adjusted Random Forest model. The blue line represents the observed cases, while the red line represents the predicted cases. The model's predictions show a closer alignment with the observed values compared to the first Random Forest model, indicating improved performance.

Evaluate the model's performance improvement using RMSE:

```
# Calculate RMSE
rmse <- sqrt(mean((test$positive - test$pred_rf2)^2))
cat("RMSE:", rmse, "\n")
#> RMSE: 231.7169
```

To visualise the improvement in model's performance, we can plot the observed vs predicted for both models:

In conclusion, the model's performance can be further improved by adjusting hyperparameters, adding additional features, or using more advanced algorithms. The iterative process of model refinement and evaluation is essential for developing accurate predictions of malaria transmission dynamics.

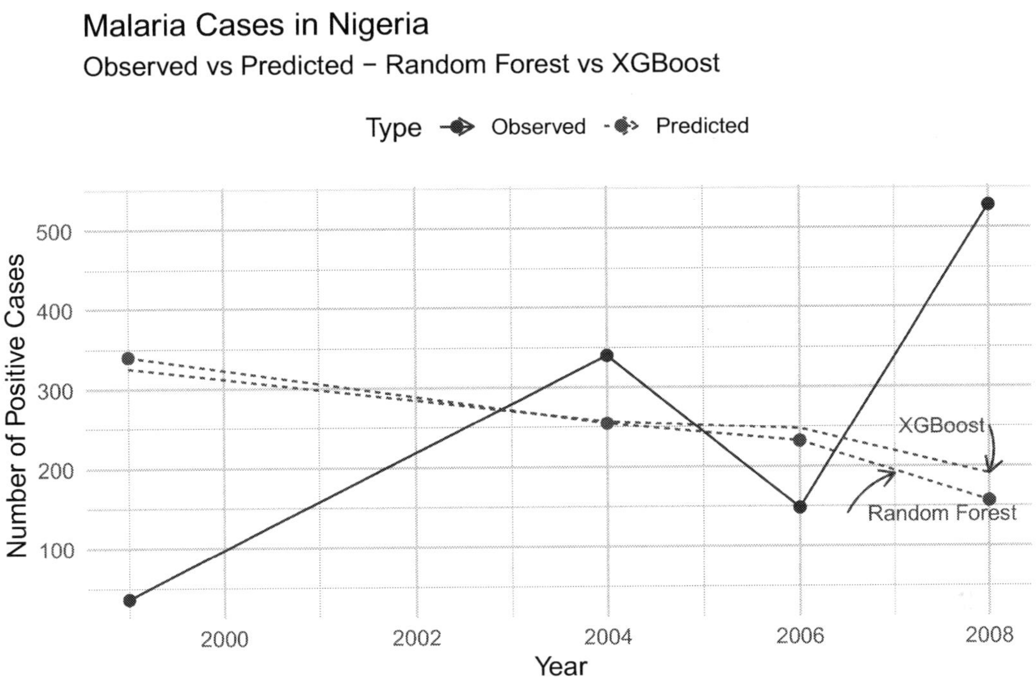

Figure 16.7 The plot shows the observed vs predicted malaria positive cases in Nigeria made with both Random Forest and XGBoost models. The blue line represents the observed cases, while the red line represents the predicted cases from the Random Forest and XGBoost models.

16.5 Summary

In this chapter, we explored the dynamics of malaria transmission and emphasized the importance of mapping outbreaks to guide public health interventions. Using the `malariaAtlas` package, we downloaded malaria data for Nigeria and visualized the spatial distribution of cases across the country. Additionally, and demonstrated how machine learning techniques can analyse historical data to predict future trends in malaria transmission.

17

Summary: The State of Health

Learning Objectives

- How health metrics vary across different countries
- Gain insights from the Global Burden of Disease (GBD) study on health metrics at the country level
- Evaluate the implications of health metrics for global public health policy and interventions

In the previous sections, we explored various aspects of health metrics, including tailored case studies, data sources, modelling, and visualisation techniques. We discussed key health metrics such as mortality rates, life expectancy, Disability-Adjusted Life Years (DALYs), Years of Life Lost (YLLs), and Years Lived with Disability (YLDs). We also examined the role of risk factors, disease burdens, and health outcomes in shaping population health profiles.

In this final chapter, we will focus on visualising health metrics across countries to understand the state of health globally. We will explore the implications of cross-country comparisons of health metrics for public health policy and interventions. We will use data from the **Global Burden of Disease (GBD)** study and the **OECD's Health at a Glance** report to compare health indicators, disease burdens, and risk factors across different countries. By analysing health metrics at the country level, we can gain insights into public health priorities, identify areas for improvement, and inform global public health policy.

17.1 Data Sources for Health Metrics Comparison

Data availability is crucial for comparing health metrics across countries and regions. The **OECD's Health at a Glance** report and the **Global Burden of Disease (GBD)** study offer comprehensive data on health indicators, disease burdens, and risk factors, enabling cross-country comparisons and insights into public health priorities.

17.1.1 Example of OECD Health at a Glance Data

The **OECD's Health at a Glance** report offers a comparative overview of health indicators among member countries. The report examines metrics such as life expectancy, health expenditures, and major health trends. It also provides accessible insights into public health priorities and performance indicators, facilitating comparisons and helping to identify areas for improvement (www.oecd-ilibrary.org).

In this example, we will download data from the OECD's Health at a Glance report website (https://data-explorer.oecd.org/) to compare **Disability-adjusted life years (DALYs)**

DOI: 10.1201/9781032625935-17

due to Ambient Particulate Matter as a risk exposure per 1 000 inhabitants (accessed Nov 2024).

We can use the `url` for DALYs due to Ambient Particulate Matter found by searching for the keyword `DALYs` in the search box of the OECD report website.

The url is broken down into the following components:

- sdmx.oecd.org/public/rest/data/
- OECD.ENV.EPI,DSD_EXP_MORSC@DF_EXP_MORSC,1.0/
- .A.DALY.10P3HB.PM_2_5_OUT._T._T?startPeriod=2010

Data are available to download in the `SDMX` format, which is a standard for exchanging statistical data. We will use the `{rsdmx}` package to download the data and convert it to a data frame for analysis.

```
install.packages("rsdmx")
library(rsdmx)
```

```
library(tidyverse)
```

```
# Read the data
sdmx_data <- readSDMX(url)

# Convert SDMX data to a data frame
df <- as.data.frame(sdmx_data)
```

A glimpse of the data shows the structure of the data frame, including the column names and data types.

```
df %>%
  janitor::clean_names() %>%
  head(3) %>%
  glimpse()
#> Rows: 3
#> Columns: 14
#> $ ref_area        <chr> "PRI", "PRI", "PRI"
#> $ freq            <chr> "A", "A", "A"
#> $ measure         <chr> "DALY", "DALY", "DALY"
#> $ unit_measure    <chr> "10P3HB", "10P3HB", "10P3HB"
#> $ risk            <chr> "PM_2_5_OUT", "PM_2_5_OUT", "PM_2_5_OUT"
#> $ age             <chr> "_T", "_T", "_T"
#> $ sex             <chr> "_T", "_T", "_T"
#> $ unit_mult       <chr> "0", "0", "0"
#> $ decimals        <chr> "2", "2", "2"
#> $ conversion_type <chr> "_Z", "_Z", "_Z"
#> $ price_base      <chr> "_Z", "_Z", "_Z"
#> $ obs_time        <chr> "2017", "2018", "2019"
#> $ obs_value       <dbl> 3.199, 3.417, 3.667
#> $ obs_status      <chr> "A", "A", "A"
```

Observation time spans from 2010 to 2019 for 212 countries. We filter the data to include only the relevant columns and arrange it by observation time to get a better understanding of the data.

```
dalys_pm25 <- df %>%
  janitor::clean_names() %>%
  select(ref_area, measure, risk, obs_time, obs_value) %>%
  arrange(obs_time)

dalys_pm25 %>%
  head()
#>   ref_area measure        risk obs_time obs_value
#> 1      PRI    DALY PM_2_5_OUT     2010     2.474
#> 2      DZA    DALY PM_2_5_OUT     2010    14.680
#> 3      CHL    DALY PM_2_5_OUT     2010     6.758
#> 4    OECDA    DALY PM_2_5_OUT     2010     5.516
#> 5      NPL    DALY PM_2_5_OUT     2010    14.249
#> 6      MWI    DALY PM_2_5_OUT     2010     4.211
```

Then, to make the data more interpretable, we convert the `ref_area` column from `ISO3` codes to `country names` using the `{countrycode}` package. Data provides information for various regions and groups, which we exclude from the analysis.

```
library(countrycode)
dalys_pm25 <- dalys_pm25 %>%
   filter(!ref_area %in% c("A9", "ASEAN", "EA19", "EU27",
                           "EU28", "F98", "G20", "OECD",
                           "OECDA", "OECDE", "OECDSO", "W")) %>%
  mutate(ref_area = countrycode::countrycode(ref_area,
                                             origin = "iso3c",
                                             destination = "country.name"))
```

Finally, to visualise the data we use a line plot to compare Disability-adjusted life years (DALYs) due to Ambient Particulate Matter as a risk exposure per 1 000 inhabitants for Egypt, Serbia, Morocco, Italy, and Iceland. These countries were selected based on their geographical location and varying levels of DALYs due to Ambient Particulate Matter.

We can conclude that the Disability-adjusted life years (DALYs) due to Ambient Particulate Matter varied across countries from 2010 to 2019. This variation may be due to differences in environmental policies, air quality, and public health interventions aimed at reducing exposure to particulate matter. In particular, countries like Egypt and Serbia experienced higher DALYs due to Ambient Particulate Matter compared to countries like Iceland and Italy.

In general, the data shows that regions with high air pollution, such as parts of East Asia, see increased DALYs from respiratory conditions. This is due to the high levels of particulate matter in the air, which can lead to respiratory diseases like asthma and **chronic obstructive pulmonary disease (COPD)**. Countries with stringent air quality regulations, such as those in Western Europe, tend to have lower DALYs from air pollution-related conditions.

17.1.2 Example of GBD Data Cross-Country Comparisons

The **Global Burden of Disease GBD** study by the **Institute for Health Metrics and Evaluation (IHME)** provides comprehensive data on various health metrics covering a vast array of diseases, injuries, and risk factors across 204 countries. To access the GBD data (<www.healthdata.org>), we can use the **Sustainable Development Goals (SDG) API**

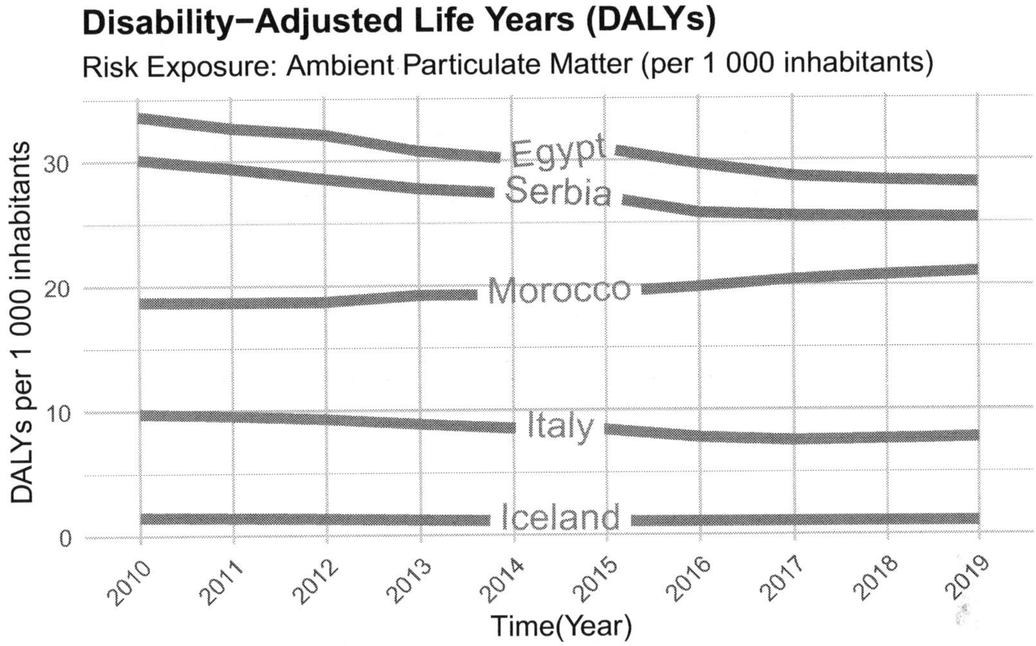

Figure 17.1 Disability-adjusted life years (DALYs) due to Ambient Particulate Matter as a risk exposure per 1 000 inhabitants in selected countries from 2010 to 2019.

provided by the IHME. The API allows users to access GBD data for specific indicators, locations, and years, enabling cross-country comparisons. In Section A.3 is provided a detailed guide on how to access and use the **SDG API**.

In this example, we will compare the **Tuberculosis** Incidence Rate in 2019 for selected countries using the Sustainable Development Goals (SDG) API data. We will use the `{hmsidwR}` package to download the data and visualise the results using a bar plot.

```
# Install the hmsidwR package
install.packages("hmsidwR")
# or the development version
devtools::install_github("fgazzelloni/hmsidwR")
```

```
# Load the libraries
library(hmsidwR)
```

We download the data using the `gbd_get_data` function from the `{hmsidwR}` package. The function requires the URL, API key, endpoint, indicator ID, location ID, and year as input parameters, as shown below:

```
data_1001 <- hmsidwR::gbd_get_data(
  url = "https://api.healthdata.org/sdg/v1",
  key = "YOUR-KEY",
  endpoint = "GetResultsByIndicator",
  indicator_id = "1001",
  location_id = c("29","86","102"),
  year = "2019"
```

```
)
```

Filter the data by both gender and subset to include only the relevant columns:

```
data_1001 %>%
  filter(sex_label=="Both sexes") %>%
  select(location_name, indicator_short, mean_estimate)
#>              location_name indicator_short      mean_estimate
#> 1                    Tonga        TB Incid 31.80181440147271
#> 2                    Italy        TB Incid 5.277028727101566
#> 3 United States of America        TB Incid  2.52029721501685
```

To compare the cross-countries results to identify disparities in Tuberculosis Incidence Rate in 2019 for selected countries, we can use a bar plot.

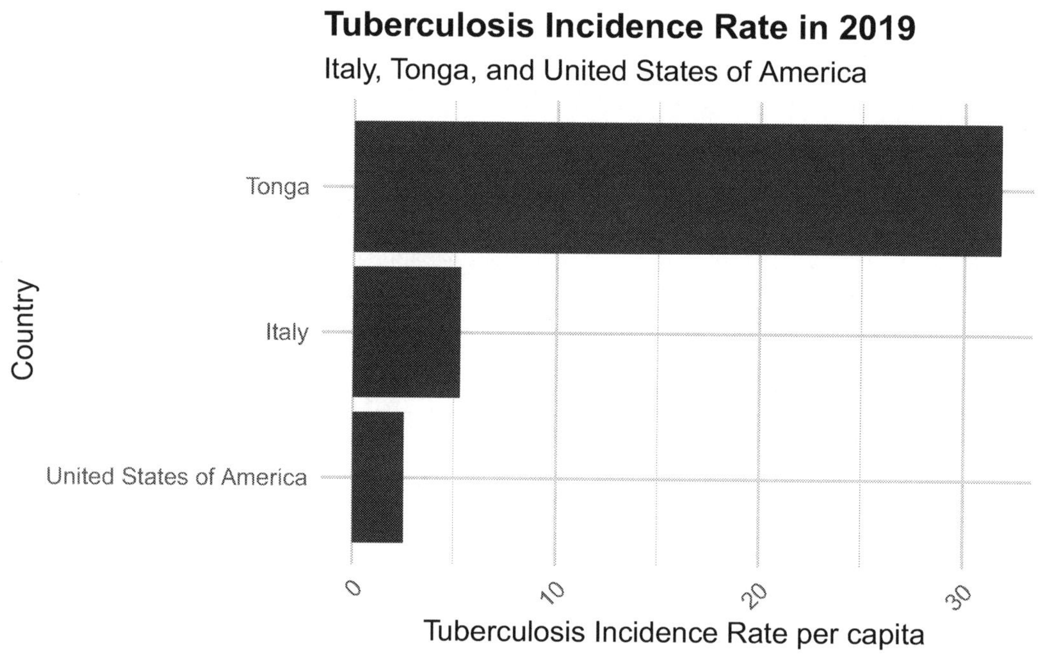

Figure 17.2 A bar plot showing Tuberculosis Incidence Rate in 2019 for selected countries. Tonga is a country located in the South Pacific, east of Australia, and north of New Zealand. It is part of the region known as Oceania, being situated east of Fiji, south of Samoa, and west of the Cook Islands. Tonga is made up of 170 islands, where four-fifths of them are uninhabited.

Tuberculosis can still be a significant concern, even in smaller island nations, due to factors like limited healthcare infrastructure, high prevalence of co-morbidities, and socio-economic conditions. Tonga, a country located in the South Pacific, east of Australia, and north of New Zealand, part of the region known as Oceania, is made up of 170 islands, where four-fifths of them are uninhabited. The country faces challenges in managing infectious diseases like tuberculosis due to its geographical location and limited resources. The comparison of Tuberculosis Incidence Rate in 2019 for Italy, Tonga, and the United States of America highlights the disparities in disease burden and health outcomes across countries.

17.2 Key Determinants of Health Metrics Variation

Health metrics can vary significantly across countries due to a combination of factors that influence population health outcomes. Some of the key determinants of health metrics variation include:

- Healthcare Infrastructure and Access
- Socioeconomic Status
- Environmental Factors
- Lifestyle and Behavioral Factors
- Public Health Policies and Interventions
- Cultural and Social Norms

These determinants influence health outcomes and disease burdens in different populations, shaping the overall health profile of a country. The availability and quality of healthcare services, income level, employment status, and education, are strongly linked to health outcomes. Geographic factors, such as climate, also influence disease patterns; tropical regions may have higher rates of vector-borne diseases like malaria and for this reason have higher DALYs due to these diseases. Countries that prioritize preventive health measures often see long-term benefits in population health metrics.

17.3 Example: Years Lived with Disability (YLDs) due to Injuries

The **Global Burden of Disease (GBD)** study provides detailed data on a wide range of health metrics, including Years Lived with Disability (YLDs) due to injuries. Considered non fatal outcomes, YLDs measure the impact of injuries on population health by quantifying the years lived with a disability caused by an injury. By comparing YLDs due to injuries across countries with different Sustainable Development Index (SDI) levels, we can identify disparities in injury-related health outcomes and inform public health interventions to reduce the burden of injuries.

In this example we will use the GBD data to compare the **Years Lived with Disability (YLDs) due to Injuries** for high, middle, and low **Sustainable Development Index (SDI)** countries from 1990 to 2021. Data are available on the GBD website at www.healthdata.org[1], and we will use the {ggplot2} package to create a line plot visualising the YLDs due to Injuries by country and SDI level.

```
ylds_injuries %>% head(3) %>% glimpse()
#> Rows: 3
#> Columns: 4
#> $ year          <int> 1990, 1990, 1990
#> $ sex_name      <chr> "Both", "Both", "Both"
#> $ location_name <chr> "High SDI", "High-middle SDI", "Low SDI"
#> $ avg           <dbl> 0.8681205, 0.9437509, 0.5304269
```

[1]For reproducibility a copy of the "injuries" data are stored on the GitHub Repository of this book (https://github.com/Fgazzelloni/hmsidR) in the data/inst/extdata folder.

```
ylds_injuries %>%
  filter(!str_detect(location_name, "-middle")) %>%
  ggplot(aes(x = year, y = avg,
             group = location_name)) +
  geomtextpath::geom_textline(aes(label = location_name),
                               hjust = 0.5,
                               vjust = 0.5,
                               size = 2) +
  facet_wrap(~ sex_name, scales = "free") +
  labs(title = "GBD-YLDs due to Injuries (1990 - 2021)",
       caption = "IHME Data | Graphic: @fgazzelloni",
       x = "Time (Year)", y = "Average Value") +
  theme_minimal()
```

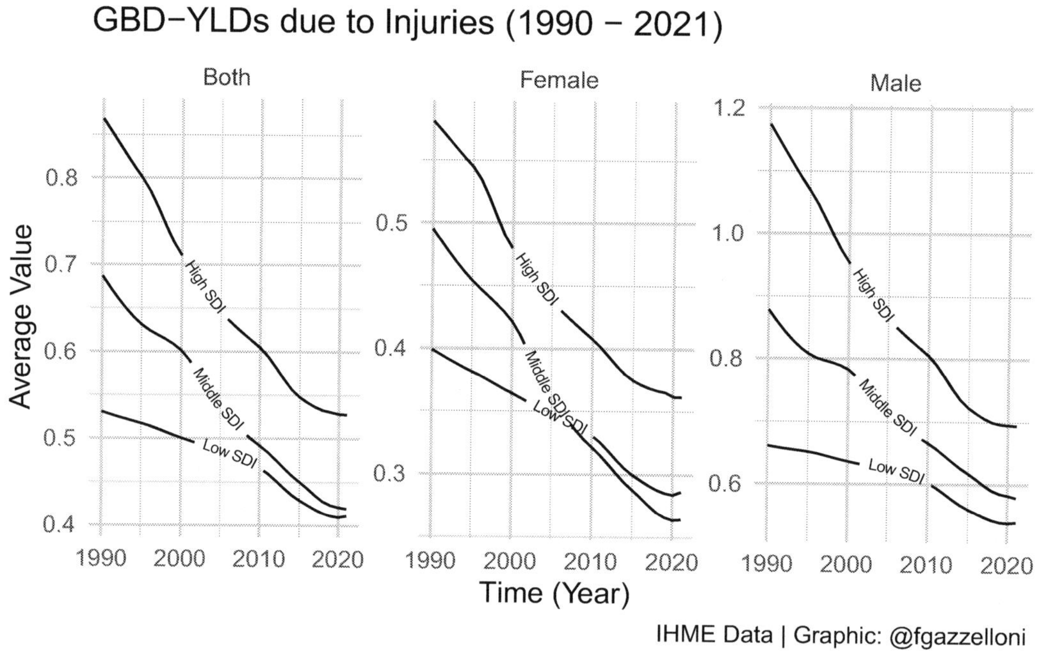

Figure 17.3 GBD-YLDs due to Injuries (1990 - 2021) by country and SDI level.

We can conclude that the Years Lived with Disability (YLDs) due to Injuries varied across countries with different Sustainable Development Index (SDI) levels from 1990 to 2021. High SDI countries generally had lower YLDs due to Injuries compared to middle and low SDI countries. This variation may be due to differences in healthcare infrastructure, access to preventive services, and public health interventions aimed at reducing injuries and their impact on population health.

Additionally, the data reveals a consistent decline in YLD rates due to injuries across all SDI levels (High, Middle, and Low) from 1990 to 2021. This trend reflects advancements in injury prevention, improved healthcare access, and enhanced living conditions, which have collectively reduced the disability burden of injuries among females. However, there is a notable crossover in injury-related YLD rates for females between middle and low SDI countries over time. This shift suggests changing dynamics in injury risk and healthcare access, with middle SDI countries achieving greater reductions in disability from injuries, while low SDI countries experience a rising burden.

17.4 Example: Injuries Cross-Country Variation by Type

In this example, we will use the GBD data to compare the types of injuries contributing to the burden of disease in high, middle, and low SDI countries from 1990 to 2021[2]. For example, we can compare the average number of injuries by type (e.g., road injuries, falls, self-harm) in high, middle, and low SDI countries. This comparison can help identify the most common types of injuries and inform targeted public health interventions to reduce the burden of injuries in different populations.

```
injuries_types %>% head(2) %>% glimpse()
#> Rows: 2
#> Columns: 3
#> $ location_name <chr> "High SDI", "High SDI"
#> $ cause_name    <chr> "Cyclist road injuries", "Foreign body in eyes"
#> $ avg           <dbl> 1.2603803, 0.2409338
```

To compare the types of injuries contributing to the burden of disease in different countries, we can use a **treemap visualisation**. A treemap is a hierarchical chart that displays data in nested rectangles, with each rectangle representing a different category or subcategory. In this example, we will create a treemap to visualise the average number of injuries by type in high, middle, and low SDI countries.

```
library(treemapify)
# ?geom_treemap
```

```
injuries_types %>%
  filter(!str_detect(location_name, "-middle")) %>%
  ggplot(aes(area = avg,
             label = cause_name,
             fill = cause_name)) +
  geom_treemap(show.legend = F) +
  geom_treemap_text(fontface = "bold",
                    reflow = T,
                    min.size = 1,
                    color = "white",
                    place = "centre",
                    grow = TRUE) +
  facet_wrap(~location_name, scales = "free") +
  labs(title = "GBD-YLDs due to Injuries types - Treemap (1990 - 2021)",
       subtitle = "Average values",
       caption = "IHME Data | Graphic: @fgazzelloni")
```

[2]For reproducibility a copy of the "injuries" data are stored on the GitHub Repository of this book (https://github.com/Fgazzelloni/hmsidR) in the data/inst/extdata folder.

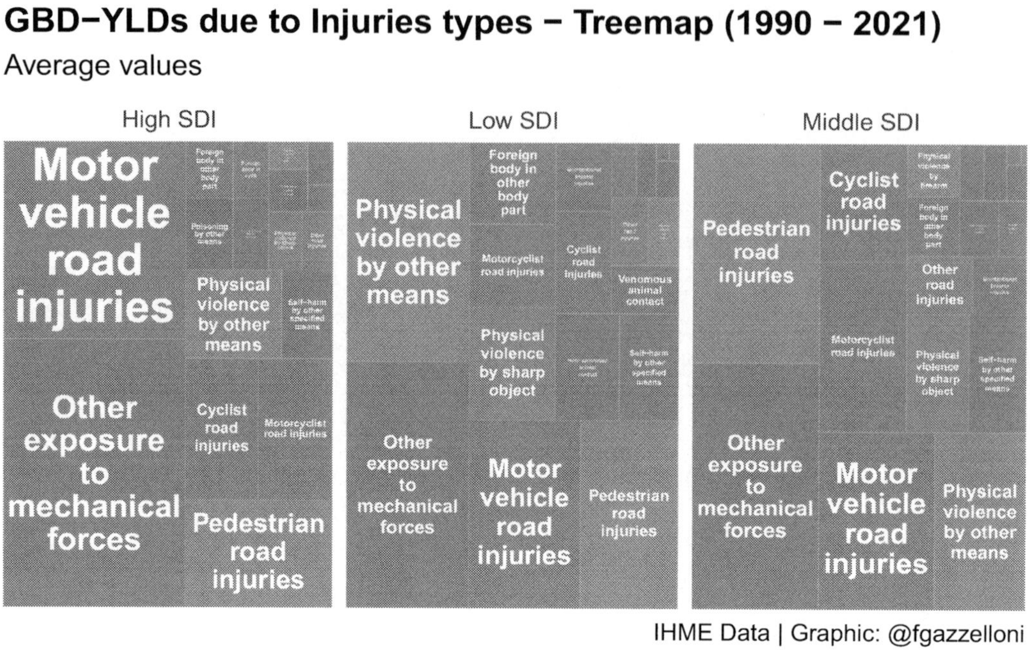

Figure 17.4 GBD-Injuries Treemap (1990 - 2021)

We can conclude that the types of injuries contributing to the burden of disease varied across high, middle, and low SDI countries from 1990 to 2021. Road injuries, falls, and self-harm were common types of injuries in all countries, with variations in the average number of injuries by type. This information can help inform targeted public health interventions to reduce the burden of injuries and improve population health outcomes.

17.5 Example: All Causes DALYs Rate by Country

In this example, we will visualise the **Disability Adjusted Life Years (DALYs) Rate by Country** for all causes using the GBD data. We will use data from the `{hmsidwR}` package, `spatialdalys2021`, to create a *choropleth* map showing the DALYs rate per 100,000 population for each country. The map will provide a visual representation of the burden of disease across different countries, highlighting disparities in health outcomes and disease burdens.

```
hmsidwR::spatialdalys2021 %>%
  ggplot(mapping=aes(x=long, y=lat,
                     fill = value, map_id = location)) +
  geom_polygon(aes(group=group)) +
  # change the values of the fill scale
  scale_fill_viridis_c(option = "plasma",
                       labels = scales::number_format(scale = 1e-3),
                       name = "DALYs") +
  coord_sf() +
```

```
labs(title = "All Causes | DALYs Rate by Country (per 100,000)",
     subtitle = "Values in thousands",
     caption = "IHME Data 2021 | Graphic: @fgazzelloni") +
theme_void()
```

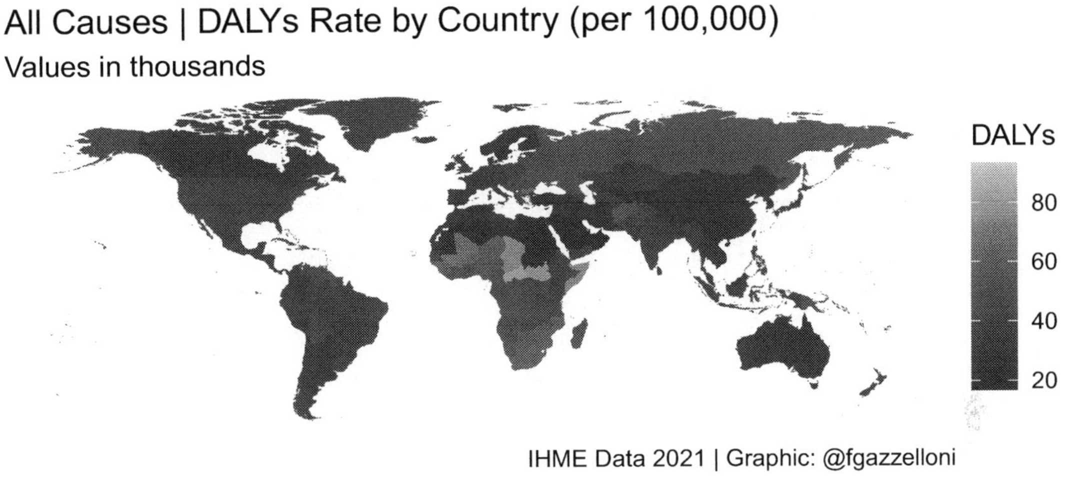

Figure 17.5 All Causes | DALYs Rate by Country (per 100,000)

We can conclude that the Disability Adjusted Life Years (DALYs) Rate varied across countries, with some countries experiencing higher DALYs rates compared to others. This variation reflects differences in disease burdens, health outcomes, and the impact of different health conditions on population health. The choropleth map provides a visual representation of the burden of disease, highlighting disparities in health outcomes and informing public health interventions to improve population health.

In general, what emerges from the GBD 2021 data is that low-income countries, particularly in sub-Saharan Africa, often exhibit the highest DALYs per capita. This is primarily due to a heavy burden of infectious diseases (e.g., malaria, HIV/AIDS, tuberculosis), maternal and neonatal health issues, and malnutrition-related conditions. Countries like the Central African Republic, South Sudan, and Lesotho consistently report some of the highest DALYs per capita.

On the other hand, high-income countries, particularly in Western Europe, North America, and parts of East Asia (e.g., Japan, Singapore), tend to have the lowest DALYs per capita. These countries benefit from well-developed healthcare systems, lower prevalence of infectious diseases, and greater control over non-communicable diseases through early detection and lifestyle interventions. Countries like Iceland, Switzerland, and Singapore consistently report some of the lowest DALYs per capita.

Additionally, lifestyle-related factors like smoking and dietary habits play a significant role in the burden of cardiovascular diseases and cancers globally.

17.6 Implications for Global Public Health Policy

In summary, comparing health metrics across countries is essential for understanding the state of health globally. Resources like the GBD study and the OECD's Health at a Glance report provide valuable insights into health metrics, enabling comparisons and identifying areas for improvement. By analysing health metrics across countries, we can gain insights into public health priorities, disease burdens, and health outcomes, which are crucial for informing global public health policy and interventions.

Analysing health metrics at a global level reveals key patterns in disease prevalence, mortality rates, and risk factors, offering insights into how socio-economic, environmental, and policy variables influence health outcomes. Such comparative analyses are critical for setting international health priorities and targeting interventions in regions with the greatest need.

Regional studies play an equally significant role in contextualizing global insights. For instance, **The State of Health in the European Union in 2019 (Santos et al., 2019)**[3] highlights the importance of tailoring health policies to regional contexts. By focusing on EU countries, the study identifies unique challenges and opportunities, providing a blueprint for targeted interventions and efficient resource allocation. These findings underscore that while global frameworks are valuable, effective public health strategies often require adaptation to local circumstances, cultures, and health systems. Investing in health metric comparisons strengthens global collaboration by fostering data sharing, capacity building, and the exchange of best practices among nations.

[3] J Vasco Santos et al., "The State of Health in the European Union in 2019," *European Journal of Public Health* 31, no. Supplement_3 (October 1, 2021): ckab164.043, doi:10.1093/eurpub/ckab164.043.

Conclusions

This book represents more than just an academic effort—it is the result of a deeply personal journey to bridge the gap between traditional health metrics and advanced machine learning approaches in tackling global health challenges. The process of writing this book has been an exploration of not only the methodologies and tools that define health analytics but also the human stories and challenges embedded in the numbers. It has been a privilege to assemble insights that illuminate the profound impact of diseases on populations and to shape them into a resource for those working to make a difference in public health.

At its core, this work reflects countless hours of research, analysis, and synthesis—navigating datasets, refining models, and translating complex concepts into practical applications. Disability-Adjusted Life Years (DALYs) and related metrics form the foundation of the book. These measures are more than statistics; they reflect the human toll of diseases and injuries, capturing the burden of ill health on individuals and societies in ways that drive meaningful action.

Machine learning has emerged as a game-changing approach during this journey. Applying techniques like transfer learning—where models are adapted to new, data-limited scenarios—has demonstrated the immense potential of these methods in forecasting health trends and designing targeted interventions. Witnessing these techniques in action was both challenging and rewarding, as they redefine how we approach complex health issues and open new pathways for innovation.

The process of writing this book required meticulous attention to every stage—data collection, preprocessing, exploratory analysis, model selection, and evaluation. Drawing on trusted sources such as the Global Burden of Disease (GBD) study, the World Health Organization (WHO), and the Institute for Health Metrics and Evaluation (IHME), the work reflects a commitment to credibility and depth. At times, it was overwhelming to navigate the wide range of global health data while uncovering patterns and connections that matter most. Yet the result is a comprehensive, adaptable framework for understanding health dynamics and confronting the challenges posed by infectious diseases.

Reflecting on this journey, I am inspired by the increasing significance of these tools and methodologies in today's interconnected world. Pandemics, emerging diseases, and the effects of climate change underscore the urgent need for accurate predictions and informed responses. This work highlights the power of machine learning not only to refine health metrics but also to expand our capacity to address crises with agility, precision, and foresight.

This book also exemplifies the importance of collaboration and curiosity. Every dataset, case study, and insight included here is part of a larger puzzle—one that invites readers to take these tools further. Whether you are a policymaker seeking to allocate resources effectively, a researcher developing the next innovative model, or a student eager to make an impact, the findings provide a foundation for enhancing public health strategies and fostering meaningful change. Above all, this work demonstrates the profound value of evidence-based decision-making in improving health outcomes and achieving greater equity in global health.

As I reflect on this journey, I am reminded of the challenges and rewards of exploring such a complex and evolving field. This book is not just a resource but a reflection of a personal mission to contribute meaningfully to global health. My hope is that it equips readers with practical tools, sparks new ideas, and inspires future advancements that continue to push the boundaries of health metrics and analytics. The journey continues, with this work serving as a foundation for future efforts to improve innovation and data-driven insights in addressing the world's most pressing challenges.

Formulary

Statistical Distributions

Normal (Gaussian) Distribution

- **Formula**:

$$f(x) = \frac{1}{\sqrt{2\pi\sigma^2}} e^{-\frac{(x-\mu)^2}{2\sigma^2}}$$

- **Description**: The normal distribution is a continuous probability distribution characterized by a bell-shaped curve. It is defined by the mean (μ) and standard deviation (σ).

Binomial Distribution

- **Formula**:

$$P(X = k) = \binom{n}{k} p^k (1-p)^{n-k}$$

- **Description**: The binomial distribution represents the number of successes in a fixed number of independent Bernoulli trials, with a constant probability of success p in each trial. Here, n is the number of trials and k is the number of successes.

Poisson Distribution

- **Formula**:

$$P(X = k) = \frac{\lambda^k e^{-\lambda}}{k!}$$

- **Description**: The Poisson distribution represents the probability of a given number of events occurring in a fixed interval of time or space, given the average number of times the event occurs over that interval. Here, λ is the average number of events, k is the number of occurrences, and e is Euler's number.

Exponential Distribution

- **Formula**:

$$f(x) = \lambda e^{-\lambda x} \quad \text{for } x \geq 0$$

- **Description**: The exponential distribution represents the time between events in a Poisson process. It is defined by the rate parameter λ.

Uniform Distribution

- **Formula**:

$$f(x) = \begin{cases} \frac{1}{b-a} & a \leq x \leq b \\ 0 & \text{otherwise} \end{cases}$$

- **Description**: The uniform distribution describes an equal probability for all values in the interval $[a, b]$. It is a continuous distribution.

Bernoulli Distribution

- **Formula**:

$$P(X = x) = p^x(1-p)^{1-x} \quad \text{for } x \in \{0, 1\}$$

- **Description**: The Bernoulli distribution is a discrete distribution representing the outcome of a single binary experiment with success probability p.

Beta Distribution

- **Formula**:

$$f(x) = \frac{x^{\alpha-1}(1-x)^{\beta-1}}{B(\alpha, \beta)} \quad \text{for } 0 \leq x \leq 1$$

- **Description**: The beta distribution is a continuous distribution defined on the interval [0, 1], parameterized by α and β, and is useful in Bayesian statistics.

Gamma Distribution

- **Formula**:

$$f(x) = \frac{\beta^\alpha x^{\alpha-1} e^{-\beta x}}{\Gamma(\alpha)} \quad \text{for } x \geq 0$$

- **Description**: The gamma distribution is a continuous distribution defined by shape parameter α and rate parameter β. It generalizes the exponential distribution.

Chi-Squared Distribution

- **Formula**:

$$f(x) = \frac{1}{2^{k/2}\Gamma(k/2)} x^{k/2-1} e^{-x/2} \quad \text{for } x \geq 0$$

- **Description**: The chi-squared distribution is a special case of the gamma distribution with $\alpha = k/2$ and $\beta = 1/2$, often used in hypothesis testing and confidence intervals.

Student's t-Distribution

- **Formula**:

$$f(t) = \frac{\Gamma\left(\frac{\nu+1}{2}\right)}{\sqrt{\nu\pi}\,\Gamma\left(\frac{\nu}{2}\right)} \left(1 + \frac{t^2}{\nu}\right)^{-\frac{\nu+1}{2}}$$

- **Description**: The t-distribution is used to estimate population parameters when the sample size is small and the population variance is unknown. It is defined by the degrees of freedom ν.

F-Distribution

- **Formula:**

$$f(x) = \frac{\left(\frac{d_1}{d_2}\right)^{d_1/2} x^{d_1/2-1}}{B\left(\frac{d_1}{2}, \frac{d_2}{2}\right)\left(1 + \frac{d_1}{d_2}x\right)^{(d_1+d_2)/2}}$$

- **Description:** The F-distribution is used to compare two variances and is defined by two degrees of freedom, d_1 and d_2.

Multinomial Distribution

- **Formula:**

$$P(X_1 = x_1, \ldots, X_k = x_k) = \frac{n!}{x_1! \cdots x_k!} p_1^{x_1} \cdots p_k^{x_k}$$

- **Description:** The multinomial distribution generalizes the binomial distribution to more than two outcomes. It describes the probabilities of counts among categories.

Geometric Distribution

- **Formula:**

$$P(X = k) = (1 - p)^{k-1} p \quad \text{for } k \in \{1, 2, 3, \ldots\}$$

- **Description:** The geometric distribution represents the number of trials needed to get the first success in a sequence of independent Bernoulli trials with success probability p.

Hypergeometric Distribution

- **Formula:**

$$P(X = k) = \frac{\binom{K}{k}\binom{N-K}{n-k}}{\binom{N}{n}}$$

- **Description:** The hypergeometric distribution describes the probability of k successes in n draws from a finite population of size N containing K successes, without replacement.

Log-Normal Distribution

- **Formula:**

$$f(x) = \frac{1}{x\sigma\sqrt{2\pi}} e^{-\frac{(\ln x - \mu)^2}{2\sigma^2}} \quad \text{for } x > 0$$

- **Description:** The log-normal distribution describes a variable whose logarithm is normally distributed. It is useful in modeling positively skewed data.

Machine Learning Models

Linear Regression

- **Formula:**

$$y = \beta_0 + \beta_1 x_1 + \beta_2 x_2 + \cdots + \beta_n x_n + \epsilon$$

- **Description**: Predicts a continuous target variable based on linear relationships between the target and one or more predictor variables.

Logistic Regression

- **Formula**:

$$\text{logit}(P(Y=1)) = \ln\left(\frac{P(Y=1)}{1-P(Y=1)}\right) = \beta_0 + \beta_1 x_1 + \beta_2 x_2 + \cdots + \beta_n x_n$$

- **Description**: Predicts a binary outcome based on linear relationships between the predictor variables and the log-odds of the outcome.

Generalized Linear Model (GLM)

- **Formula**:

$$g(E(Y)) = \beta_0 + \beta_1 x_1 + \beta_2 x_2 + \cdots + \beta_n x_n$$

- **Description**: A generalized linear model is a flexible generalization of ordinary linear regression that allows for the dependent variable Y to have a distribution other than normal. The link function g relates the expected value of the response variable $E(Y)$ to the linear predictors. β_0 is the intercept, and β_i are the coefficients for the predictor variables x_i.

Generalized Additive Model (GAM)

- **Formula**:

$$g(E(Y)) = \beta_0 + f_1(x_1) + f_2(x_2) + \cdots + f_n(x_n)$$

- **Description**: A generalized additive model is an extension of generalized linear models where the linear predictor depends linearly on unknown smooth functions of some predictor variables, and it allows for non-linear relationships between the dependent and independent variables. Here, g is the link function, $E(Y)$ is the expected value of the response variable Y, β_0 is the intercept

Decision Tree

- **Formula**: Recursive binary splitting
- **Description**: Splits the data into subsets based on the value of input features. Each internal node represents a "test" on an attribute, each branch represents the outcome of the test, and each leaf node represents a class label or continuous value.

Random Forest

- **Formula**: Aggregated decision trees
- **Description**: Combines the predictions of multiple decision trees to improve accuracy and control over-fitting. Each tree is trained on a bootstrapped sample of the data and uses a random subset of features.

Support Vector Machine (SVM)

- **Formula**:

$$f(x) = \text{sign}(\mathbf{w} \cdot \mathbf{x} + b)$$

- **Description**: Finds the hyperplane that best separates the classes in the feature space. The formula represents the decision boundary, where $\mathbf{w}$ is the weight vector and b is the bias.

K-Nearest Neighbors (KNN)

- **Formula**:

$$\hat{y} = \frac{1}{k}\sum_{i=1}^{k} y_i$$

- **Description**: Classifies a data point based on the majority class among its k nearest neighbors. For regression, it predicts the average of the k nearest neighbors' values.

Naive Bayes

- **Formula**:

$$P(Y|X) = \frac{P(X|Y)P(Y)}{P(X)}$$

- **Description**: Assumes independence between predictors. It uses Bayes' theorem to predict the probability of a class given the predictors.

Principal Component Analysis (PCA)

- **Formula**:

$$Z = XW$$

- **Description**: Reduces the dimensionality of the data by transforming the original variables into new uncorrelated variables (principal components), ordered by the amount of variance they capture.

K-Means Clustering

- **Formula**:

$$\arg\min_{S} \sum_{i=1}^{k} \sum_{x \in S_i} \|x - \mu_i\|^2$$

- **Description**: Partitions the data into k clusters by minimizing the sum of squared distances between the data points and the cluster centroids μ_i.

Neural Networks

- **Formula**:

$$a^{(l)} = \sigma(z^{(l)})$$
$$z^{(l)} = W^{(l)}a^{(l-1)} + b^{(l)}$$

- **Description**: Composed of layers of interconnected nodes (neurons). Each neuron's output is a weighted sum of its inputs passed through an activation function σ. The parameters $W^{(l)}$ and $b^{(l)}$ are the weights and biases of layer l.

Convolutional Neural Networks (CNN)

- **Formula**:
$$(f * g)(t) = \int_{-\infty}^{\infty} f(\tau)g(t-\tau)\,d\tau$$
- **Description**: Uses convolutional layers to apply filters to the input, which helps in capturing spatial hierarchies in data, particularly useful for image and video processing.

Recurrent Neural Networks (RNN)

- **Formula**:
$$h_t = \sigma(W_h h_{t-1} + W_x x_t + b)$$
- **Description**: Designed to recognize patterns in sequences of data by maintaining a hidden state h_t that captures information from previous time steps.

Gradient Boosting Machines (GBM)

- **Formula**:
$$F_m(x) = F_{m-1}(x) + \eta \cdot h_m(x)$$
- **Description**: Builds an additive model in a forward stage-wise manner. Each base learner h_m is trained to reduce the residual error of the ensemble's previous predictions.

Long Short-Term Memory Networks (LSTM)

- **Formula**:
$$\begin{aligned}
f_t &= \sigma(W_f \cdot [h_{t-1}, x_t] + b_f)\\
i_t &= \sigma(W_i \cdot [h_{t-1}, x_t] + b_i)\\
\tilde{C}_t &= \tanh(W_C \cdot [h_{t-1}, x_t] + b_C)\\
C_t &= f_t * C_{t-1} + i_t * \tilde{C}_t\\
o_t &= \sigma(W_o \cdot [h_{t-1}, x_t] + b_o)\\
h_t &= o_t * \tanh(C_t)
\end{aligned}$$
- **Description**: A type of RNN that can learn long-term dependencies by using gates to control the flow of information.

A

Life Tables, Markov Chain, and APIs

A.1 Life Tables and Life Expectancy

Back in the 1700s the Swiss mathematician and physicist Daniel Bernoulli (1700 - 1782) developed the use of a life table model by differentiating life tables based on specific causes of death.[1]

Originally made by the English scientist **John Graunt** (1620-1674), for the analysis of the mortality of the population of London and the impact of different diseases. Life tables contain fundamental statistics for the calculation of probabilities of deaths and the computation of life expectancy at birth and at different ages.

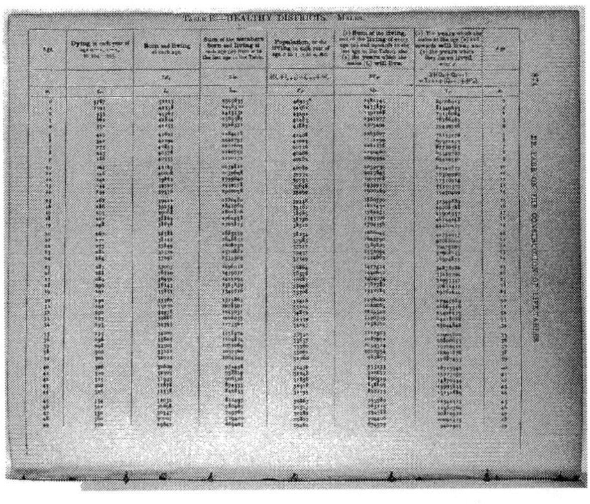

Figure A.1 "Life tables", William Farr (England 1859)

A.1.1 Life Tables Components

More recent life tables are standardized to be used for a population of 100 000 at age 0.

> l_x survivors at age x it starts with a value of 100 000
> d_x deceased at age x
> q_x probability of deaths

[1] "Life Table - an Overview | ScienceDirect Topics," n.d., https://www.sciencedirect.com/topics/medicine-and-dentistry/life-table.

DOI: 10.1201/9781032625935-A

p_x probability of survival

The probability of survival is given by:

$$p_x = 1 - q_x$$

Let's start constructing a life table

The **Global Life Tables** are included in the `{hmsidwR}` package as `gho_lifetables` dataset. This dataset has been released by the WHO, and contains various indicators.

The construction of the Global Life Tables takes consideration of age-specific mortality patterns, which is the main improvements made on life tables construction since the first set of model life tables published by the United Nations in 1955, see[2] for more information about a detailed procedure.

To have a look at the package documentation for this dataset, use:

```
?hmsidwR::gho_lifetables
```

```
library(tidyverse)
hmsidwR::gho_lifetables %>%
  count(indicator) %>%
  select(-n)
#> # A tibble: 7 x 1
#>   indicator
#>   <chr>
#> 1 Tx
#> 2 ex
#> 3 lx
#> 4 nLx
#> 5 nMx
#> 6 ndx
#> 7 nqx
```

The indicator of interest for re-building a life table are:

- `lx` - number of people left alive at age x
- `age`

These two key elements are crucial for building the life tables.

```
lx <- hmsidwR::gho_lifetables %>%
  distinct() %>%
  filter(
    indicator == "lx",
    year == "2019"
  )
```

```
x <- lx %>%
  filter(sex == "female") %>%
  select(x = age)
```

[2]"Modified Logit Life Table System: Principles, Empirical Validation, and Application: Population Studies: Vol 57, No 2," n.d., https://www.tandfonline.com/doi/abs/10.1080/0032472032000097083.

```
lx_f <- lx %>%
  filter(sex == "female") %>%
  select(lx = value)

lx_m <- lx %>%
  filter(sex == "male") %>%
  select(lx = value)
```

The probability of survival is calculated as follow:

$$p_x = \frac{l_x}{l_{x+1}}$$

```
px <- lx_f$lx / lag(lx_f$lx)
```

```
data.frame(
  x,
  lx = round(lx_f),
  dx = round(c(-diff(lx_f$lx), 0)),
  px,
  qx = 1 - lead(px),
  Lx = c(
    (lx_f$lx[1] + (lx_f$lx[2])) / 2,
    5 * (lx_f$lx[-1] + lead(lx_f$lx[-1])) / 2
  )
) %>%
  head()
#>       x     lx   dx        px          qx        Lx
#> 1    <1 100000 2584        NA 0.025843406  98707.83
#> 2 01-04  97416  915 0.9741566 0.009393050 484790.72
#> 3 05-09  96501  366 0.9906069 0.003790526 481588.68
#> 4 10-14  96135  249 0.9962095 0.002588600 480052.07
#> 5 15-19  95886  305 0.9974114 0.003185671 478666.28
#> 6 20-24  95581  399 0.9968143 0.004179281 476903.98
```

```
hmsidwR::gho_lifetables %>%
  distinct() %>%
  mutate(indicator = gsub(" .*", "", indicator)) %>%
  filter(
    indicator == "nLx",
    year == "2019",
    sex == "female"
  ) %>%
  head()
#> # A tibble: 6 x 5
#>   indicator  year age   sex     value
#>   <chr>     <dbl> <ord> <chr>   <dbl>
#> 1 nLx        2019 <1    female  97857.
#> 2 nLx        2019 01-04 female 387467.
#> 3 nLx        2019 05-09 female 481589.
#> 4 nLx        2019 10-14 female 480052.
```

```
#> 5 nLx         2019 15-19 female 478666.
#> 6 nLx         2019 20-24 female 476904.
```

A.1.2 Life Expectancy

Life expectancy is the expected number of years a person will live, based on current age and prevailing mortality rates. There are several methods to calculate life expectancy, but one common approach is to use the actuarial life table, which is a statistical table that provides the mortality rates for a population at different ages. The following steps can be used to calculate life expectancy using a life table:

Identify the relevant mortality rates for the population and time period of interest. Calculate the probability of surviving to each age, given the mortality rates. Multiply the probability of surviving to each age by the remaining life expectancy at that age to obtain the expected number of years of life remaining at each age. Sum the expected number of years of life remaining at each age to obtain the total life expectancy. Note that life expectancy is a statistical estimate and can be influenced by many factors, such as lifestyle, health, and environmental factors, so actual individual life expectancy can vary widely.

Here are some key references for calculating life expectancy:

1. United Nations World Population Prospects - The UN provides detailed life tables and population data, including life expectancy, for countries and regions around the world.
2. Centers for Disease Control and Prevention (CDC) - The CDC provides life tables for the United States, as well as information on how life expectancy is calculated and factors that affect it.
3. World Health Organization (WHO) - The WHO provides information on global health and life expectancy, including data and reports on trends in life expectancy and mortality.
4. Actuarial Science textbooks - Books such as "Actuarial Mathematics" by Bowers, Gerber, Hickman, Jones, and Nesbitt, or "An Introduction to Actuarial Mathematics" by Michel Millar, provide comprehensive coverage of the methods and mathematics used in calculating life expectancy.
5. Journal articles - Articles in actuarial and demographic journals, such as the North American Actuarial Journal or Demographic Research, often provide in-depth coverage of the latest research and methods for calculating life expectancy.

A.2 Markov Chain

A Markov chain is a stochastic model describing a sequence of possible events in which the probability of each event depends only on the state attained in the previous event. The state space of a Markov chain is the set of all possible states of the system. The transition probabilities are the probabilities of moving from one state to another. The transition matrix is a square matrix that describes the transition probabilities between states.

The code for this replication of the **Markov Chain** is from Dobrow - **Bayesian analysis of infectious diseases** book (chapter4). It shows clearly how to create a Markov chain and calculate the transition probabilities.

```
set.seed(000)
markov <- function(init, mat, n, labels) {
  if (missing(labels)) labels <- 1:length(init)
  simlist <- numeric(n + 1)
  states <- 1:length(init)
  simlist[1] <- sample(states, 1, prob = init)

  for (i in 2:(n + 1)) {
    simlist[i] <- sample(states, 1, prob = mat[simlist[i - 1], ])
  }

  labels[simlist]
}
```

```
P <- matrix(c(.51, .49, .49, .51),
  nrow = 2, ncol = 2, byrow = TRUE
)
init <- c(1, 0)
```

```
markov(init = init, mat = P, n = 100)
```

```
# Define the number of transitions
n_transitions <- 10000

# Simulate Markov chain
simulated_chain <- markov(init, P, n_transitions)

# Calculate the transition probabilities
transition_counts <- table(
  simulated_chain[-1],
  simulated_chain[-(n_transitions + 1)]
)
transition_probabilities <- transition_counts / rowSums(transition_counts)
transition_probabilities
#>
#>             1         2
#>    1 0.5140224 0.4859776
#>    2 0.4844249 0.5155751
```

```
# Calculate prior probabilities
prior_probabilities <- table(
  simulated_chain[-n_transitions]) / n_transitions
prior_probabilities
#>
#>      1      2
#> 0.4992 0.5008
```

```
# Calculate posterior probabilities
posterior_probabilities <- transition_probabilities %*% prior_probabilities
```

```
posterior_probabilities
#>
#>          [,1]
#>   1 0.4999776
#>   2 0.5000249
```

A.3 Collecting Data with APIs

Collecting data for research analysis involves selecting sources and methods to optimize computational time when downloading and reading files. Once the data are prepared and ready to use, an additional step is required to make them suitable for the selected model. The source of the data is a critical variable. Generally, data can be downloaded using an API (application programming interface), which allows users to access data directly from the source through specified back-end computations.

There are alternatives to using an API; data can be downloaded directly to a computer or loaded through library packages. Available files are usually provided in various formats, such as delimited files (.csv), spreadsheets (.xls), JSON files (.json), and others. Below is an example of how to use an API to download a file directly to your computer.

```
library(httr)
url <- ""
httr::GET(url = url)
```

A.3.1 Download Data with APIs

A.3.1.1 IHME Data APIs

Head over https://ghdx.healthdata.org/ihme-api to get access to the IHME API's page. The page provides IHME APIs for Sustainable Development Goals (SDG) data. Then, click on https://api.healthdata.org/sdg to login and request an API key. More information on the methodology and data can be found at https://www.gatesfoundation.org/goalkeepers/report/2024-report/data-sources/#ExploretheData.

Load necessary libraries:

```
library(httr)
library(jsonlite)
library(tidyverse)
```

The IHME API provides the following queries. These queries might be updated in the future, so it is important to check the API documentation for the most recent queries.

- SDG Query Input:
  - GetGoal
  - GetIndicator
  - GetTarget
  - GetLocation
  - GetAgeGroup
  - GetScenario

  - GetSex
  - GetResultsByTarget

- Query Input for Results:

  - GetResultsByTarget
  - GetResultsByIndicator
  - GetResultsByLocation
  - GetResultsByYear

Use the function `gbd_get_data` to download data from the IHME API. The function requires the following arguments in quotation marks:

- The `url` where to download the data, such as: `"https://api.healthdata.org/sdg/v1"`
- An `API key` = "YOUR-KEY"
- A `sdg-endpoint`, such as:

  "GetResultsByLocation?location_id=86&indicator_id=1002&year=2019"

The function returns a data frame with the results.

```
gbd_get_data <- function(url, key, sdg) {
  library(httr)
  library(jsonlite)
  url <- paste0(url, "/", sdg)
  headers <- c("Authorization" = key)
  res <- GET(url, add_headers(headers))
  data <- fromJSON(rawToChar(res$content))
  data <- data$results
}
```

Build the query to download results by adding specification of the data. Let's start with:

- `GetIndicator`

```
indicator <- gbd_get_data(
  url = "https://api.healthdata.org/sdg/v1",
  key = "YOUR-KEY",
  sdg = "GetIndicator"
)
```

As an example, let's see the first 6 indicators.

```
library(tidyverse)
indicator %>%
  select(indicator_id, indicator_name) %>%
  arrange(indicator_id) %>%
  head()
```

Then use the `indicator_id` to download the data for a specific indicator.

```
agegroup <- gbd_get_data(
  url = "https://api.healthdata.org/sdg/v1",
  key = "YOUR-KEY",
  sdg = "GetAgeGroup"
)
```

Description: df [6 x 2]

	indicator_id <int>	indicator_name <chr>
1	1000	HIV incidence rate
2	1001	Tuberculosis incidence rate
3	1002	Malaria incidence rate
4	1004	Prevalence of 15 neglected tropical diseases
5	1035	Met need for family planning with modern contraception methods
6	1037	Coverage of essential health services, as defined by the UHC service coverage index

6 rows

Figure A.2 GBD-SDG Indicators

```
agegroup %>%
  select(age_group_id, age_group_name) %>%
  arrange(age_group_id) %>%
  head()
```

Description: df [6 x 2]

	age_group_id <int>	age_group_name <chr>
1	1	Under 5
2	2	Early Neonatal
3	3	Late Neonatal
4	4	Post Neonatal
5	5	1 to 4
6	6	5 to 9

6 rows

Figure A.3 GBD-SDG Age Groups

```
dat19 <- gbd_get_data(
  url = "https://api.healthdata.org/sdg/v1",
  key = "YOUR-KEY",
  sdg = "GetResultsByIndicator?indicator_id=1001&location_id=86&year=2019"
)

dat19%>%
  select(location_name, indicator_name, sex_label, mean_estimate)
```

Description: df [3 x 4]

	location_name <chr>	indicator_name <chr>	sex_label <chr>	mean_estimate <chr>
1	Italy	Tuberculosis incidence rate	Males	6.7275038464861465
2	Italy	Tuberculosis incidence rate	Females	3.901111779672232
3	Italy	Tuberculosis incidence rate	Both sexes	5.277028727101566

3 rows

Figure A.4 GBD-SDG Tuberculosis Data 2019

The same data can be downloaded using the `httr` package. The following code downloads the data for the indicator with `indicator_id = 1001`, `location_id = 86`, and `year = 2019`.

We can use the `GET()` function with this url = https://api.healthdata.org/sdg/v1/GetResultsByIndicator?indicator_id=1001&location_id=86&year=2019

```
headers <- c("Authorization" = "YOUR-KEY")
res <- GET(url= url,
           add_headers(headers))

res$content%>%
  rawToChar() %>%
  fromJSON()
```

An advanced version of the `gbd_get_data()` function can be found in the `{hmsidwR}` package. The function `hmsidwR::gbd_get_data()` allows the user to endpoint customisation, instead of using `sdg` argument with the long query string, an `endpoint` is used to specify the starting point of the quesry, such as `GetResultsByIndicator`. Then, the user can specify the `indicator_id`, `location_id`, and `year` to download the data for specific indicator, location, and year.

The function requires the arguments to be within quotation marks:

```
hmsidwR::gbd_get_data(
  url = "https://api.healthdata.org/sdg/v1",
  key = "YOUR-KEY",
  endpoint = "GetResultsByIndicator",
  indicator_id = "1001",
  location_id = "86",
  year = "2019"
)
```

The output is still the same as Figure A.4 in the previous example.

A.3.2 Package References

The {hmsidwR} package is available at https://github.com/Fgazzelloni/hmsidwR. The package provides data and functions to support this book.

Download the package from CRAN or for the development version use GitHub:

```
# Download from CRAN
install.packages("hmsidwR")

# Download from GitHub
# install.packages("devtools")
devtools::install_github("Fgazzelloni/hmsidwR")
```

B

Tools Used to Make This Book

This appendix provides a comprehensive guide to replicating the environment and code used in this book. To get started, you'll need to install the **R programming language** along with **RStudio IDE**. Additionally, we'll walk through the steps for setting up a **Quarto book project**, integrating it with **GitHub** for version control, and ensuring reproducibility with the `{renv}` package. This setup will allow you to restore the project's environment exactly as it was during the book's creation, ensuring that all code examples run seamlessly.

B.1 RStudio Installation

First, you'll need to download and install R and RStudio Desktop. You can do this by visiting the following link: RStudio Desktop Download.

B.2 How to Set Up This Project with Quarto

Quarto is the next-generation version of RMarkdown, designed for a wide range of publishing tasks, including creating notes, presentations, websites, and books. This book has been developed using Quarto, with the project versioned on GitHub. For more details on how to publish a Quarto book, refer to the official Quarto documentation.

To set up your project:

1. In RStudio, create a new project in a new directory.
2. Enable Git for version control.
3. Select "Quarto Book Project" as the project type. This will automatically generate a `_quarto.yml` file with the following structure:

```
---
project:
  type: book
---
```

4. To preview your book, use the terminal to run `quarto preview`. This command will generate a `_book` directory containing the compiled book files.

DOI: 10.1201/9781032625935-B

B.2.0.1 GitHub Useful Commands

You can manage your project using GitHub directly from RStudio or via command line. To connect your project with GitHub:

1. After creating your project, initiate a Git repository with:

```
git init
git remote add origin https://github.com/yourusername/your-repo.git
```

2. Commit your files and push them to the GitHub repository:

```
git branch -M main
git push -u origin main
```

B.2.0.2 Publish Your Book on GitHub Pages

To publish your Quarto book on GitHub Pages:

1. Modify the `_quarto.yml` file to specify the output directory as `docs`:

```
---
project:
  type: book
  output-dir: docs
---
```

2. Add a `.nojekyll` file to prevent GitHub Pages from ignoring files:

```
touch .nojekyll
```

3. Render your book with:

```
quarto render
```

   This command will create a `docs` folder where the compiled book will be stored.

B.2.0.3 Adding a Package

If you want to add a custom R package to your book project, follow these steps:

1. Create a new package using `devtools`:

```
devtools::create("yourpkg")
```

2. Add raw data processing scripts:

```
usethis::use_data_raw()
```

   This command creates a `.R` script in the `data-raw` directory for processing your data.

3. Save processed data for use in the package:

```
usethis::use_data(yourdata)
```

4. Document your package functions and datasets:

```
usethis::use_r("yourdataset")
devtools::document()
```

Use vignettes for additional documentation:

```
vignette("rd-other") # For datasets
vignette("rd")
```

Finally, build your package to include all new data and functions:

```
devtools::load_all(".")
```

B.2.0.4 Ensuring Reproducibility with renv

To ensure that all analyses and code examples in the book are reproducible, we've utilized the **renv** package. This package captures the specific versions of all R packages used in the project, storing them in an **renv.lock** file located in the root directory of the book's GitHub repository.

To restore the project environment to its original state:

1. Clone the project repository.
2. Run the following command in your R console:

```
renv::restore()
```

This command reads the **renv.lock** file and reinstalls all packages with the exact versions used during the book's development.

Using **renv** ensures that all code examples work as intended, regardless of future package updates, making it easier for readers to replicate analyses or adapt the code to their datasets.

C

Tips on Converting to Python

Translating R code into Python can be a smooth transition with the right approach. Let's start with the basics, from installing packages to loading libraries, and compare the equivalents between R and Python, including the popular tidyverse in R and its counterparts in Python.

C.1 Packages and Libraries

1. **Installing Packages:**

   - **R:**

   ```
   install.packages("package_name")
   ```

   - **Python (using pip):**

   ```
   !pip install package_name
   ```

   - **Python (using conda):**

   ```
   !conda install package_name
   ```

2. **Loading Libraries:**

   - **R:**

   ```
   library(package_name)
   ```

   - **Python:**

   ```
   import package_name
   ```

C.2 Comparing tidyverse with its Python Equivalents

- **tidyverse (R):** tidyverse is a collection of R packages designed for data science, including dplyr for data manipulation, ggplot2 for data visualization, tidyr for data tidying, etc.

```
library(tidyverse)
```

- **Python Equivalents:**
  - **pandas:** Similar to dplyr, pandas provides powerful data manipulation tools.

DOI: 10.1201/9781032625935-C

```
import pandas as pd
```

- **matplotlib/seaborn:** Comparable to ggplot2, these libraries are used for data visualization.

```
import matplotlib.pyplot as plt
import seaborn as sns
```

- **numpy:** While not a direct equivalent to tidyr, numpy offers functionalities for array manipulation and numerical computing, which can be handy for data tidying tasks.

```
import numpy as np
```

- **scikit-learn:** Provides tools for data preprocessing, modelling, and evaluation, resembling some functionalities of tidyverse packages like modelr.

```
from sklearn import ...
```

- **tidyverse-like package:** There isn't a single package in Python that encompasses the entire functionality of tidyverse, but you can combine pandas, matplotlib/seaborn, numpy, and scikit-learn to achieve similar results.

By understanding these equivalences and leveraging the rich ecosystem of Python libraries, you can effectively translate your R code into Python, ensuring a smooth transition while retaining the analytical power and flexibility you need for your projects.

C.3 Creating Data Making Statistics

1. **Creating Basic Data:**

   - **R:**

```
# Create a data frame
data <- data.frame(
  x = c(1, 2, 3, 4, 5),
  y = c(2, 3, 4, 5, 6)
)
```

   - **Python (using pandas):**

```
import pandas as pd

# Create a DataFrame
data = pd.DataFrame({
    'x': [1, 2, 3, 4, 5],
    'y': [2, 3, 4, 5, 6]
})
```

2. **Basic Statistics:**

   - **R:**

```
# Summary statistics
summary(data)
```

- **Python (using pandas):**

```
# Summary statistics
print(data.describe())
```

C.4 Building a Linear Regression Model

- **R:**

```
# Load the lm function from the stats package
library(stats)

# Fit a linear regression model
lm_model <- lm(y ~ x, data = data)

# Summary of the model
summary(lm_model)
```

- **Python (using statsmodels):**

```
import statsmodels.api as sm

# Add a constant term for intercept
X = sm.add_constant(data['x'])

# Fit a linear regression model
lm_model = sm.OLS(data['y'], X).fit()

# Summary of the model
print(lm_model.summary())
```

- **Python (using scikit-learn):**

```
from sklearn.linear_model import LinearRegression

# Initialize the model
lm_model = LinearRegression()

# Fit the model
lm_model.fit(data[['x']], data['y'])

# Coefficients
print("Intercept:", lm_model.intercept_)
print("Coefficient:", lm_model.coef_)
```

While the syntax and libraries may differ slightly, the overall process remains conceptually similar. By understanding these comparisons, you can effectively transition between R and Python for data analysis and modelling tasks.

C.5 Example of a Model Workflow

1. **Data Preprocessing**:

```
import pandas as pd
from sklearn.preprocessing import StandardScaler
data = pd.read_csv('data.csv')
data.fillna(method='ffill', inplace=True)
scaler = StandardScaler()
scaled_data = scaler.fit_transform(
  data[['feature1', 'feature2', 'feature3']]
  )
```

2. **Model Selection and Training**:

```
from sklearn.model_selection import train_test_split
from sklearn.linear_model import LinearRegression
from sklearn.metrics import mean_squared_error

X = data[['feature1', 'feature2', 'feature3']]
y = data['DALYs']
X_train,
X_test,
y_train,
y_test = train_test_split(X, y, test_size=0.2, random_state=42)

model = LinearRegression()
model.fit(X_train, y_train)
y_pred = model.predict(X_test)

mse = mean_squared_error(y_test, y_pred)
print(f'Mean Squared Error: {mse}')
```

3. **Time Series Forecasting Example**:

```
from fbprophet import Prophet
ts_data = data[['date', 'DALYs']]
ts_data.rename(columns={'date': 'ds', 'DALYs': 'y'}, inplace=True)
model = Prophet()
model.fit(ts_data)
future = model.make_future_dataframe(periods=365)
forecast = model.predict(future)
model.plot(forecast)
```

4. **The SIR Model Example**:

   Set-up the environment for running python in RStudio by loading the `{reticulate}` package and the following commands:

```
library(reticulate)
```

This is to configurate python and for installing necessary packages:

```
py_config()

# type <pip3 install scipy> on terminal
# type <pip3 install matplotlib> on terminal
```

```
import matplotlib
matplotlib.use('TkAgg')  # Ensure you have an interactive backend
import matplotlib.pyplot as plt
import scipy.integrate as spi
import numpy as np
```

Set-up the parameters:

```
beta = 1.4247
gamma = 0.14286
TS = 1.0
ND = 70.0
S0 = 1 - 1e-6
I0 = 1e-6
INPUT = (S0, I0, 0.0)
```

Define differential equations:

```
def diff_eqs(INP, t):
    Y = np.zeros((3))
    V = INP
    Y[0] = - beta * V[0] * V[1]
    Y[1] = beta * V[0] * V[1] - gamma * V[1]
    Y[2] = gamma * V[1]
    return Y

t_start = 0.0; t_end = ND; t_inc = TS
t_range = np.arange(t_start, t_end + t_inc, t_inc)
RES = spi.odeint(diff_eqs, INPUT, t_range)
```

```
#Plotting
# Ensure interactive mode is on and plot
plt.ion()
plt.subplot(211)
plt.plot(RES[:, 0], '-g', label='Susceptibles')
plt.plot(RES[:, 2], '-k', label='Recovereds')
plt.legend(loc=0)
plt.title('SIR Model')
plt.xlabel('Time')
plt.ylabel('Susceptibles and Recovereds')
```

```
plt.subplot(212)
plt.plot(RES[:, 1], '-r', label='Infectious')
plt.xlabel('Time')
plt.ylabel('Infectious')

plt.show()
```

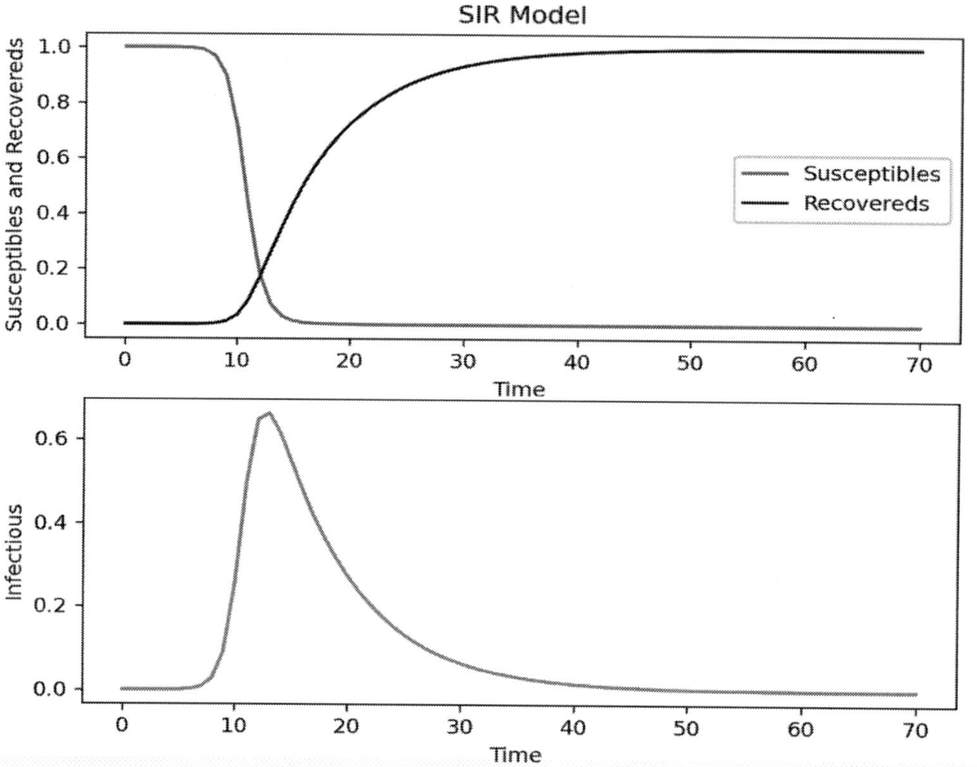

Figure C.1 SIR Model with Python

The code for this example is adapted from: Modeling Infectious Diseases in Humans and Animals Matt J. Keeling & Pejman Rohani.

By following these steps, you can analyze DALYs and infectious diseases, drawing trends, understanding relationships, and predicting future outcomes effectively.

References

Ahmad, Hammad, Asad Ali, Syeda Hira Fatima, Farrah Zaidi, Muhammad Khisroon, Syed Basit Rasheed, Ihsan Ullah, Saleem Ullah, and Muhammad Shakir. "Spatial Modeling of Dengue Prevalence and Kriging Prediction of Dengue Outbreak in Khyber Pakhtunkhwa (Pakistan) Using Presence Only Data." *Stochastic Environmental Research and Risk Assessment* 34, no. 7 (July 1, 2020): 1023–36. doi:10.1007/s00477-020-01818-9.

"Alan Lopez," December 11, 2023. https://en.wikipedia.org/w/index.php?title=Alan_Lopez&oldid=1189335406.

"Analytic Hierarchy Process." *Wikipedia*, March 2024. https://en.wikipedia.org/w/index.php?title=Analytic_hierarchy_process&oldid=1214553274.

"Approximate Bayesian Inference for Latent Gaussian Models by Using Integrated Nested Laplace Approximations - Rue - 2009 - Journal of the Royal Statistical Society: Series b (Statistical Methodology) - Wiley Online Library," n.d. https://rss.onlinelibrary.wiley.com/doi/full/10.1111/j.1467-9868.2008.00700.x.

Baker, Ruth E., Jose-Maria Peña, Jayaratnam Jayamohan, and Antoine Jérusalem. "Mechanistic Models Versus Machine Learning, a Fight Worth Fighting for the Biological Community?" *Biology Letters* 14, no. 5 (May 16, 2018): 20170660. doi:10.1098/rsbl.2017.0660.

Bourke, Joanna. *Fear: A Cultural History.* Catapult, 2007.

Broemeling, Lyle D. *Bayesian Analysis of Infectious Diseases: COVID-19 and Beyond.* New York: Chapman; Hall/CRC, 2021. doi:10.1201/9781003125983.

Butcher, Brandon, and Brian J. Smith. *The American Statistician* 74, no. 3 (July 2020): 308–9. doi:10.1080/00031305.2020.1790217.

CDC. "About Rabies," May 14, 2024. https://www.cdc.gov/rabies/about/index.html.

Chowell, Gerardo, Sushma Dahal, Amna Tariq, Kimberlyn Roosa, James M. Hyman, and Ruiyan Luo. "An Ensemble n-Sub-Epidemic Modeling Framework for Short-Term Forecasting Epidemic Trajectories: Application to the COVID-19 Pandemic in the USA." *PLOS Computational Biology* 18, no. 10 (October 6, 2022): e1010602. doi:10.1371/journal.pcbi.1010602.

"Christopher J. L. Murray," January 1, 2024. https://en.wikipedia.org/w/index.php?title=Christopher_J._L._Murray&oldid=1192936044.

"Constitution of the World Health Organization," n.d. https://www.who.int/about/accountability/governance/constitution.

"Coronaviridae - Wikipedia," n.d. https://en.wikipedia.org/wiki/Coronaviridae.

Dempsey, Mary. "Decline in Tuberculosis." *American Review of Tuberculosis*, April 23, 2019. https://www.atsjournals.org/doi/epdf/10.1164/art.1947.56.2.157?role=tab.

———. "Decline in Tuberculosis." *American Review of Tuberculosis*, April 23, 2019. https://www.atsjournals.org/doi/epdf/10.1164/art.1947.56.2.157?role=tab.

Devleesschauwer, Brecht, Scott A. McDonald, Niko Speybroeck, and Grant M. A. Wyper. "Valuing the Years of Life Lost Due to COVID-19: The Differences and Pitfalls." *International Journal of Public Health* 65, no. 6 (2020): 719–20. doi:10.1007/s00038-020-01430-2.

"Disability-Adjusted Life Year," December 8, 2023. https://en.wikipedia.org/w/index.php?title=Disability-adjusted_life_year&oldid=1188922629.

"Disability-Adjusted Life Year," December 8, 2023. https://en.wikipedia.org/w/index.php?title=Disability-adjusted_life_year&oldid=1188922629.

Dobrow, Robert P. *Introduction to Stochastic Processes with R*. John Wiley & Sons, 2016.

Dubos, R. "The State of Health and the Quality of Life." *Western Journal of Medicine* 125, no. 1 (July 1976): 8–9. https://www.ncbi.nlm.nih.gov/pmc/articles/PMC1237171/.

———. "The State of Health and the Quality of Life." *Western Journal of Medicine* 125, no. 1 (July 1976): 8–9. https://www.ncbi.nlm.nih.gov/pmc/articles/PMC1237171/.

"Echoutcome," October 8, 2016. https://web.archive.org/web/20161008010513/http://echoutcome.eu/.

Ferrari, Alize J., Damian Francesco Santomauro, Amirali Aali, Yohannes Habtegiorgis Abate, Cristiana Abbafati, Hedayat Abbastabar, Samar Abd ElHafeez, et al. "Global Incidence, Prevalence, Years Lived with Disability (YLDs), Disability-Adjusted Life-Years (DALYs), and Healthy Life Expectancy (HALE) for 371 Diseases and Injuries in 204 Countries and Territories and 811 Subnational Locations, 1990–2021: A Systematic Analysis for the Global Burden of Disease Study 2021." *The Lancet* 403, no. 10440 (May 18, 2024): 2133–61. doi:10.1016/S0140-6736(24)00757-8.

"FES/Data_Sets/Ischemic_Stroke at Master · Topepo/FES," n.d. https://github.com/topepo/FES/tree/master/Data_Sets/Ischemic_Stroke.

Forecasting: Principles and Practice (3rd Ed), n.d. https://otexts.com/fpp3/.

Foreman, Kyle J., Rafael Lozano, Alan D. Lopez, and Christopher JL Murray. "Modeling Causes of Death: An Integrated Approach Using CODEm." *Population Health Metrics* 10, no. 1 (January 2012): 1. doi:10.1186/1478-7954-10-1.

Gilks, W. R., S. Richardson, and David Spiegelhalter, eds. *Markov Chain Monte Carlo in Practice*. Chapman; Hall/CRC, 1995. doi:10.1201/b14835.

"Global Health Estimates," n.d. https://www.who.int/data/global-health-estimates.

Haenszel, William. "A Standardized Rate for Mortality Defined in Units of Lost Years of Life." *American Journal of Public Health and the Nations Health* 40, no. 1 (January 1950): 17–26. https://www.ncbi.nlm.nih.gov/pmc/articles/PMC1528498/.

Hampson, Katie, Laurent Coudeville, Tiziana Lembo, Maganga Sambo, Alexia Kieffer, Michaël Attlan, Jacques Barrat, et al. "Estimating the Global Burden of Endemic Canine Rabies." *PLOS Neglected Tropical Diseases* 9, no. 4 (April 2015): e0003709. doi:10.1371/journal.pntd.0003709.

"Healthy Life Expectancy (HALE)," n.d. https://www.who.int/data/gho/data/themes/topics/indicator-groups/indicator-group-details/GHO/healthy-life-expectancy-(hale).

"Healthy Life Years," January 26, 2024. https://en.wikipedia.org/w/index.php?title=Healthy_Life_Years&oldid=1199224227.

Holmes, David. "Report Triggers Quibbles over QALYs, a Staple of Health Metrics." *Nature Medicine* 19, no. 3 (March 1, 2013): 248–48. doi:10.1038/nm0313-248.

Huang, Xing-Yao, Qi Chen, Meng-Xu Sun, Hang-Yu Zhou, Qing Ye, Wu Chen, Jin-Yu Peng, et al. "A Pangolin-Origin SARS-CoV-2-Related Coronavirus: Infectivity, Pathogenicity, and Cross-Protection by Preexisting Immunity." *Cell Discovery* 9, no. 1 (June 17, 2023): 1–13. doi:10.1038/s41421-023-00557-9.

Hult, Marja, Olli Halminen, Miika Linna, Sakari Suominen, and Mari Kangasniemi. "Cost-Effectiveness Calculators for Health, Well-Being and Safety Promotion: A Systematic Review." *The European Journal of Public Health* 31, no. 5 (May 10, 2021): 997–1003. doi:10.1093/eurpub/ckab068.

Hyder, Adnan A., Prasanthi Puvanachandra, and Richard H. Morrow. "Measuring the Health of Populations: Explaining Composite Indicators." *Journal of Public Health Research* 1, no. 3 (December 2012): 222–28. doi:10.4081/jphr.2012.e35.

Ihmeuw/Ihme-Modeling. Institute for Health Metrics; Evaluation, 2024. https://github.com/ihmeuw/ihme-modeling.

"Indicator Metadata Registry Details," n.d. https://www.who.int/data/gho/indicator-metadata-registry/imr-details/158.

"Ipc2021," n.d. https://ipc2021.popconf.org/abstracts/210817.

"John Graunt," January 24, 2024. https://en.wikipedia.org/w/index.php?title=John_Graunt&oldid=1198718407.

"John Graunt," January 24, 2024. https://en.wikipedia.org/w/index.php?title=John_Graunt&oldid=1198718407.

Johnson, Max Kuhn, and Kjell. *2 Illustrative Example: Predicting Risk of Ischemic Stroke | Feature Engineering and Selection: A Practical Approach for Predictive Models*, n.d. https://bookdown.org/max/FES/stroke-tour.html.

Keeling, M. J., and L. Danon. "Mathematical Modelling of Infectious Diseases." *British Medical Bulletin* 92, no. 1 (December 1, 2009): 33–42. doi:10.1093/bmb/ldp038.

Kolokolnikov, Theodore, and David Iron. "Law of Mass Action and Saturation in SIR Model with Application to Coronavirus Modelling." *Infectious Disease Modelling* 6 (November 16, 2020): 91–97. doi:10.1016/j.idm.2020.11.002.

Kovacheva, Ts. P. "Life Tables - Key Parameters and Relationships Between Them." *International Mathematical Forum* 12 (2017): 469–79. doi:10.12988/imf.2017.7225.

"KPSS Test," October 12, 2023. https://en.wikipedia.org/w/index.php?title=KPSS_test&oldid=1179751435.

"Kriging," July 18, 2024. https://en.wikipedia.org/w/index.php?title=Kriging&oldid=1235203584.

"Kriging Best Fit: Kbfit - Fit Variogram Models and Kriging Models to Spatial Data and Select the Best Model Based on the Metrics Values — Kbfit," n.d. https://fgazzelloni.github.io/hmsidwR/reference/kbfit.html.

Kuhn, Max. *The Caret Package*, n.d. https://topepo.github.io/caret/.

Laura H. Kahn, M. D. *One Health and the Politics of COVID-19*. Johns Hopkins University Press, 2024. doi:10.56021/9781421449326.

Li, Ying, Thomas Hills, and Ralph Hertwig. "A Brief History of Risk." *Cognition* 203 (October 2020): 104344. doi:10.1016/j.cognition.2020.104344.

"Life Expectancy for CP, VS, TBI and SCI," n.d. https://www.lifeexpectancy.org/lifetable.shtml.

"Life Table - an Overview | ScienceDirect Topics," n.d. https://www.sciencedirect.com/topics/medicine-and-dentistry/life-table.

Liu, Xiaoxue, Yan Guo, Fang Wang, Yong Yu, Yaqiong Yan, Haoyu Wen, Fang Shi, et al. "Disability Weight Measurement for the Severity of Different Diseases in Wuhan, China." *Population Health Metrics* 21 (May 2023): 5. doi:10.1186/s12963-023-00304-y.

Lugnér, Anna K., and Paul F. M. Krabbe. "An Overview of the Time Trade-Off Method: Concept, Foundation, and the Evaluation of Distorting Factors in Putting a Value on Health." *Expert Review of Pharmacoeconomics & Outcomes Research* 20, no. 4 (August 2020): 331–42. doi:10.1080/14737167.2020.1779062.

"Machine Learning." *Wikipedia*, April 2024. https://en.wikipedia.org/w/index.php?title=Machine_learning&oldid=1220758567.

"Meningitis," n.d. https://www.who.int/news-room/fact-sheets/detail/meningitis.

"Mlr-Org," n.d. https://mlr-org.com/.

"Modified Logit Life Table System: Principles, Empirical Validation, and Application: Population Studies: Vol 57, No 2," n.d. https://www.tandfonline.com/doi/abs/10.1080/0032472032000097083.

Moraga, Paula. *Chapter 14 Kriging | Spatial Statistics for Data Science: Theory and Practice with R*, n.d. https://www.paulamoraga.com/book-spatial/kriging.html?q=kri#kriging.

Murray, C. J. "Quantifying the Burden of Disease: The Technical Basis for Disability-Adjusted Life Years." *Bulletin of the World Health Organization* 72, no. 3 (1994): 429–45. https://www.ncbi.nlm.nih.gov/pmc/articles/PMC2486718/.

Murray, C. J., A. D. Lopez, and D. T. Jamison. "The Global Burden of Disease in 1990: Summary Results, Sensitivity Analysis and Future Directions." *Bulletin of the World Health Organization* 72, no. 3 (1994): 495–509. https://www.ncbi.nlm.nih.gov/pmc/articles/PMC2486716/.

Murray, Christopher J. L., Aleksandr Y. Aravkin, Peng Zheng, Cristiana Abbafati, Kaja M. Abbas, Mohsen Abbasi-Kangevari, Foad Abd-Allah, et al. "Global Burden of 87 Risk Factors in 204 Countries and Territories, 1990–2019: A Systematic Analysis for the Global Burden of Disease Study 2019." *The Lancet* 396, no. 10258 (October 17, 2020): 1223–49. doi:10.1016/S0140-6736(20)30752-2.

Murray, Christopher J. L., Joshua A. Salomon, Colin D. Mathers, Alan D. Lopez, and Weltgesundheitsorganisation, eds. *Summary Measures of Population Health: Concepts, Ethics, Measurement and Applications*. World Health Organization, 2002.

Murray, Christopher JL, and Julio Frenk. "Health Metrics and Evaluation: Strengthening the Science." *The Lancet* 371, no. 9619 (April 5, 2008): 1191–99. doi:10.1016/S0140-6736(08)60526-7.

Muszyńska-Spielauer, Magdalena, and Marc Luy. "Well-Being Adjusted Health Expectancy: A New Summary Measure of Population Health." *European Journal of Population* 38, no. 5 (December 2022): 1009–31. doi:10.1007/s10680-022-09628-1.

null, null. "Ebola Virus Disease in West Africa — the First 9 Months of the Epidemic and Forward Projections." *New England Journal of Medicine* 371, no. 16 (October 16, 2014): 1481–95. doi:10.1056/NEJMoa1411100.

Ock, Minsu, Bomi Park, Hyesook Park, In-Hwan Oh, Seok-Jun Yoon, Bogeum Cho, and Min-Woo Jo. "Disability Weights Measurement for 289 Causes of Disease Considering Disease Severity in Korea." *Journal of Korean Medical Science* 34, no. Suppl 1 (February 2019): e60. doi:10.3346/jkms.2019.34.e60.

Onovo, Amobi Andrew, Akinyemi Atobatele, Abiye Kalaiwo, Christopher Obanubi, Ezekiel James, Pamela Gado, Gertrude Odezugo, Dolapo Ogundehin, Doreen Magaji, and Michele Russell. "Using Supervised Machine Learning and Empirical Bayesian Kriging to Reveal Correlates and Patterns of COVID-19 Disease Outbreak in Sub-Saharan Africa: Exploratory Data Analysis," n.d. doi:10.1101/2020.04.27.20082057.

"Pandemic - Wikipedia," n.d. https://en.wikipedia.org/wiki/Pandemic.

Pebesma, Edzer J. "Multivariable Geostatistics in s: The Gstat Package." *Computers & Geosciences* 30, no. 7 (August 1, 2004): 683–91. doi:10.1016/j.cageo.2004.03.012.

Porst, Michael, Elena von der Lippe, Janko Leddin, Aline Anton, Annelene Wengler, Jan Breitkreuz, Katrin Schüssel, et al. "The Burden of Disease in Germany at the National and Regional Level." *Deutsches Ärzteblatt International* 119, no. 46 (November 2022): 785–92. doi:10.3238/arztebl.m2022.0314.

"Q–Q Plot," March 20, 2025. https://en.wikipedia.org/w/index.php?title=Q%E2%80%93Q_plot&oldid=1281381233.

"Quality-Adjusted Life Year," December 27, 2023. https://en.wikipedia.org/w/index.php?title=Quality-adjusted_life_year&oldid=1192021016.

"Rabies," n.d. https://www.who.int/news-room/fact-sheets/detail/rabies.

Rehm, Jürgen, and Ulrich Frick. "Establishing Disability Weights from Pairwise Comparisons for a US Burden of Disease Study." *International Journal of Methods in Psychiatric Research* 22, no. 2 (May 2013): 144–54. doi:10.1002/mpr.1383.

Reiner, Robert C., and Simon I. Hay. "The Overlapping Burden of the Three Leading Causes of Disability and Death in Sub-Saharan African Children." *Nature Communications* 13, no. 1 (December 6, 2022): 7457. doi:10.1038/s41467-022-34240-6.

"R-INLA Project - What Is INLA?" n.d. https://www.r-inla.org/what-is-inla.

Roster, Kirstin, Colm Connaughton, and Francisco A. Rodrigues. "Forecasting New Diseases in Low-Data Settings Using Transfer Learning." *Chaos, Solitons, and Fractals* 161 (August 2022): 112306. doi:10.1016/j.chaos.2022.112306.

Santangelo, Omar Enzo, Vito Gentile, Stefano Pizzo, Domiziana Giordano, and Fabrizio Cedrone. "Machine Learning and Prediction of Infectious Diseases: A Systematic Review." *Machine Learning and Knowledge Extraction* 5, no. 1 (March 2023): 175–98. doi:10.3390/make5010013.

Selemani, Majige, Amina S. Msengwa, Sigilbert Mrema, Amri Shamte, Michael J. Mahande, Karen Yeates, Maurice C. Y. Mbago, and Angelina M. Lutambi. "Assessing the Effects of Mosquito Nets on Malaria Mortality Using a Space Time Model: A Case Study of Rufiji and Ifakara Health and Demographic Surveillance System Sites in Rural Tanzania." *Malaria Journal* 15, no. 1 (May 4, 2016): 257. doi:10.1186/s12936-016-1311-9.

Silge, Max Kuhn, and Julia. *Tidy Modeling with r*, n.d. https://www.tmwr.org/.

Stanaway, Jeffrey D, Ashkan Afshin, Emmanuela Gakidou, Stephen S Lim, Degu Abate, Kalkidan Hassen Abate, Cristiana Abbafati, et al. "Global, Regional, and National Comparative Risk Assessment of 84 Behavioural, Environmental and Occupational, and Metabolic Risks or Clusters of Risks for 195 Countries and Territories, 1990–2017: A Systematic Analysis for the Global Burden of Disease Study 2017." *The Lancet* 392, no. 10159 (November 2018): 1923–94. doi:10.1016/s0140-6736(18)32225-6.

Tiemersma, Edine W., Marieke J. van der Werf, Martien W. Borgdorff, Brian G. Williams, and Nico J. D. Nagelkerke. "Natural History of Tuberculosis: Duration and Fatality of Untreated Pulmonary Tuberculosis in HIV Negative Patients: A Systematic Review." *PLOS ONE* 6, no. 4 (April 4, 2011): e17601. doi:10.1371/journal.pone.0017601.

Tsugane, Shoichiro. "Why Has Japan Become the World's Most Long-Lived Country: Insights from a Food and Nutrition Perspective." *European Journal of Clinical Nutrition* 75, no. 6 (2021): 921–28. doi:10.1038/s41430-020-0677-5.

Vasco Santos, J, A Padron Monedero, B Bikbov, DA Grad, D Plass, E-A Mechili, F Gazzelloni, et al. "The State of Health in the European Union in 2019." *European Journal of Public Health* 31, no. Supplement_3 (October 1, 2021): ckab164.043. doi:10.1093/eurpub/ckab164.043.

Volz, Erik M., Joel C. Miller, Alison Galvani, and Lauren Ancel Meyers. "Effects of Heterogeneous and Clustered Contact Patterns on Infectious Disease Dynamics." *PLoS Computational Biology* 7, no. 6 (June 2, 2011): e1002042. doi:10.1371/journal.pcbi.1002042.

Vos, Theo, Stephen S. Lim, Cristiana Abbafati, Kaja M. Abbas, Mohammad Abbasi, Mitra Abbasifard, Mohsen Abbasi-Kangevari, et al. "Global Burden of 369 Diseases and Injuries in 204 Countries and Territories, 1990–2019: A Systematic Analysis for the Global Burden of Disease Study 2019." *The Lancet* 396, no. 10258 (October 2020): 1204–22. doi:10.1016/S0140-6736(20)30925-9.

Vos, Theo, Stephen S Lim, Cristiana Abbafati, Kaja M Abbas, Mohammad Abbasi, Mitra Abbasifard, Mohsen Abbasi-Kangevari, et al. "Global Burden of 369 Diseases and Injuries in 204 Countries and Territories, 1990–2019: A Systematic Analysis for the Global Burden of Disease Study 2019." *The Lancet* 396, no. 10258 (October 2020): 1204–22. doi:10.1016/s0140-6736(20)30925-9.

Wackernagel, Hans. "Linear Regression and Simple Kriging." edited by Hans Wackernagel, 15–26. Berlin, Heidelberg: Springer, 2003. doi:10.1007/978-3-662-05294-5_3.

"Well-Being Adjusted Health Expectancy - a New Summary Measure of Population Health | Population Europe," n.d. https://population-europe.eu/research/books-and-reports/well-being-adjusted-health-expectancy-new-summary-measure-population.

"WHO-Convened Global Study of Origins of SARS-CoV-2: China Part," n.d. https://www.who.int/publications/i/item/who-convened-global-study-of-origins-of-sars-cov-2-china-part.

"William Playfair," March 9, 2025. https://en.wikipedia.org/w/index.php?title=William_Playfair&oldid=1279573846.

"World Malaria Report 2022," n.d. https://www.who.int/publications-detail-redirect/9789240064898.

Wyper, Grant M. A., Ian Grant, Eilidh Fletcher, Neil Chalmers, Gerry McCartney, and Diane L. Stockton. "Prioritising the Development of Severity Distributions in Burden of Disease Studies for Countries in the European Region." *Archives of Public Health* 78, no. 1 (January 2020): 3. doi:10.1186/s13690-019-0385-6.

"Zoonosis - Wikipedia," n.d. https://en.wikipedia.org/wiki/Zoonosis.

Index

FSC
www.fsc.org
MIX
Papier | Fördert
gute Waldnutzung
FSC® C083411

Kolibri 360 GmbH
Ferdinand-Jühlke-Straße 7
99095 Erfurt, Deutschland
produktsicherheit@kolibri360.de